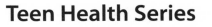

Teen Health Series

Diabetes Information For Teens, Second Edition

Diabetes Information For Teens, Second Edition

Health Tips About Managing Diabetes And Preventing Related Complications

Including Facts About Insulin, Glucose Control, Healthy Eating, Physical Activity, And Learning To Live With Diabetes

Edited by Karen Bellenir

Omnigraphics

155 W. Congress, Suite 200
Detroit, MI 48226

Bibliographic Note

Because this page cannot legibly accommodate all the copyright notices, the Bibliographic Note portion of the Preface constitutes an extension of the copyright notice.

Edited by Karen Bellenir

Teen Health Series

Karen Bellenir, *Managing Editor*
David A. Cooke, M.D., *Medical Consultant*
Elizabeth Collins, *Research and Permissions Coordinator*
Cherry Edwards, *Permissions Assistant*
EdIndex, *Services for Publishers, Indexers*

* * *

Omnigraphics, Inc.

Matthew P. Barbour, *Senior Vice President*
Kevin M. Hayes, *Operations Manager*

* * *

Peter E. Ruffner, *Publisher*

Copyright © 2012 Omnigraphics, Inc.

ISBN 978-0-7808-1218-5

Library of Congress Cataloging-in-Publication Data

Diabetes information for teens : health tips about managing diabetes and preventing related complications, including facts about insulin, glucose control, healthy eating, physical activity, and learning to live with diabetes / edited by Karen Bellenir. -- 2nd ed.
     p. cm. -- (Teen health series)
  Includes bibliographical references and index.
  Summary: "Provides basic consumer health information for teens about managing diabetes and preventing complications, making healthy diet and exercise choices, and coping with emotional and lifestyle concerns. Includes index and resource information"-- Provided by publisher.
   ISBN 978-0-7808-1218-5 (hardcover : alk. paper) 1. Diabetes--Juvenile literature. 2. Diabetes in adolescence--Juvenile literature. I. Bellenir, Karen.
  RC660.5.D53 2011
  616.4'62--dc23
                                                                                                2011038652

∞

Table of Contents

Part Three: Nutrition, Physical Activity, And Weight Management

Part Four: Mental Health And Lifestyle Issues

Part Five: The Physical Complications Of Diabetes

Part Six: If You Need More Information

Preface

About This Book

The teen years are especially important in the battle against diabetes. As young people begin to take more personal responsibility for managing their health, they make their own choices about what to eat and what activities to pursue. These decisions can have consequences that impact well-being throughout the adult years.

Currently, efforts to overcome diabetes are making little progress. According to recent U.S. statistics, the prevalence of type 1 diabetes appears to be increasing among children and adolescents. Researchers suspect that a combination of genetic and environmental factors may be involved in a process that causes the body's autoimmune system to destroy insulin-producing pancreatic beta-cells. In addition, type 2 diabetes, which used to occur almost exclusively in adults, is now appearing with greater frequency among young people. Evidence suggests the trend is related to a tendency for children and adolescents to be more overweight and less active. Furthermore, racial and ethnic minority groups are disproportionately affected.

But the news is not all bleak. Medical advancements are helping people with diabetes better manage the disease, forestalling its complications. In addition, new insights into the disease's development are leading to more focused prevention efforts. In some cases, these involve lifestyle changes that can help delay—or even prevent—diabetes from developing. For people in whom the disease does appear, proper care and health management can help patients avoid its most serious long-term complications, such as nerve damage, loss of vision, amputation, kidney failure, and even premature death.

Diabetes Information For Teens, Second Edition examines the alarming trends in diabetes prevalence, and it provides information about positive steps that can be taken. The book provides facts about the different types of diabetes, its medical management, and the roles of nutrition and physical activity in averting its consequences. Suggestions are included for handling problematic situations, such as caring for diabetes at school or dealing with the emotional ups and downs associated with having a chronic disease, and a special section describes related health concerns and the prevention of complications. For readers seeking more information, the book provides a directory of diabetes resources and information about finding diabetes-friendly recipes and cookbooks.

How To Use This Book

This book is divided into parts and chapters. Parts focus on broad areas of interest; chapters are devoted to single topics within a part.

Part One: Understanding Diabetes explains how the metabolic processes that fuel the body can sometimes go awry and lead to the disease known as diabetes. It describes the differences between the many forms of diabetes, and it summarizes what researchers have learned and what they hope to discover.

Part Two: Medical Management Of Diabetes talks about the importance of working with a health care team and self-monitoring blood glucose. It explains commonly used diabetes medications and discusses the different roles played by oral diabetes medications and insulin. Problems related to blood sugar levels that are too high or too low are also addressed.

Part Three: Nutrition, Physical Activity, And Weight Management includes facts about meal planning and dietary strategies that can help keep blood sugar levels within a target range. It also discusses the importance of physical activity as a disease-management tool, and it explains how achieving a healthy body weight can help keep diabetes better controlled.

Part Four: Mental Health And Lifestyle Issues looks at the emotional aspects of dealing with diabetes and how disease management practices interact with daily life. It explains how depression and eating disorders are of special concern to people with diabetes, and it offers tips for dealing with diabetes in particular situations, such as at school, while traveling, or when sick.

Part Five: The Physical Complications of Diabetes explains how the metabolic processes that lead to diabetes can also damage the heart, blood vessels, nerves, eyes, kidneys, and other organs and systems of the body. Suggestions for preventing—or at least delaying—these health consequences are also included.

Part Six: If You Need More Information offers a directory of resources for more information about diabetes and suggestions for finding diabetes-friendly recipes and cookbooks.

Bibliographic Note

This volume contains documents and excerpts from publications issued by the following government agencies: Agency for Healthcare Research and Quality; Centers for Disease Control and Prevention (CDC); Federal Trade Commission (FTC); National Center for Complementary and Alternative Medicine; National Diabetes Education Program; National Diabetes Information Clearinghouse; National Eye Institute; National Highway Traffic Safety Administration; National Institute of Child Health and Human Development; National Institute of Diabetes and Digestive and Kidney Diseases; National Institutes of Health; Office of Minority Health; U.S. Food and Drug Administration (FDA); and the Weight-Control Information Network.

In addition, this volume contains copyrighted documents and articles produced by the following organizations and publications: A.D.A.M., Inc.; American Association of Diabetes Educators; American Diabetes Association; BD Consumer Healthcare (Becton, Dickinson and Company); International Diabetes Federation; Joslin Diabetes Center; LifeMed Media, Inc.; and Nemours Foundation.

The photograph on the front cover is © Mark Hatfield/iStockphoto.

Full citation information is provided on the first page of each chapter. Every effort has been made to secure all necessary rights to reprint the copyrighted material. If any omissions have been made, please contact Omnigraphics to make corrections for future editions.

Acknowledgements

In addition to the organizations listed above, special thanks are due to Liz Collins, research and permissions coordinator; Cherry Edwards, permissions assistant; and WhimsyInk, prepress services provider.

About The Teen Health Series

At the request of librarians serving today's young adults, the *Teen Health Series* was developed as a specially focused set of volumes within Omnigraphics' *Health Reference Series*. Each volume deals comprehensively with a topic selected according to the needs and interests of people in middle school and high school.

Teens seeking preventive guidance, information about disease warning signs, medical statistics, and risk factors for health problems will find answers to their questions in the *Teen*

Health Series. The *Series*, however, is not intended to serve as a tool for diagnosing illness, in prescribing treatments, or as a substitute for the physician/patient relationship. All people concerned about medical symptoms or the possibility of disease are encouraged to seek professional care from an appropriate health care provider.

If there is a topic you would like to see addressed in a future volume of the *Teen Health Series*, please write to:

Editor
Teen Health Series
Omnigraphics, Inc.
155 W. Congress, Suite 200
Detroit, MI 48226

A Note About Spelling And Style

Teen Health Series editors use *Stedman's Medical Dictionary* as an authority for questions related to the spelling of medical terms and the *Chicago Manual of Style* for questions related to grammatical structures, punctuation, and other editorial concerns. Consistent adherence is not always possible, however, because the individual volumes within the *Series* include many documents from a wide variety of different producers and copyright holders, and the editor's primary goal is to present material from each source as accurately as is possible following the terms specified by each document's producer. This sometimes means that information in different chapters or sections may follow other guidelines and alternate spelling authorities. For example, occasionally a copyright holder may require that eponymous terms be shown in possessive forms (Crohn's disease vs. Crohn disease) or that British spelling norms be retained (leukaemia vs. leukemia).

Locating Information Within The Teen Health Series

The *Teen Health Series* contains a wealth of information about a wide variety of medical topics. As the *Series* continues to grow in size and scope, locating the precise information needed by a specific student may become more challenging. To address this concern, information about books within the *Teen Health Series* is included in *A Contents Guide to the Health Reference Series*. The *Contents Guide* presents an extensive list of more than 16,000 diseases, treatments, and other topics of general interest compiled from the Tables of Contents and major index headings from the books of the *Teen Health Series* and *Health Reference Series*. To access *A Contents Guide to the Health Reference Series*, visit www.healthreferenceseries.com.

Our Advisory Board

We would like to thank the following advisory board members for providing guidance to the development of this Series:

Medical Consultant

Medical consultation services are provided to the *Teen Health Series* editors by David A. Cooke, M.D. Dr. Cooke is a graduate of Brandeis University, and he received his M.D. degree from the University of Michigan. He completed residency training at the University of Wisconsin Hospital and Clinics. He is board-certified in internal medicine. Dr. Cooke currently works as part of the University of Michigan Health System and practices in Ann Arbor, MI. In his free time, he enjoys writing, science fiction, and spending time with his family.

Part One
Understanding Diabetes

Chapter 1

Facts And Statistics About Diabetes

What Is Diabetes?

Diabetes means that your blood glucose, also called blood sugar, is too high. Glucose comes from the food you eat and is needed to fuel our bodies. Glucose is also stored in our liver and muscles. Your blood always has some glucose in it because your body needs glucose for energy. But having too much glucose in your blood is not healthy.

An organ called the pancreas makes insulin. Insulin helps glucose get from your blood into your cells. Cells take the glucose and turn it into energy.

If you have diabetes, the pancreas makes little or no insulin or your cells cannot use insulin very well. Glucose builds up in your blood and cannot get into your cells. If your blood glucose stays too high, it can damage many parts of the body such as the heart, eyes, kidneys, and nerves.

There are three main types of diabetes.

In type 1 diabetes, the cells in the pancreas that make insulin are destroyed. If you have type 1 diabetes, you need to get insulin from shots or a pump everyday. Most teens can learn to adjust the amount of insulin they take according to their physical activity and eating patterns. This makes it easier to manage your diabetes when you have a busy schedule. Type 1 used to be called "insulin dependent" or "juvenile" diabetes.

In type 2 diabetes, the pancreas still makes some insulin but cells cannot use it very well. If you have type 2 diabetes, you may need to take insulin or pills to help your body's supply of

---

About This Chapter: This chapter begins with information from "Tips for Teens with Diabetes: What Is Diabetes?" National Diabetes Education Program (www.ndep.nih.gov), January 11, 2007. Text under the heading "Diabetes Is Common, Disabling, And Deadly" is from "Diabetes," Centers for Disease Control and Prevention (CDC), April 8, 2010.

insulin work better. Type 2 used to be called "adult onset diabetes." Now more teens are getting type 2, especially if they are overweight.

Gestational diabetes is a type of diabetes that occurs when women are pregnant. Having it raises their risk for getting diabetes, mostly type 2, for the rest of their lives. It also raises their child's risk for being overweight and for getting type 2 diabetes.

What's It Mean?

- **Type 1 diabetes** usually is first diagnosed in children and young adults, although the disease can occur at any age. Type 1 may be autoimmune, genetic, or environmental and accounts for 5% of diabetes cases. There is no known way to prevent this type of diabetes.

- **Type 2 diabetes,** which is linked to obesity and physical inactivity, accounts for 90%–95% of diabetes cases and most often occurs in people older than 40. Type 2 is associated with older age, obesity, family history of diabetes, history of gestational diabetes, impaired glucose metabolism, physical inactivity, race, and ethnicity. Type 2 diabetes in children and adolescents, although still rare, is being diagnosed more frequently among American Indians, African Americans, Hispanics/Latinos, and Asians/Pacific Islanders.

- **Prediabetes** is a condition in which a person has blood glucose levels higher than normal but not high enough to be classified as diabetes. An estimated 57 million American adults had prediabetes in 2007. People with this condition have an increased risk of developing type 2 diabetes, heart disease, and stroke.

- **Gestational diabetes** is a form of glucose intolerance diagnosed during pregnancy. Gestational diabetes occurs more frequently among African Americans, Hispanics/Latinos, and American Indians. It is also more common in obese women and women with a family history of diabetes. Gestational diabetes requires treatment to normalize maternal blood glucose levels to avoid complications in the infant. Women who have had gestational diabetes have a 35%–60% chance of developing diabetes during the 10–20 years following their pregnancy.

- Other types of diabetes result from specific genetic conditions (such as maturity-onset diabetes of youth), surgery, medications, infections, pancreatic disease, and other illnesses. Other types of diabetes account for 1%–5% of all diagnosed cases.

Source: Excerpted from "Diabetes," Centers for Disease Control and Prevention (www.cdc.gov), April 8, 2010.

Why do teens get diabetes?

Genes and things like viruses and toxins may cause a person to get type 1 diabetes. Studies are being done to identify the causes of type 1 diabetes and to stop the process that destroys the pancreas. Researchers can now predict who is at risk for developing type 1 diabetes and in the future may be able to prevent or delay the onset of the disease.

Being overweight increases the risk for type 2 diabetes. Teens who make unhealthy food choices, are not physically active, or who have a family member with diabetes are more likely to get type 2 diabetes. Some racial groups have a greater chance of getting diabetes—American Indians, Alaska Natives, African Americans, Hispanics/Latinos, Asian Americans, and Pacific Islanders. It is not true that eating too much sugar causes diabetes.

What do I need to do to take care of my diabetes?

The key to taking care of your diabetes is to keep your blood glucose as close to normal as possible. The best way to do this is to make healthy food choices, eat the right amounts of food, and be active everyday. It is important to stay at a healthy weight and take your medicines and check your blood glucose as planned with your health care team.

Your doctor will tell you what blood glucose level is right for you. Your goal is to keep your blood glucose as close to this level as you can. Your doctor or diabetes educator will teach you how to check your blood glucose with a glucose meter.

It helps to know what affects your blood glucose level. Food, illness, and stress raise your blood glucose. Insulin or pills and being physically active lower your blood glucose. Talk with your doctor or diabetes educator about how these things change your blood glucose levels and how you can make changes in your diabetes plan.

Carbohydrates, or carbs for short, are a good source of energy for our bodies. But if you eat too many carbs at one time, your blood glucose can get too high. Many foods contain carbs. Great carb choices include whole grain foods, nonfat or low-fat milk, and fresh fruits and vegetables. Eat more of them rather than white bread, whole milk, sweetened fruit drinks, regular soda, potato chips, sweets, and desserts.

Why do I need to take care of my diabetes?

If you take care of your diabetes you can lower your risk for other health problems. High blood glucose can harm blood vessels and cause heart attacks or strokes. It can also damage organs in the body and cause blindness, kidney failure, loss of toes or feet, gum problems, or loss of teeth.

The good news is that when you take care of your diabetes, you can reduce or avoid these problems.

Do not let diabetes stop you! You can do all the things your friends do and live a long and healthy life.

Diabetes Is Common, Disabling, And Deadly

- 23.6 million people in the United States (7.8% of the total population) have diabetes. Of these, 5.7 million have undiagnosed diabetes.

- In 2007, about 1.6 million new cases of diabetes were diagnosed in people aged 20 years or older.

- African American, Hispanic, American Indian, and Alaska Native adults are twice as likely as white adults to have diabetes.

- If current trends continue, one in three Americans will develop diabetes sometime in their lifetime, and those with diabetes will lose, on average, 10–15 years of life.

- Diabetes is the leading cause of new cases of blindness, kidney failure, and nontraumatic lower-extremity amputations among adults.

- Diabetes was the sixth leading cause of death on U.S. death certificates in 2006. Overall, the risk for death among people with diabetes is about twice that of people without diabetes of similar age.

- In 1999–2000, 7% of U.S. adolescents aged 12–19 years had impaired fasting glucose (prediabetes), putting them at increased risk of developing type 2 diabetes, heart disease, and stroke.

Diabetes Is Costly

- Total costs (direct and indirect) of diabetes: $174 billion.

- Direct medical costs: $116 billion.

- Indirect costs (related to disability, work loss, premature death): $58 billion.

- People with diagnosed diabetes have medical expenditures that are about 2.3 times higher than medical expenditures for people without diabetes

Diabetes Is Preventable and Controllable

Recent studies show that lifestyle changes can prevent or delay the onset of type 2 diabetes among people at high risk.

- For people with prediabetes, lifestyle changes, including a 5%–7% weight loss and at least 150 minutes of physical activity per week, can reduce the rate of onset of type 2 diabetes by 58%.

- Disability and premature death are not inevitable consequences of diabetes. By working with their support network and health care providers, people with diabetes can prevent premature death and disability by controlling their blood glucose, blood pressure, and blood lipids and by receiving other preventive care in a timely manner.

- Blood glucose control reduces the risk for eye, kidney, and nerve diseases among people with diabetes by about 40%.

- Blood pressure control reduces the risk for heart disease and stroke among people with diabetes by 33%–50%. It reduces the risk for eye, kidney, and nerve diseases by about 33%.

- Detecting and treating diabetic eye disease with laser therapy can reduce the risk for loss of eyesight by 50%–60%. Comprehensive foot care programs can reduce amputation rates by 45%–85%.

Number Of U.S. Adults Treated For Diabetes More Than Doubled

Approximately 19 million U.S. adults reported receiving treatment for diabetes in 2007, more than double the 9 million who said they received care in 1996, according to the latest *News and Numbers* from the Agency for Healthcare Research and Quality (AHRQ). AHRQ also identified these statistical trends between 1996 and 2007:

- The number of people age 65 and older treated for diabetes increased from 4.3 million to 8 million; for people age 45 to 64, the increase was 3.6 million to 8.9 million; and for 18 to 44 year olds, the increase went from 1.2 million to 2.4 million.

- Treatment costs for diabetes, paid by all sources, more than doubled, rising from $18.5 billion in 1996 (in 2007 dollars) to $41 billion in 2007.

- Outpatient care costs also doubled from about $5 billion to roughly $10 billion.

- Total prescription drug costs nearly increased fourfold from $4 billion to $19 billion over the 11-year period. Per patient, the cost of prescription medicines more than doubled, rising from $495 in 1996 to $1,048 a year in 2007.

Source: Excerpted from "The Number of U.S. Adults Treated for Diabetes More Than Doubled Between 1996 and 2007," Agency for Healthcare Research and Quality (AHRQ), January 5, 2011.

Chapter 2

Diabetes In Children And Adolescents

Type 1 diabetes in U.S. children and adolescents may be increasing, and many more new cases of type 2 diabetes are being reported in young people.

Type 1 Diabetes

Type 1 diabetes mostly has an acute onset, with children and adolescents usually able to pinpoint when symptoms began. Onset can occur at any age, but it most often occurs in children and young adults.

Since the pancreas can no longer produce insulin, people with type 1 diabetes are required to take insulin daily, either by injection or via an insulin pump. Other methods to deliver insulin are being investigated. Children with type 1 diabetes are at risk for long-term complications (damage to the cardiovascular system, kidneys, eyes, nerves, blood vessels, skin, gums, and teeth).

Type 1 diabetes accounts for five to ten percent of all diagnosed cases of diabetes, but it is the leading cause of diabetes in children of all ages, and in those less than 10 years of age, type 1 accounts for almost all diabetes. A diabetes management plan for young people includes insulin therapy, self-monitoring of blood glucose, healthy eating, and physical activity. The plan is designed to ensure proper growth and prevention of hypoglycemia. New management strategies are helping children with type 1 diabetes live long and healthy lives.

About This Chapter: Excerpted from "Overview of Diabetes in Children and Adolescents," a fact sheet from the National Diabetes Education Program, August 2008. The complete text, including references, is available online at http://ndep.nih.gov/media/Youth_FactSheet.pdf.

Symptoms

The immunologic process that leads to type 1 diabetes can begin years before the symptoms of type 1 diabetes develop. Symptoms become apparent when most of the beta-cell population is destroyed and develop over a short period of time. Early symptoms, which are mainly due to hyperglycemia, include increased thirst and urination, constant hunger, weight loss, and blurred vision. Children also may feel very tired.

As insulin deficiency worsens, ketoacids (formed from the breakdown of fat) build up in the blood and are excreted in the urine and breath. They cause the feeling of shortness of breath and abdominal pain, vomiting, and worsening dehydration. Elevation of blood glucose, acidosis, and dehydration comprise the condition known as diabetic ketoacidosis or DKA. If diabetes is not diagnosed and treated with insulin at this point, the individual can lapse into a life-threatening diabetic coma. Often, children with vomiting are mistakenly diagnosed as having gastroenteritis. New-onset diabetes can be differentiated from a GI infection by the frequent urination that accompanies continued vomiting, as opposed to decreased urination due to dehydration if the vomiting is caused by a GI "bug."

Risk Factors

A combination of genetic and environmental factors put people at increased risk for type 1 diabetes. Researchers are working to identify these factors so that targeted treatments can be designed to stop the autoimmune process that destroys the pancreatic beta-cells.

Autoimmune diseases such as celiac disease and autoimmune thyroiditis are associated with type 1 diabetes.

Type 2 Diabetes

Type 2 diabetes used to occur mainly in adults who were overweight and older than 40 years. Now, as more children and adolescents in the United States become overweight, obese, and inactive, type 2 diabetes is occurring more often in young people. Type 2 diabetes is more common in certain racial and ethnic groups such as African Americans, American Indians, Hispanic/Latino Americans, and some Asian and Pacific Islander Americans. The increased incidence of type 2 diabetes in youth is a "first consequence" of the obesity epidemic among young people, and is a significant and growing public health problem. Overweight and obese children are at increased risk for developing type 2 diabetes during childhood, adolescence, and later in life.

Symptoms

Type 2 diabetes usually develops slowly and insidiously in children. Symptoms may be similar to those of type 1 diabetes. A child or teen can feel very tired, thirsty, or nauseated and have to urinate often. Other symptoms may include weight loss, blurred vision, frequent infections, and slow healing of wounds or sores. Some children or adolescents with type 2 diabetes may show no symptoms at all when they are diagnosed, and others may present with vaginal yeast infection or burning on urination due to yeast infection. Some children may have extreme elevation of the blood glucose level associated with severe dehydration and coma. Therefore, it is important for health care providers to identify and test children or teens who are at high risk for the disease.

Physical signs of insulin resistance include acanthosis nigricans, where the skin around the neck or in the armpits appears dark and thick, and feels velvety. High blood pressure and dyslipidemia also are associated with insulin resistance. Girls can have polycystic ovary syndrome with infrequent or absent periods, and excess hair and acne.

Risk Factors

Being overweight, having a family member who has type 2 diabetes, being a member of a high risk racial or ethnic group, having signs of insulin resistance, being older than 10 years of age, and experiencing puberty are risk factors for the disease.

Children with type 2 diabetes also are at risk for the long-term complications of diabetes and the co-morbidities associated with insulin resistance (lipid abnormalities and hypertension).

Timely diagnosis and treatment of type 2 diabetes can prevent or delay the onset of diabetes complications. The cornerstone of diabetes management for children with type 2 diabetes is healthy eating, with portion control, and increased physical activity. To control their diabetes, children with type 2 diabetes also may need to take glucose-lowering medications. However, few of the available medications have been approved for use in children and youth.

Other Types Of Diabetes

Gestational Diabetes: Gestational diabetes mellitus (GDM) is a form of diabetes that is diagnosed in about seven percent of all pregnancies, at a rate of about 200,000 per year. The children of women with a history of GDM are at increased risk for obesity and diabetes compared to other children.

"Hybrid" Or "Mixed" Diabetes: While for the most part it is easy to determine if a child or teenager has type 1 or type 2 diabetes, some teens have elements of both kinds of diabetes. This phenomenon may be called "hybrid" or "mixed" diabetes. It is not surprising that some youth have elements of both type 1 and type 2 diabetes, given the fact that more children are becoming overweight and obese. Youth with "hybrid" diabetes are likely to have both of the following: insulin resistance that is associated with obesity and type 2 diabetes, and antibodies against the pancreatic islet cells that are associated with autoimmunity and type 1 diabetes. The signs and symptoms are the same as those for type 1 and type 2 diabetes.

Maturity-Onset Diabetes Of The Young: Maturity-onset diabetes of the young (MODY), due to one of six gene defects, is a rare form of diabetes in children that is caused by a single gene defect that results in faulty insulin secretion. MODY is defined by its early onset (usually before age 25), absence of ketosis, and autosomal dominant inheritance. Thus, each child of a parent with MODY has a 50 percent chance of inheriting the same type of diabetes. MODY is thought to account for two to five percent of all cases of diabetes and often goes unrecognized. Treatment of MODY varies. Some children respond to diet therapy, exercise, and/or oral anti-diabetes medications that enhance insulin release. Others may require insulin therapy.

Secondary Diabetes: Diabetes can occur in children with other diseases such as cystic fibrosis or those using glucocorticoid drugs. These causes may account for one to five percent of all diagnosed cases of diabetes.

Statistics About Diabetes In Children And Adolescents

Diabetes is one of the most common diseases in school-aged children. According to the National Diabetes Fact Sheet, about 186,300 young people in the US under age 20 had diabetes in 2007. This represents 0.2% of all people in this age group. Based on data from 2002–2003, the SEARCH for Diabetes in Youth study reported that approximately 15,000 U.S.

Less Than One Percent Of Kids Have Diabetes

It's estimated that less than one percent of kids have diabetes—about one in every four or five hundred kids. Overall in the United States, nearly eight percent of people have the disease, and most people with diabetes are over 50. But, until the last decade or so, it was very rare to see someone under 35 with type 2 diabetes. Now, doctors are seeing a lot more kids with this kind of diabetes. That's one reason why you hear a lot about kids and diabetes lately—people are trying to figure out why kids are suddenly getting this kind of the disease. Doctors think it's probably because kids get less exercise and are more likely to be overweight than before.

Source: Excerpted from "Diabetes: Test Your Smarts," BAM! (Body and Mind), Centers for Disease Control and Prevention, 2005. Reviewed by David A. Cooke, MD, FACP, August 2011.

---

youth under 20 years of age are diagnosed annually with type 1 diabetes, while 3,700 are newly diagnosed with type 2 diabetes. Type 2 diabetes is rare in children younger than 10 years of age, regardless of race or ethnicity. After 10 years of age, type 2 diabetes becomes increasingly common, especially in minority populations, representing 14.9% of newly diagnosed cases of diabetes in non-Hispanic whites, 46.1% in Hispanic youth, 57.8% in African Americans, 69.7 % in Asian/Pacific Islanders, and 86.2% in American Indian youth.

Results from the 2005–2006 National Health and Nutrition Examination Survey (NHANES), using measured heights and weights, indicate that an estimated 16–17 percent of children and adolescents ages 2–19 years had a BMI greater than or equal to 95th percentile of the age- and sex-specific BMI—about double the number of two decades ago. Overweight in youth contributes to the increasing numbers of young people who have type 2 diabetes.

Chapter 3

Minorities Disproportionately Affected By Diabetes

Diabetes Data And Statistics

More than 23.6 million people have diabetes in the United States, and pre-diabetes is far more common than previously believed. About 26 percent of U.S. adults aged 20 years or older, or 57 million people, currently have pre-diabetes. Racial and ethnic minority groups, especially the elderly among these populations, are disproportionately affected by diabetes.

On average, African Americans are twice as likely to have diabetes as whites. The highest incidence of diabetes in African Americans occurs between 65–75 years of age. African American women are especially affected. When adjusted for age, African American women are more likely to be diagnosed with diabetes than non-Hispanic whites, African American men, or Hispanics. African Americans with diabetes are more likely to experience complications of diabetes. End-stage renal disease and amputations of lower extremities (legs and feet) are also more common in African Americans with diabetes. In 2007, the CDC estimated that 14.7% of non-Hispanic blacks were diagnosed with diabetes.

As of 2008, 2.5 million Hispanic adults, 18 years and older, about 11 percent of that population, have diabetes. Diabetes is more prevalent in older Hispanics with the highest rates in Hispanics 65 and older. On average, Hispanics are 1.5 times as likely to have diabetes as whites. Mexican Americans, the largest Hispanic subgroup, are almost twice as likely to have diagnosed diabetes than U.S. non-Hispanic whites. And, in 2006 the death rate from diabetes in Hispanics was 50 percent higher than the death rate of non-Hispanic whites.

About This Chapter: This chapter includes excerpts from the following documents produced by the Office of Minority Health (http://minorityhealth.hhs.gov) in September 2010: "Diabetes Data/Statistics," "African Americans and Diabetes," "Hispanic Americans and Diabetes," "American Indians/Alaska Natives and Diabetes," "Asian Americans/Pacific Islanders and Diabetes," and "Native Hawaiians/Pacific Islanders and Diabetes."

On average, American Indians and Alaska Natives are twice as likely as non-Hispanic whites of similar age to have diabetes. As of 2005, 14.2 percent of the American Indian and Alaska Natives aged 20 years or older and receiving care by the Indian Health Service had been diagnosed with diabetes. At the regional level, diabetes is least common among Alaska Natives (6%) and most common among American Indians in southern Arizona (29.3%).

Diabetes is the fifth leading cause of death in the Asian American and Pacific Islander population. Prevalence data for diabetes among this group are limited, but some subpopulations are at increased risk for diabetes. Native Hawaiians, Japanese, and Filipino adults, 20 years of older living in Hawaii were about two times more likely to have been diagnosed with diabetes compared to white residents. An estimated 7.5% of Asian Americans have diabetes.

Diabetes And African Americans

African Americans are twice as likely to be diagnosed with diabetes as non-Hispanic whites. In addition, they are more likely to suffer complications from diabetes, such as end-stage renal disease and lower extremity amputations. Although African Americans have the same or lower rate of high cholesterol as their non-Hispanic white counterparts, they are more likely to have high blood pressure.

- African American adults are twice as likely than non-Hispanic white adults to have been diagnosed with diabetes by a physician.

- In 2006, African American men were 2.2 times as likely to start treatment for end-stage renal disease related to diabetes, as compared to non-Hispanic white men.

Quick Facts

- African American adults were twice as likely than non-Hispanic white adults to have been diagnosed with diabetes by a physician.
- American Indian/Alaska Native adults were 2.1 times as likely as white adults to be diagnosed with diabetes.
- In Hawaii, Native Hawaiians are more than 5.7 times as likely as whites living in Hawaii to die from diabetes.
- Mexican American adults were 1.9 times more likely than non-Hispanic white adults to have been diagnosed with diabetes by a physician.

Source: "Diabetes Data/Statistics," Office of Minority Health, September 2010.

- In 2006, diabetic African Americans were 1.5 times as likely as diabetic whites to be hospitalized.

- In 2006, African Americans were 2.3 times as likely as non-Hispanic whites to die from diabetes.

Age-adjusted percentages of persons 18 years of age and over with diabetes, 2008 (National Health Interview Survey, NHIS)

- Non-Hispanic Black: 11.4

- Non-Hispanic White: 7.1

Age-adjusted prevalence of visual impairment per 100 adults with diabetes (2008)

- African Americans: Men: 14.1; Women 21.1; Total: 18.3

- White: Men: 15.5; Women: 23.2; Total: 19.3

Rate of initiation of treatment for end-stage renal disease related to diabetes per 100,000 diabetic population (2006)

- African Americans: Men: 417.3; Women: 322.3; Total: 362.8

- White: Men: 196.8; Women: 134.2; Total: 164.4

Age-adjusted rate for lower extremity amputation per 1,000 diabetic population, 2005

- African Americans: 5.7

- White: 2.5

Age-adjusted diabetes death rates per 100,000 (2006)

- African Americans: Male: 50.6; Female: 42.4; Total: 45.9

- Non-Hispanic White: Male: 24.7; Female: 17.0; Total 20.4

Diabetes And Hispanic Americans

According to a national examination survey, Mexican Americans are almost twice as likely as non-Hispanic whites to be diagnosed with diabetes by a physician. They have higher rates of end-stage renal disease, caused by diabetes, and they are 50% more likely to die from diabetes as non-Hispanic whites.

Mexican American adults are 1.9 times more likely than non-Hispanic white adults to have been diagnosed with diabetes by a physician.

In 2006, Hispanics were 1.7 times as likely to start treatment for end-stage renal disease related to diabetes, compared to non-Hispanic white men.

In 2006, Hispanics were 1.5 times as likely as non-Hispanic whites to die from diabetes.

Age-adjusted percentages of persons 18 years of age and over with diabetes, 2008 (National Health Interview Survey, NHIS)

- Hispanics/Latinos: 11.0
- Non-Hispanic White: 7.1

Age-adjusted percentage of visual impairment per 100 adults with diabetes (2008)

- Hispanics/Latinos: Men: 17.1; Women: 18.5; Total: 17.9
- White: Men: 15.5; Women: 23.2; Total: 19.3

Rate of initiation of treatment for end-stage renal disease related to diabetes per 100,000 diabetic population (2006)

- Hispanics/Latinos: Men: 319.8; Women: 233.7; Total: 273.2
- White: Men: 196.8; Women: 134.2; Total: 164.4

Age-adjusted diabetes death rates per 100,000 (2006)

Hispanics: Male: 33.7; Female: 26.8; Total: 29.9

Non-Hispanic White: Male: 24.7; Female: 17.0; Total: 20.4

Diabetes And American Indians And Alaska Natives

American Indians/Alaska Natives are twice as likely to be told by a physician that they have diabetes as their non-Hispanic white counterparts. They are also almost twice as likely to die from diabetes as non-Hispanic whites. Data is limited for this population.

- American Indian/Alaska Native adults were 2.1 times as likely as white adults to be diagnosed with diabetes.

- American Indians/Alaska Natives were almost twice as likely as non-Hispanic whites to die from diabetes.

Age-Adjusted Percentage of persons 18 years of age and over with diabetes, 2008 (National Health Interview survey, NHIS)

- American Indian/Native American: 15.0

- Non-Hispanic White: 7.1

Age-Adjusted Diabetes Death Rates per 100,000 (2006)

- American Indian/Alaska Native: 39.6

- Non-Hispanic White: 20.4

Diabetes And Asians and Pacific Islanders

Asians, in general, have the same rate of diabetes as non-Hispanic whites. However, there are differences within this population.

- In Hawaii, Native Hawaiians have more than twice the rate of diabetes as whites.

- Asians are 20% less likely than non-Hispanic whites to die from diabetes.

- In Hawaii, Native Hawaiians are 5.7 times as likely as whites living in Hawaii to die from diabetes.

- Filipinos living in Hawaii have more than three times the death rate as whites living in Hawaii.

Age-adjusted percentages of persons 18 years of age and over with diabetes, 2008

- Asians: 8.0

- Non-Hispanic White: 7.1

Age-adjusted diabetes death rates per 100,000 (2006)

- Asians/Pacific Islanders: 15.8

- Non-Hispanic White: 20.4

Diabetes And Native Hawaiians And Pacific Islanders

While Asian Americans, in general, have the same rate of diabetes as non-Hispanic whites, there are differences within the Native Hawaiian/Pacific Islander population.

- Native Hawaiians/Pacific Islanders are more than three times more likely to be diagnosed with diabetes.

- In 2006, Native Hawaiians/Pacific Islanders were 40 percent less likely to have had a foot examination within the past 12 months, as compared to non-Hispanic whites.

Age-adjusted percentage of persons 18 years of age and over with diabetes, 2007

- Native Hawaiian/Pacific Islanders: 20.6 (estimate considered unreliable)

- Non-Hispanic White: 6.4

Percent of adults diagnosed with diabetes, 2000–2002

- Hawaiian: 7.9
- Japanese: 6.6
- Filipino: 7.5
- White: 3.4

Percent of retinopathy among adults with diabetes, 2000–2002

- Hawaiian state population: 21.9
- Filipino: 18.3
- White: 16.5
- Hawaiian: 28.7
- Japanese: 19.8

Age-adjusted diabetes death rates per 100,000, 2000–2002

- Hawaiian: 216
- Japanese: 100
- Filipino: 116
- White: 38

Chapter 4

Metabolic Syndrome: An Early Warning Sign

Choices. Life is full of them. And many choices affect our health: Will you choose pizza at that post-game dinner or salad with grilled chicken? Do you flop down in front of the TV after school or work out?

Every year scientists discover more about how the choices we make today have a direct impact on the way our bodies function in future. This definitely applies to a condition known as metabolic syndrome.

Metabolic Syndrome Is An Early Warning Sign

Metabolic syndrome isn't a disease. In fact, people who have it usually feel perfectly fine. But metabolic syndrome is a signal that someone could be on the road to serious health problems.

Diagnosing metabolic syndrome helps health professionals figure out a person's risk of developing heart disease, type 2 diabetes, or other diseases. It's kind of like a storm warning: If you hear a hurricane is headed your way, you're going to tune in to weather alerts and do what you can to stay safe. In the same way, finding out that you have metabolic syndrome can help you take steps to prevent diseases like heart disease or type 2 diabetes down the road.

About This Chapter: "Metabolic Syndrome," March 2010, reprinted with permission from www.kidshealth.org. Copyright © 2010 The Nemours Foundation. This information was provided by KidsHealth, one of the largest resources online for medically reviewed health information written for parents, kids, and teens. For more articles like this one, visit www.KidsHealth.org, or www.TeensHealth.org.

What Exactly Is Metabolic Syndrome?

Metabolic syndrome is a collection of problems that health experts call "risk factors." People need to have three or more of the following risk factors before doctors consider them to have metabolic syndrome:

- Excessive belly fat (having an "apple-shaped" body)

- High blood pressure

- Abnormal levels of blood fats, including cholesterol and triglycerides

- High blood sugar

High blood pressure and cholesterol problems might seem like things only old people grumble about. But that's not so anymore. The chances of developing these problems go up if someone is overweight, and many kids and teens fall into this category. Nearly one in ten teens—and more than a third of obese teens—have metabolic syndrome.

How Do I Know If I Have It?

If you have metabolic syndrome, you probably won't know about it until a health professional tells you.

Doctors don't evaluate everyone for metabolic syndrome. Your doctor is less likely to be concerned about it if you are fit and healthy. But if your health provider thinks you're overweight or gaining weight too fast, he or she may consider metabolic syndrome a possibility. That's especially true if you have family members with heart problems or other weight-related diseases.

If someone has one of the risk factors for metabolic syndrome, like high blood pressure, a doctor may check for the others, too.

Checking for metabolic syndrome mostly involves stuff your doctor would be doing anyway, like taking your blood pressure and calculating your body mass index (BMI). If these are high, the doctor also might run blood tests to check out blood sugar and fat levels.

Why Do People Get Metabolic Syndrome?

Being overweight seems to play a major role in metabolic syndrome. Genes do, too. Some people have a genetic tendency to some metabolic syndrome risk factors, like high cholesterol or high blood pressure.

The risk of developing metabolic syndrome appears to be highest around puberty. That may be because body fat, blood pressure, and lipids are all affected by the hormones that bring about growth and development.

The good news is that you can do many things to help keep yourself from getting the health problems that metabolic syndrome can lead to.

Changing Your Course

In the case of metabolic syndrome, making a couple of lifestyle changes is the best way to keep yourself on a track to good health. Here are the top ones:

- **Drop Excess Pounds:** If you're overweight, even a moderate amount of weight loss can bring about big improvements in your blood pressure, blood lipid levels, and your body's ability to use insulin.

- **Stop Sitting And Start Moving:** Take one of those hours you spend in front of a screen and spend it on something that gets your blood flowing. Even a 30-minute walk each day can cause dramatically improve how insulin works in your body, and help your blood pressure and blood lipid levels.

- **Eat Mindfully:** Don't just chow down—think of food as fuel. That doesn't mean boring eating, it just means making an effort to get the right foods into your diet. For example: Choose complex instead of simple carbs (that is, whole-grain bread instead of white bread, brown rice instead of white rice). Get more fiber by eating more beans, fruits, and vegetables. Choose more foods with "healthy" fats like olive oil and nuts, and avoid too many empty calories from soda and sweets.

Insulin Resistance

Many people with metabolic syndrome have insulin resistance, which means insulin doesn't work in their bodies as well as it should. Insulin is a hormone made by the pancreas (located near the stomach). It helps turn the sugar your body gets from food into energy. Most people with insulin resistance are overweight. Being overweight makes the pancreas work harder to make enough insulin to help the body handle sugar as it should. Eventually, the pancreas can become exhausted and make less and less insulin. Because insulin is needed to regulate sugar levels in the blood, a person's blood sugar starts to go up. This can lead to type 2 diabetes.

- **Don't Smoke:** No surprise here—it's just about the worst thing you can do for your heart and lungs.

It can be hard to take this stuff seriously when your thirties and forties seem like a world away. But think about what you want your life to look like then. Maybe you see a family, good friends, a home, a career, perhaps a pet or two. What you probably don't see is having to live with the daily effects of diabetes or heart disease. So why not do whatever you can now to keep those problems from happening later?

Today's a good day to start.

Chapter 5

Insulin Resistance And Pre-Diabetes

What is insulin resistance?

Insulin resistance is a condition in which the body produces insulin but does not use it properly. Insulin, a hormone made by the pancreas, helps the body use glucose for energy. Glucose is a form of sugar that is the body's main source of energy.

The body's digestive system breaks food down into glucose, which then travels in the bloodstream to cells throughout the body. Glucose in the blood is called blood glucose, also known as blood sugar. As the blood glucose level rises after a meal, the pancreas releases insulin to help cells take in and use the glucose.

When people are insulin resistant, their muscle, fat, and liver cells do not respond properly to insulin. As a result, their bodies need more insulin to help glucose enter cells. The pancreas tries to keep up with this increased demand for insulin by producing more. Eventually, the pancreas fails to keep up with the body's need for insulin. Excess glucose builds up in the bloodstream, setting the stage for diabetes. Many people with insulin resistance have high levels of both glucose and insulin circulating in their blood at the same time.

Insulin resistance increases the chance of developing type 2 diabetes and heart disease. Learning about insulin resistance is the first step toward making lifestyle changes that can help prevent diabetes and other health problems.

About This Chapter: From "Insulin Resistance and Pre-diabetes," National Institute of Diabetes and Digestive and Kidney Diseases, October 2008.

What causes insulin resistance?

Scientists have identified specific genes that make people more likely to develop insulin resistance and diabetes. Excess weight and lack of physical activity also contribute to insulin resistance.

Many people with insulin resistance and high blood glucose have other conditions that increase the risk of developing type 2 diabetes and damage to the heart and blood vessels, also called cardiovascular disease. These conditions include having excess weight around the waist, high blood pressure, and abnormal levels of cholesterol and triglycerides in the blood. Having several of these problems is called metabolic syndrome or insulin resistance syndrome, formerly called syndrome X (for more information about metabolic syndrome, see Chapter 4).

What is pre-diabetes?

Pre-diabetes is a condition in which blood glucose levels are higher than normal but not high enough for a diagnosis of diabetes. This condition is sometimes called impaired fasting glucose (IFG) or impaired glucose tolerance (IGT), depending on the test used to diagnose it. The U.S. Department of Health and Human Services estimates that about one in four U.S. adults aged 20 years or older—or 57 million people—had pre-diabetes in 2007.

People with pre-diabetes are at increased risk of developing type 2 diabetes, formerly called adult-onset diabetes or noninsulin-dependent diabetes. Type 2 diabetes is sometimes defined as the form of diabetes that develops when the body does not respond properly to insulin, as opposed to type 1 diabetes, in which the pancreas makes little or no insulin.

Studies have shown that most people with pre-diabetes develop type 2 diabetes within 10 years, unless they lose five to seven percent of their body weight—about 10 to 15 pounds for someone who weighs 200 pounds—by making changes in their diet and level of physical activity. People with pre-diabetes also are at increased risk of developing cardiovascular disease.

What are the symptoms of insulin resistance and pre-diabetes?

Insulin resistance and pre-diabetes usually have no symptoms. People may have one or both conditions for several years without noticing anything. People with a severe form of insulin resistance may have dark patches of skin, usually on the back of the neck. Sometimes people have a dark ring around their neck. Other possible sites for dark patches include elbows, knees, knuckles, and armpits. This condition is called acanthosis nigricans.

How are insulin resistance and pre-diabetes diagnosed?

Health care providers use blood tests to determine whether a person has pre-diabetes but do not usually test for insulin resistance. Insulin resistance can be assessed by measuring the level of insulin in the blood. However, the test that most accurately measures insulin resistance, called the euglycemic clamp, is too costly and complicated to be used in most doctors' offices. The clamp is a research tool used by scientists to learn more about glucose metabolism. If tests indicate pre-diabetes or metabolic syndrome, insulin resistance most likely is present.

Diabetes and pre-diabetes can be detected with one of the following tests:

- **Fasting Glucose Test:** This test measures blood glucose in people who have not eaten anything for at least eight hours. This test is most reliable when done in the morning. Fasting glucose levels of 100 to 125 mg/dL are above normal but not high enough to be called diabetes. This condition is called pre-diabetes or IFG. People with IFG often have had insulin resistance for some time. They are much more likely to develop diabetes than people with normal blood glucose levels.

- **Glucose Tolerance Test:** This test measures blood glucose after people fast for at least eight hours and two hours after they drink a sweet liquid provided by a doctor or laboratory. A blood glucose level between 140 and 199 mg/dL means glucose tolerance is not normal but is not high enough for a diagnosis of diabetes. This form of pre-diabetes is called IGT and, like IFG, it points toward a history of insulin resistance and a risk for developing diabetes.

People whose test results indicate they have pre-diabetes should have their blood glucose levels checked again in one to two years.

Can insulin resistance and pre-diabetes be reversed?

Yes. Physical activity and weight loss help the body respond better to insulin. By losing weight and being more physically active, people with insulin resistance or pre-diabetes may avoid developing type 2 diabetes.

The Diabetes Prevention Program (DPP) and other large studies have shown that people with pre-diabetes can often prevent or delay diabetes if they lose a modest amount of weight by cutting fat and calorie intake and increasing physical activity—for example, walking 30 minutes a day five days a week. Losing just five to seven percent of body weight prevents or delays diabetes by nearly 60 percent. In the DPP, people aged 60 or older who made lifestyle changes lowered their chances of developing diabetes by 70 percent. Many participants in the lifestyle intervention group returned to normal blood glucose levels and lowered their risk for developing heart disease and other problems associated with diabetes. The DPP also showed that the diabetes drug metformin reduced the risk of developing diabetes by 31 percent.

People with insulin resistance or pre-diabetes can help their body use insulin normally by being physically active, making wise food choices, and reaching and maintaining a healthy weight. Physical activity helps muscle cells use blood glucose for energy by making the cells more sensitive to insulin.

Risk Factors For Pre-Diabetes And Type 2 Diabetes

The American Diabetes Association recommends that testing to detect pre-diabetes and type 2 diabetes be considered in adults without symptoms who are overweight or obese and have one or more additional risk factors for diabetes. In those without these risk factors, testing should begin at age 45.

Risk factors for pre-diabetes and diabetes—in addition to being overweight or obese or being age 45 or older—include the following:

- Being physically inactive
- Having a parent or sibling with diabetes
- Having a family background that is African American, Alaska Native, American Indian, Asian American, Hispanic/Latino, or Pacific Islander
- Giving birth to a baby weighing more than nine pounds or being diagnosed with gestational diabetes—diabetes first found during pregnancy
- Having high blood pressure—140/90 or above—or being treated for high blood pressure
- Having an HDL, or "good," cholesterol level below 35 mg/dL or a triglyceride level above 250 mg/dL
- Having polycystic ovary syndrome, also called PCOS
- Having impaired fasting glucose (IFG) or impaired glucose tolerance (IGT) on previous testing
- Having other conditions associated with insulin resistance, such as severe obesity or acanthosis nigricans
- Having a history of cardiovascular disease

If test results are normal, testing should be repeated at least every three years. Health care providers may recommend more frequent testing depending on initial results and risk status.

Points To Remember

- Insulin resistance is a condition in which the body's cells do not use insulin properly. Insulin helps cells use blood glucose for energy.

- Insulin resistance increases the risk of developing pre-diabetes, type 2 diabetes, and cardiovascular disease.

- Pre-diabetes is a condition in which blood glucose levels are higher than normal but not high enough for a diagnosis of diabetes.

- Causes of insulin resistance and pre-diabetes include genetic factors, excess weight, and lack of physical activity.

- Being physically active, making wise food choices, and reaching and maintaining a healthy weight can help prevent or reverse insulin resistance and pre-diabetes.

- The Diabetes Prevention Program (DPP) study confirmed that people at risk for developing type 2 diabetes can prevent or delay the onset of diabetes by losing five to seven percent of their body weight through regular physical activity and a diet low in fat and calories.

Can medicines help reverse insulin resistance or pre-diabetes?

Clinical trials have shown that people at high risk for developing diabetes can be given treatments that delay or prevent onset of diabetes. The first therapy should always be an intensive lifestyle modification program because weight loss and physical activity are much more effective than any medication at reducing diabetes risk.

Several drugs have been shown to reduce diabetes risk to varying degrees. No drug is approved by the U.S. Food and Drug Administration to treat insulin resistance or pre-diabetes or to prevent type 2 diabetes. The American Diabetes Association recommends that metformin is the only drug that should be considered for use in diabetes prevention. Other drugs that have delayed diabetes have side effects or haven't shown long-lasting benefit. Metformin use was recommended only for very high-risk individuals who have both forms of pre-diabetes (IGT and IFG), have a body mass index (BMI) of at least 35, and are younger than age 60. In the DPP, metformin was shown to be most effective in younger, heavier patients.

What research is underway?

Researchers continue to follow DPP participants to learn about the long-term effects of the study. Other research sponsored by the National Institutes of Health builds on the findings from the DPP, including research focusing on lowering diabetes risk in children. Once considered an adult disease, type 2 diabetes is becoming more common in children, and researchers are seeking ways to reverse this trend.

The National Institute of Diabetes and Digestive and Kidney Diseases (NIDDK) also sponsors the TODAY (Treatment Options for Type 2 Diabetes in Adolescents and Youth) study, which focuses on treatment of type 2 diabetes in children and teens at 13 sites. The TODAY study will evaluate the effects of three treatment approaches on control of blood glucose levels, insulin production, insulin resistance, and other outcomes. Each approach involves medication, but one of the three treatment groups will also receive an intensive lifestyle intervention to help the participants lose weight and increase physical fitness. More information about the TODAY study is available at http://www.todaystudy.org.

Chapter 6

Type 1 Diabetes

Introduction

The two major forms of diabetes are type 1, previously called insulin-dependent diabetes mellitus (IDDM) or juvenile-onset diabetes, and type 2, previously called non-insulin-dependent diabetes mellitus (NIDDM) or maturity-onset diabetes.

Both type 1 and type 2 diabetes share one central feature: elevated blood sugar (glucose) levels due to absolute or relative insufficiencies of insulin, a hormone produced by the pancreas. Insulin is a key regulator of the body's metabolism. It works in the following way:

- During and immediately after a meal, digestion breaks carbohydrates down into sugar molecules (of which glucose is one) and proteins into amino acids.

- Right after the meal, glucose and amino acids are absorbed directly into the bloodstream, and blood glucose levels rise sharply. (Glucose levels after a meal are called postprandial levels.)

- The rise in blood glucose levels signals important cells in the pancreas, called beta cells, to secrete insulin, which pours into the bloodstream. Within 20 minutes after a meal insulin rises to its peak level.

- Insulin enables glucose to enter cells in the body, particularly muscle and liver cells. Here, insulin and other hormones direct whether glucose will be burned for energy or stored for future use.

- When insulin levels are high, the liver stops producing glucose and stores it in other forms until the body needs it again.

About This Chapter: Excerpted from "Diabetes: Type 1," © 2011 A.D.A.M., Inc. Reprinted with permission.

- As blood glucose levels reach their peak, the pancreas reduces the production of insulin.

- About two to four hours after a meal both blood glucose and insulin are at low levels, with insulin being slightly higher. The blood glucose levels are then referred to as fasting blood glucose concentrations.

The pancreas is located behind the liver and stomach. In addition to secreting digestive enzymes, the pancreas secretes the hormones insulin and glucagon into the bloodstream. The release of insulin into the blood lowers the level of blood glucose (simple sugars from food) by enhancing glucose to enter the body cells, where it is metabolized. If blood glucose levels get too low, the pancreas secretes glucagon to stimulate the release of glucose from the liver.

In type 1 diabetes, the pancreas does not produce insulin. Onset is usually in childhood or adolescence. Type 1 diabetes is considered an autoimmune disorder that involves:

- Beta cells in the pancreas that produce insulin are gradually destroyed. Eventually insulin deficiency is absolute.

- Without insulin to move glucose into cells, blood glucose levels become excessively high, a condition known as hyperglycemia.

- Because the body cannot utilize the sugar, it spills over into the urine and is lost.

- Weakness, weight loss, frequent urination, and excessive hunger and thirst are among the initial symptoms.

- Patients with type 1 diabetes need to take daily insulin for survival.

Causes

Autoimmune Response

Type 1 diabetes is considered a progressive autoimmune disease, in which the beta cells that produce insulin are slowly destroyed by the body's own immune system. It is unknown what first starts this process, but evidence suggests that both a genetic predisposition and environmental factors, such as a viral infection, are involved.

Genetic Factors

Researchers have found at least 18 genetic locations, labeled IDDM1–IDDM18, which are related to type 1 diabetes. The IDDM1 region contains the HLA genes that encode proteins called major histocompatibility complex. The genes in this region affect the immune response. Other chromosomes and genes continue to be identified.

Most people who develop type 1 diabetes, however, do not have a family history of the disease. The odds of inheriting the disease are only 10% if a first-degree relative has diabetes and, even in identical twins, one twin has only a 33% chance of having type 1 diabetes if the other twin has it. Children are more likely to inherit the disease from a father with type 1 diabetes than from a mother with the disorder.

Genetic factors cannot fully explain the development of diabetes. Over the past 40 years, a major increase in the incidence of type 1 diabetes has been reported in certain European countries, and the incidence has tripled in the U.S.

Viruses

Some research suggests that viral infections may trigger the disease in genetically susceptible individuals.

Among the viruses under scrutiny are enteric viruses, which attack the intestinal tract. Coxsackie viruses are a family of enteric viruses of particular interest. Epidemics of Coxsackie virus, as well as mumps and congenital rubella, have been associated with type 1 diabetes.

Risk Factors

Type 1 diabetes is much less common than type 2 diabetes, consisting of only 5–10% of all cases of diabetes. Nevertheless, like type 2 diabetes, new cases of type 1 diabetes have been rising over the past few decades. While type 2 diabetes has been increasing among African-American and Hispanic adolescents, the highest rates of type 1 diabetes are found among Caucasian youth.

Type 1 diabetes can occur at any age but usually appears between infancy and the late 30s, most typically in childhood or adolescence. Males and females are equally at risk. Studies report the following may be risk factors for developing type 1 diabetes:

- Being ill in early infancy

- Having a parent with type 1 diabetes (the risk is greater if a father has the condition)

- Having an older mother

- Having a mother who had preeclampsia during pregnancy

- Having other autoimmune disorders such as Grave's disease, Hashimoto's thyroiditis (a form of hypothyroidism), Addison's disease, multiple sclerosis (MS), or pernicious anemia

Diabetic Ketoacidosis

Diabetic ketoacidosis (DKA) is a life-threatening complication caused by a complete (or almost complete) lack of insulin. In DKA, the body produces abnormally high levels of blood acids called ketones. Ketones are byproducts of fat breakdown that build up in the blood and appear in the urine. They are produced when the body burns fat instead of glucose for energy. The buildup of ketones in the body is called ketoacidosis. Extreme stages of diabetic ketoacidosis can lead to coma and death.

For some people, DKA may be the first sign that someone has diabetes. In type 1 diabetes, it usually occurs when a patient is not compliant with insulin therapy or intentionally reduces insulin doses in order to lose weight. It can also be triggered by a severe illness or infection.

Symptoms and complications include:

- Thirst and dry mouth
- Frequent urination
- Fatigue
- Dry warm skin
- Nausea and vomiting and stomach pain
- Deep and rapid breathing sometimes with frequent sighing
- Fruity breath odor
- Confusion and decreased consciousness
- Cerebral edema, or brain swelling, is a rare but very dangerous complication that can result in coma, brain damage, or death.
- Other serious complications from DKA include aspiration pneumonia and adult respiratory distress syndrome.

Life-saving treatment uses rapid replacement of fluids with a salt (saline) solution followed by low-dose insulin and potassium replacement.

Symptoms

The process that destroys the insulin-producing beta cells can be long and invisible. At the point when insulin production bottoms out, however, type 1 diabetes usually appears suddenly and progresses quickly. Warning signs of type 1 diabetes include:

- Frequent urination (in children, a recurrence of bed-wetting after toilet training has been completed)

- Unusual thirst, especially for sweet, cold drinks

- Extreme hunger

- Sudden, sometimes dramatic, weight loss

- Weakness

- Extreme fatigue

- Blurred vision or other changes in eyesight

- Irritability

- Nausea and vomiting

Children with type 1 diabetes may also be restless, apathetic, and have trouble functioning at school. In severe cases, diabetic coma may be the first sign of type 1 diabetes.

Diagnosis

Fasting Plasma Glucose Test: The fasting plasma glucose (FPG) test has been the standard test for diagnosing diabetes. It is a simple blood test taken after eight hours of fasting. FPG levels indicate:

- Normal: 100 mg/dL (or 5.5 mmol/L) or below

- Pre-diabetes (a risk factor for type 2 diabetes): Between 100–125 mg/dL (5.5–7.0 mmol/L)

- Diabetes: 126 mg/dL (7.0 mmol/L) or higher

The FPG test is not always reliable, so a repeat test is recommended if the initial test suggests the presence of diabetes, or if the tests are normal in people who have symptoms or risk factors for diabetes. Widespread screening of patients to identify those at higher risk for diabetes type 1 is not recommended.

Specific Problems For Adolescents With Type 1 Diabetes

Lack of Blood Glucose Control: Control of blood glucose levels is generally very poor in adolescents and young adults. Adolescents with diabetes are at higher risk than adults for ketoacidosis resulting from noncompliance. Young people who do not control glucose are also at high risk for permanent damage in small vessels, such as those in the eyes.

Eating Disorders: Up to a third of young women with type 1 diabetes have eating disorders and under-use insulin to lose weight. Anorexia and bulimia pose significant health risks in any young person, but they can be especially dangerous for people with diabetes.

Oral Glucose Tolerance Test: The oral glucose tolerance test (OGTT) is more complex than the FPG and may over-diagnose diabetes in people who do not have it. Some doctors recommend it as a follow-up after FPG, if the latter test results are normal but the patient has symptoms or risk factors of diabetes. The test uses the following procedures: It first uses an FPG test. A blood test is then taken two hours later after drinking a special glucose solution. OGTT levels indicate:

- Normal: 140 mg/dL or below

- Pre-diabetes: Between 140–199 mg/dL

- Diabetes: 200 mg/dL or higher

Patients who have the FPG and OGTT tests must not eat for at least eight hours prior to the test.

Hemoglobin A1C Test: This test examines blood levels of glycosylated hemoglobin, also known as hemoglobin A1C (HbA1c). The results are given in percentages and indicate a person's average blood glucose levels over the past two to three months. (The FPG and OGTT show a person's glucose level for only the time of the test.) The A1C test is not affected by recent food intake so patients do not need to fast to prepare for it.

In 2010, the American Diabetes Association advised that the A1C test can be used as another option for diagnosing diabetes.

A1C levels indicate:

- Normal: Less than 5.7 percent

- Pre-diabetes: Between 5.7 - 6.4 percent

- Diabetes. 6.5 percent or higher

In general, most adult patients with diabetes should aim for A1C levels below or around 7%. Your doctor may adjust this goal depending on your individual health profile.

Goal A1C levels for children are:

- Between 7.5–8.5% for children under age 6 years

- Less than 8% for children age 6–12 years

- Less than 7.5% for children age 13–19 years

The American Diabetes Association recommends that results from the A1C test be used as to calculate estimated Average Glucose (eAG). EAG is a relatively new term that patients may see on lab results from their A1C tests. It converts the A1C percentages into the same mg/dL units that patients are familiar with from their daily home blood glucose tests. For example, an A1C of 7% is equal to an eAG of 154 mg/dL. The eAG terminology can help patients better interpret the results of their A1C tests, and make it easier to correlate A1C with results from home blood glucose monitoring.

Autoantibody Tests

Type 1 diabetes is characterized by the presence of a variety of antibodies that attack the islet cells. These antibodies are referred to as autoantibodies because they attack the body's own cells—not a foreign invader. Blood tests for these autoantibodies can help differentiate between type 1 and type 2 diabetes.

Treatment

Insulin is essential for strict control of blood glucose levels in type 1 diabetes. Good blood glucose control is the best way to prevent major complications in type 1 diabetes, including those that affect the kidneys, eyes, nerve pathways, and blood vessels. Intensive insulin treatment in early diabetes may even help preserve any residual insulin secretion for at least two years.

There are, however, some significant problems with intensive insulin therapy:

- There is a greater risk for low blood sugar (hypoglycemia).

- Many patients experience significant weight gain from insulin administration, which may have adverse effects on blood pressure and cholesterol levels. It is important to manage heart disease risk factors that might develop as a result of insulin treatment.

A diet plan that compensates for insulin administration and supplies healthy foods is extremely important. Pancreas transplantation may eventually be considered for patients who cannot control glucose levels without frequent episodes of severe hypoglycemia.

Insulin Treatment

Standard insulin therapy usually consists of one or two daily insulin injections, one daily blood sugar test, and visits to the health care team every three months. For strictly controlling blood glucose, however, intensive management is required. The regimen is complicated although newer insulin forms may make it easier.

There are two components to insulin administration:

Table 6.1. Glucose Goals For Patients With Diabetes

	Normal	**Goal**
Blood glucose levels before meals	Less than 100 mg/dL	70–130 mg/dL for adults
		100–180 mg/dL for children under age 6
		90–180 mg/dL for children 6–12 years old
		90–130 mg/dL for children 13–19 years old
Bedtime blood glucose levels	Less than 120 mg/dL	Less than 180 mg/dL for adults
		110–200 mg/dL for children under age 6
		100–180 mg/dL for children 6–12 years old
		90–150 mg/dL for children 13–19 years old
Glycosylated hemoglobin (A1C) levels	Less than 5.7%	Less than or around 7%

Major source: Standards of Medical Care In Diabetes–2011, American Diabetes Association.

- **Basal Insulin Administration:** The basal component of the treatment attempts to provide a steady amount of background insulin throughout the day. Basal insulin levels maintain regular blood glucose needs. Insulin glargine now offers the most consistent insulin activity level, but other intermediate and long-acting forms may be beneficial when administered twice a day. Short-acting insulin delivered continuously using a pump is proving to a very good way to provide basal rates of insulin.

- **Mealtime Insulin Administration:** Meals require a boost (a bolus) of insulin to regulate the sudden rise in glucose levels after a meal.

In achieving insulin control the patient must also take other steps:

The patient should perform four or more blood glucose tests during the day.

- Patients should coordinate insulin administration with calorie intake. In general, they should eat three meals each day at regular intervals. Snacks are often necessary.

- Insulin requirements vary depending on many non-nutritional situations during the day, including exercise and sleep. People are at increased risk for low blood sugar during exercise. Some patients experience a sudden rise in blood glucose levels in the morning—the so-called "dawn phenomenon."

- The patient must also maintain a good diet plan and should visit the health care team of doctors, nurses, and dietitians once a month.

Because of the higher risk for hypoglycemia in children, doctors recommend that intensive treatment be used very cautiously in children under 13 and not at all in very young children.

Home Management

Monitoring Glucose (Blood Sugar) Levels: Both low blood sugar (hypoglycemia) and high blood sugar (hyperglycemia) are of concern for patients who take insulin. It is important, therefore, to carefully monitor blood glucose levels. In general, patients with type 1 diabetes need to take readings four or more times a day. Patients should aim for the following measurements:

- Pre-meal glucose levels of 70–130 mg/dL

- Post-meal glucose levels of less than 180 mg/dL

Different goals may be required for specific individuals, including pregnant women, very old and very young people, and those with accompanying serious medical conditions.

A typical blood sugar test includes the following: A drop of blood is obtained by pricking the finger. The blood is then applied to a chemically treated strip. Monitors read and provide results.

Home monitors are about 10–15% less accurate than laboratory monitors, and many do not meet the standards of the American Diabetes Association. Most doctors believe, however, that they are accurate enough to indicate when blood sugar is too low.

Some simple procedures may improve accuracy:

- Testing the meter once a month.

- Recalibrating it whenever a new packet of strips is used.

- Using fresh strips; outdated strips may not provide accurate results.

- Keeping the meter clean.

- Periodically comparing the meter results with the results from a laboratory.

Continuous Glucose Monitoring Systems: Continuous glucose monitoring systems (CGMs) use a needle-like sensor inserted under the skin of the abdomen to monitor glucose levels every five minutes. Depending on the system, CMGs measure glucose levels for three to seven days and sound an alarm if glucose levels are too high or low. These devices are used in addition to traditional fingerstick test kits and glucose meters but do not replace them.

Urine Tests: Urine tests are useful for detecting the presence of ketones. These tests should always be performed during illness or stressful situations, when diabetes is likely to go out of control. The patient should also undergo yearly urine tests for microalbuminuria (small amounts of protein in the urine), a risk factor for future kidney disease.

Preventing Hypoglycemia

The following tips may help avoid hypoglycemia or prepare for attacks.

- Bedtime snacks are advisable if blood glucose levels are below 180 mg/dL (10 mmol/L). Protein snacks may be best.
- Some research has suggested that children (particularly thin children) are at higher risk for hypoglycemia because the injection goes into muscle tissue. Pinching the skin so that only fat (and not muscle) tissue is gathered or using shorter needles may help.
- Various insulin regimens are available that can reduce the risk. For example, taking a fast-acting insulin (insulin lispro) before the evening meal may be particularly helpful in preventing hypoglycemia at bedtime or during the night.
- Patients who intensively control their blood sugar should monitor blood levels as often as possible, four times or more per day. This is particularly important for patients with hypoglycemia unawareness.
- In adults, it is particularly critical to monitor blood glucose levels before driving, when hypoglycemia can be very hazardous.
- Patients who are at risk for hypoglycemia should always carry hard candy, juice, sugar packets, or commercially available glucose substitutes.
- Patients at high risk for severe hypoglycemia, and their family members, should consider having on hand a glucagon emergency kit. The kit is available by prescription and contains an injection of glucagon, a hormone that helps to quickly raise blood glucose levels.

Family and friends should be aware of the symptoms and be prepared:

- If the patient is helpless (but not unconscious), family or friends should administer three to five pieces of hard candy, two to three packets of sugar, half a cup (four ounces) of fruit juice, or a commercially available glucose solution.
- If there is inadequate response within 15 minutes, the patient should receive additional sugar by mouth and may need emergency medical treatment, possibly including an intravenous glucose solution.
- Family members and friends can learn to inject glucagon.

Emergency Treatment: Patients with type 1 diabetes should always wear a medical alert ID bracelet or necklace that states that they have diabetes and take insulin.

Transplantation Procedures

Islet-Cell Transplantation

Researchers are investigating islet-cell transplantation as a way to help patients to come off insulin or reduce their use of it. Most research in recent years has focused on an islet-transplantation procedure called the Edmonton protocol.

This procedure has only been used in clinical trials, but it has helped some patients with severe type 1 diabetes to become free of insulin injections. However, many of these insulin-independent patients needed to resume insulin injections within two years. Researchers are continuing to work on refining the Edmonton protocol so that its benefits can be more sustainable and long lasting.

A major obstacle for the islet cell transplantation is the need for two or more donor pancreases to supply sufficient islet cells. Unfortunately, there are not enough pancreases available to make this procedure feasible for even 1% of patients. Researchers are looking for alternative approaches, including the use of umbilical cord cells, embryonic or adult stem cells, bone marrow transplantation, and other types of cellular therapies. These studies are still in very early stages, but researchers predict that there will be major advances in these fields in the coming years.

Organ Transplantation

Whole pancreas transplants and double transplants of pancreases and kidneys are proving to have a good long-term success rate for some patients with type 1 diabetes. The operations help to prevent further kidney damage, and long-term studies indicate that they may even eventually reverse some existing damage. There is some evidence that heart disease and diabetic neuropathy improve after pancreas transplantation (although not retinopathy).

However, organ transplantation can have significant surgical and postsurgical complications. In addition, patients need to take immunosuppressive drugs on a lifelong basis following a transplant. Doctors generally recommend transplants in cases of end-stage kidney failure or when diabetes poses more of a threat to the patient's life than the transplant itself.

Chapter 7

Type 2 Diabetes

Introduction

Type 2 diabetes is the most common form of diabetes, accounting for 90–95% of cases. In type 2 diabetes, the body does not respond properly to insulin, a condition known as insulin resistance. The disease process of type 2 diabetes involves:

- The first stage in type 2 diabetes is insulin resistance. Although insulin can attach normally to receptors on liver and muscle cells, certain mechanisms prevent insulin from moving glucose (blood sugar) into these cells where it can be used. Most patients with type 2 diabetes produce variable, even normal or high, amounts of insulin. In the beginning, this amount is usually enough to overcome such resistance.

- Over time, the pancreas becomes unable to produce enough insulin to overcome resistance. In type 2 diabetes, the initial effect of this stage is usually an abnormal rise in blood sugar after a meal (called postprandial hyperglycemia).

- Eventually, the cycle of elevated glucose further damages beta cells, thereby drastically reducing insulin production and causing full-blown diabetes. This is made evident by fasting hyperglycemia, in which glucose levels are high most of the time.

Causes

Type 2 diabetes is caused by insulin resistance, in which the body does not properly use insulin. Type 2 diabetes is thought to result from a combination of genetic factors along with lifestyle factors, such as obesity, poor diet, high alcohol intake, and being sedentary.

About This Chapter: Excerpted from "Diabetes: Type 2," © 2011 A.D.A.M., Inc. Reprinted with permission.

Genetic mutations likely affect parts of the insulin gene and various other physiologic components involved in the regulation of blood sugar. Some rare types of diabetes are directly linked to genes.

Diabetes Secondary To Other Conditions: Conditions that damage or destroy the pancreas, such as pancreatitis (inflammation), pancreatic surgery, or certain industrial chemicals, can cause diabetes. Some types of drugs can also cause temporary diabetes, including corticosteroids, beta blockers, and phenytoin. Certain genetic and hormonal disorders are associated with or increase the risk of diabetes.

Risk Factors

Nearly 26 million American children and adults have diabetes. Up to 95% of these cases are type 2. In addition, 79 million American adults have pre-diabetes, a condition that increases the risk for developing diabetes. Type 2 diabetes used to mainly develop after the age of 40, but it is now increasing in younger people and children. Obesity is likely the major factor behind this dramatic growth rate.

According to the National Institutes of Health, people have an increased risk for diabetes or pre-diabetes if they have:

- Age of 45 years or older

- Family history of diabetes

- Overweight

- Inactive lifestyle (exercise less than three times a week)

- African-American, Hispanic/Latin American, American Indian and Alaska Native, Asian-American, or Pacific Islander ethnicity

- High blood pressure (140/90 mm Hg or higher)

- HDL ("good") cholesterol less than 35 mg/dL or triglyceride level 250 mg/dL or higher

- Had diabetes during pregnancy (gestational diabetes) or have given birth to a baby that weighed more than nine pounds

- Polycystic ovary syndrome (metabolic disorder that affects female reproductive system)

- Acanthosis nigricans (dark, thickened skin around neck or armpits)

- History of disease of blood vessels to the heart, brain, or legs

- Diabetes test history of impaired fasting glucose (IFG) or impaired glucose tolerance (IGT)

Know Your Family Health History

Family health history is an important risk factor for developing a number of serious diseases, including type 2 diabetes. In fact, most people with type 2 diabetes have a family member—such as a mother, father, brother, or sister—with the disease.

A family history of type 2 diabetes is a strong risk factor for the disease. If you have a mother, father, brother, or sister with diabetes, you are at risk for type 2 diabetes. But even if you have a family history of type 2 diabetes, there are many things you can do to lower your risk. If you're overweight, losing five to seven percent of your body weight (for example, 10 pounds if you weigh 200 pounds) by exercising 30 minutes a day, five days a week and making healthy food choices can help to prevent or delay type 2 diabetes.

Source: Excerpted from "Know Your Family Health History to Prevent Diabetes in the Future," National Diabetes Education Program, 2010.

Medical Conditions Associated With Increased Risk Of Diabetes

Obesity And Metabolic Syndrome: Obesity is the number one risk factor for type 2 diabetes. Excess body fat appears to play a strong role in insulin resistance, but the way the fat is distributed is also significant. Weight concentrated around the abdomen and in the upper part of the body (apple-shaped) is associated with insulin resistance and diabetes, heart disease, high blood pressure, stroke, and unhealthy cholesterol levels. Waist circumferences greater than 35 inches in women and 40 inches in men have been specifically associated with a greater risk for heart disease and diabetes. (People with a "pear-shape"—fat that settles around the hips and flank—appear to have a lower risk for these conditions.) However, obesity does not explain all cases of type 2 diabetes.

A set of conditions referred to as metabolic syndrome is a pre-diabetic condition that is significantly associated with heart disease and higher mortality rates from all causes. The syndrome consists of obesity marked by abdominal fat, unhealthy cholesterol and triglyceride levels, high blood pressure, and insulin resistance.

Polycystic Ovary Syndrome: Polycystic ovary syndrome (PCOS) is a condition that affects about 6% of women and results in the ovarian production of high amounts of androgens (male hormones), particularly testosterone. Women with PCOS are at higher risk for insulin resistance, and about half of PCOS patients also have diabetes.

Depression: Severe clinical depression may modestly increase the risk for type 2 diabetes.

Schizophrenia: While no definitive association has been established, research has suggested an increased background risk of diabetes among people with schizophrenia. In addition, many of the new generation of antipsychotic medications may elevate blood glucose levels. Patients taking antipsychotic medications (such as clozapine, olanzapine, risperidone, aripiprazole, quetiapine fumarate, and ziprasidone) should receive a baseline blood glucose level test and be monitored for any increases during therapy.

Symptoms

Type 2 diabetes usually begins gradually and progresses slowly. Symptoms in adults include:

- Excessive thirst
- Increased urination
- Fatigue
- Blurred vision
- Weight loss
- In women, vaginal yeast infections or fungal infections under the breasts or in the groin
- Severe gum problems
- Itching
- Erectile dysfunction in men
- Unusual sensations, such as tingling or burning, in the extremities

Symptoms in children are often different:

- Most children are obese or overweight
- Increased urination is mild or even absent
- Many children develop a skin problem called acanthosis, characterized by velvety, dark colored patches of skin

Complications

Patients with diabetes have higher death rates than people who do not have diabetes regardless of sex, age, or other factors. Heart disease and stroke are the leading causes of death in these patients. All lifestyle and medical efforts should be made to reduce the risk for these conditions.

People with type 2 diabetes are also at risk for nerve damage (neuropathy) and abnormalities in both small and large blood vessels (vascular injuries) that occur as part of the diabetic disease process. Such abnormalities produce complications over time in many organs and structures in the body. Although these complications tend to be more serious in type 1 diabetes, they still are of concern in type 2 diabetes.

Diagnosis

Healthy adults age 45 and older should get tested for diabetes every three years. Patients who have certain risk factors should ask their doctors about testing at an earlier age and more frequently. These risk factors include:

- A weight that is 20% more than ideal body weight
- Sedentary lifestyle
- High blood pressure (greater than 140/90) or unhealthy cholesterol levels—especially for patients with low HDL ("good") cholesterol and high triglyceride levels
- History of heart disease, stroke, or peripheral artery disease
- A close relative (parent, sibling) with diabetes
- A high-risk ethnic group background (African-American, Latino, Native American, Asian American, Pacific Islander)
- Having delivered a baby weighing over nine pounds or having a history of gestational diabetes (in women)
- Polycystic ovary disease (in women)

Children age 10 and older should be tested for type 2 diabetes (even if they have no symptoms) every three years if they are overweight and have at least two risk factors.

Testing For Diabetes And Pre-Diabetes

Pre-diabetes precedes the onset of type 2 diabetes. People who have pre-diabetes have fasting blood glucose levels that are higher than normal, but not yet high enough to be classified as diabetes. (Pre-diabetes used to be referred to as "impaired glucose tolerance.") Pre-diabetes greatly increases the risk for diabetes.

There are three tests that can be used to diagnose diabetes or identify pre-diabetes:

Fasting Plasma Glucose Test: The fasting plasma glucose (FPG) test has been the standard test for diabetes. It is a simple blood test taken after eight hours of fasting. FPG levels indicate:

- Normal: 100 mg/dL (or 5.5 mmol/L) or below

- Pre-diabetes: Between 100–125 mg/dL (5.5–7.0 mmol/L)

- Diabetes:126 mg/dL (7.0 mmol/L) or higher

The FPG test is not always reliable, so a repeat test is recommended if the initial test suggests the presence of diabetes, or if the test is normal in people who have symptoms or risk factors for diabetes.

Oral Glucose Tolerance Test: The oral glucose tolerance test (OGTT) is more complex than the FPG and may over-diagnose diabetes in people who do not have it. Some doctors recommend it as a follow-up after FPG, if the latter test results are normal but the patient has symptoms or risk factors of diabetes. The test uses the following procedures: The patient first has an FPG test. The patient has a blood test two hours later, after drinking a special glucose solution.

OGTT levels indicate:

- Normal: 140 mg/dL or below

- Pre-diabetes: Between 140–199 mg/dL

- Diabetes: 200 mg/dL or higher

The patient cannot eat for at least eight hours prior to the FPG and OGTT tests.

Hemoglobin A1C Test: This test examines blood levels of glycosylated hemoglobin, also known as hemoglobin A1C (HbA1c, A1c). The results are given in percentages and indicate a person's average blood glucose levels over the past two to three months. (The FPG and OGTT show a person's glucose level for only the time of the test.) The A1C test is not affected by recent food intake so patients do not need to fast to prepare for the blood test.

In 2010, the American Diabetes Association recommended that the test be used as another option for diagnosing diabetes and identifying pre-diabetes.

A1C levels indicate:

- Normal: Less than 5.7%

- Pre-Diabetes: Between 5.7–6.4%

- Diabetes. 6.5% or higher

A1C tests are also used to help patients with diabetes monitor how well they are keeping their blood glucose levels under control. For patients with diabetes, A1C is measured periodically every two to three months, or at least twice a year. While fingerprick self-testing provides information on blood glucose for that day, the A1C test shows how well blood sugar has been controlled over the period of several months. In general, most patients with diabetes should aim for A1C levels of around 7%. Your doctor may adjust this goal depending on your individual health profile.

The American Diabetes Association recommends that results from the A1C test be used as to calculate estimated Average Glucose (eAG). EAG is a relatively new term that patients may see on lab results from their A1C tests. It converts the A1C percentages into the same mg/dL units that patients are familiar with from their daily home blood glucose tests. For example, an A1C of 7% is equal to an eAG of 154 mg/dL. The eAG terminology can help patients to better interpret the results of their A1C tests and make it easier to correlate A1C with results from home blood glucose monitoring.

Screening Tests For Complications

Screening For Heart Disease: All patients with diabetes should be tested for high blood pressure (hypertension) and unhealthy cholesterol and lipid levels and given an electrocardiogram. Other tests may be needed in patients with signs of heart disease.

ECG: The electrocardiogram (ECG or EKG) is used extensively in the diagnosis of heart disease, from congenital heart disease in infants to myocardial infarction and myocarditis in adults. Several different types of electrocardiogram exist.

Screening For Kidney Damage: The earliest manifestation of kidney damage is microalbuminuria, in which tiny amounts of a protein called albumin are found in the urine. Microalbuminuria typically shows up in patients with type 2 diabetes who have high blood pressure.

The American Diabetes Association recommends that people with diabetes receive an annual microalbuminuria urine test. Patients should also have their blood creatinine tested at least once a year. Creatinine is a waste product that is removed from the blood by the kidneys. High levels of creatinine may indicate kidney damage. A doctor uses the results from a creatinine blood test to calculate the glomerular filtration rate (GFR). The GFR is an indicator of kidney function; it estimates how well the kidneys are cleansing the blood.

Screening For Retinopathy: The American Diabetes Association recommends that patients with type 2 diabetes get an initial comprehensive eye exam by an ophthalmologist or optometrist shortly after they are diagnosed with diabetes, and once a year thereafter. (People at low risk may need follow-up exams only every two to three years.) The eye exam should include dilation to check for signs of retinal disease (retinopathy). In addition to a comprehensive eye exam, fundus photography may be used as a screening tool. Fundus photography uses a special type of camera to take images of the back of the eye.

Screening For Neuropathy: All patients should be screened for nerve damage (neuropathy), including a comprehensive foot exam. Patients who lose sensation in their feet should have a foot exam every three to six months to check for ulcers or infections.

Screening For Thyroid Abnormalities: Thyroid function tests should be performed.

Lifestyle Changes

Good nutrition and regular exercise can help prevent or manage medical complications of diabetes (such as heart disease and stroke) and help patients live longer and healthier lives.

Diet

There is no such thing as a single diabetes diet. Patients should meet with a professional dietitian to plan an individualized diet within the general guidelines that takes into consideration their own health needs.

Healthy eating habits along with good control of blood glucose are the basic goals, and several good dietary methods are available to meet them. General dietary guidelines for diabetes recommend:

- Carbohydrates should provide 45–65% of total daily calories. The type and amount of carbohydrates are both important. Best choices are vegetables, fruits, beans, and whole grains. These foods are also high in fiber. Patients at high risk for diabetes should try to get at least 14 grams of fiber in their diet each day. Patients with diabetes should monitor their carbohydrate intake either through carbohydrate counting or meal planning exchange lists.

- Fats should provide 25–35% of daily calories. Monounsaturated (olive, peanut, and canola oils; avocados; and nuts) and omega-3 polyunsaturated (fish, flaxseed oil, and walnuts) fats are the best types. Limit saturated fat (red meat, butter) to less than 7% of daily calories. Choose nonfat or low-fat dairy instead of whole milk products. Limit trans-fats (hydrogenated fat found in snack foods, fried foods, commercially baked goods) to less than 1% of total calories.

- Protein should provide 12–20% of daily calories, although this may vary depending on a patient's individual health requirements. Patients with kidney disease should limit protein intake to less than 10% of calories. Fish, soy, and poultry are better protein choices than red meat.

- Sodium (salt) intake should be limited to 1,500 mg/day or less. Reducing sodium can lower blood pressure and decrease the risk of heart disease and heart failure.

Weight Management

Being overweight is the number one risk factor for type 2 diabetes. Even modest weight loss can help prevent type 2 diabetes from developing. It can also help control or even stop progression of type 2 diabetes in people with the condition and reduce risk factors for heart disease. Patients should lose weight if their body mass index (BMI) is 25–29 (overweight) or higher (obese).

The American Diabetes Association recommends that patients aim for a small but consistent weight loss of ½–1 pound per week. Most patients should follow a diet that supplies at least 1,000–1,200 kcal/day for women and 1,200–1,600 kcal/day for men.

Source: © 2011 A.D.A.M., Inc. Reprinted with permission.

Exercise

Sedentary habits, especially watching TV, are associated with significantly higher risks for obesity and type 2 diabetes. Regular exercise, even of moderate intensity (such as brisk walking), improves insulin sensitivity and may play a role in preventing type 2 diabetes–regardless of weight loss.

Aerobic Exercise: Aerobic exercise has significant and particular benefits for people with diabetes. Regular aerobic exercise, even of moderate intensity, improves insulin sensitivity. The heart-protective effects of aerobic exercise are also important, even if patients have no risk factors for heart disease other than diabetes itself.

For improving blood sugar control, the American Diabetes Association recommends at least 150 minutes per week of moderate-intensity physical activity (50–70% of maximum heart rate) or at least 90 minutes per week of vigorous aerobic exercise (more than 70% of maximum heart rate). Exercise at least three days a week, and do not go more than two consecutive days without physical activity.

Strength Training: Strength training, which increases muscle and reduces fat, is also helpful for people with diabetes who are able to do this type of exercise. The American Diabetes Association recommends performing resistance exercise three times a week. Build up to three sets of eight to ten repetitions using weight that you cannot lift more than eight to ten times without developing fatigue. Be sure that your strength training targets all of the major muscle groups.

Exercise Precautions: The following are precautions for all people with diabetes, both type 1 and type 2:

- Because people with diabetes are at higher than average risk for heart disease, they should always check with their doctors before undertaking vigorous exercise. For fastest results, regular moderate to high-intensity (not high-impact) exercises are best for people who are cleared by their doctors. For people who have been sedentary or have other medical problems, lower-intensity exercises are recommended.

- Strenuous strength training or high-impact exercise is not recommended for people with uncontrolled diabetes. Such exercises can strain weakened blood vessels in the eyes of patients with retinopathy. High-impact exercise may also injure blood vessels in the feet.

Patients who are taking medications that lower blood glucose, particularly insulin, should take special precautions before starting a workout program:

- Monitor glucose levels before, during, and after workouts (glucose levels swing dramatically during exercise).

- Avoid exercise if glucose levels are above 300 mg/dL or under 100 mg/dL.

- Drink plenty of fluids before and during exercise; avoid alcohol, which increases the risk of hypoglycemia.

- Before exercising, avoid alcohol and if possible certain drugs, including beta-blockers, which make to difficult to recognize symptoms of hypoglycemia.

- Insulin-dependent athletes may need to decrease insulin doses or take in more carbohydrates prior to exercise; they may need to take an extra dose of insulin after exercise (stress hormones released during exercise may increase blood glucose levels). Inject insulin in sites away from the muscles used during exercise; this can help avoid hypoglycemia.

- Wear good, protective footwear to help avoid injuries and wounds to the feet.

- Some blood pressure drugs can interfere with exercise capacity. Patients who use blood pressure medication should talk to their doctors about how to balance medications and exercise. Patients with high blood pressure should also aim to breathe as normally as possible during exercise. Holding the breath can increase blood pressure, especially during strength training.

Warning On Dietary Supplements

Various fraudulent products are often sold on the internet as "cures" or treatments for diabetes. These dietary supplements have not been studied or approved. The U.S. Food and Drug Administration (FDA) warns patients with diabetes not to be duped by bogus and unproven remedies.

Source: © 2011 A.D.A.M., Inc. Reprinted with permission.

Treatment

Management Of Pre-Diabetes

Treatment of pre-diabetes is very important. Research shows that lifestyle and medical interventions can help prevent, or at least delay, the progression to diabetes, as well as lower their risk for heart disease.

- The most important lifestyle treatment for people with pre-diabetes is to lose weight through diet and regular exercise. Even a modest weight loss of 10–15 pounds can significantly reduce the risk of progressing to diabetes.

- Patients should have an exercise goal of 30–60 minutes, at least five days a week, and follow a low-fat, high-fiber diet. Quitting smoking is also essential.

- It is also important to have your doctor check your cholesterol and blood pressure levels on a regular basis. Your doctor should also check your fasting blood glucose and microalbuminuria levels every year, and your hemoglobin A1C and lipids every six months.

- In addition to lifestyle measures, the insulin-regulating drug metformin (Glucophage) may be recommended for patients who may be at very high risk for developing diabetes. High risk factors include an A1C of greater than 6%, high blood pressure, low HDL cholesterol, high levels of triglycerides, obesity, or family history of diabetes in a first-degree relative (parents, siblings, and children).

Management Of Type 2 Diabetes

The major treatment goals for people with type 2 diabetes are to control blood glucose levels and to treat all conditions that place patients at risk for heart disease, stroke, kidney disease, and other major complications.

Approaches to controlling blood glucose levels include:

- Achieving A1C levels of around 7%. (Patients who have a history of severe hypoglycemia, vascular complications or other diseases, or longstanding diabetes may benefit from looser control of blood sugar. Patients should discuss individualized treatment goals with their doctors.)

- Close monitoring of blood sugar and hemoglobin A1C levels.

- Use of oral anti-hyperglycemic drugs such as metformin as first-line drug treatments, and insulin if needed.

Approaches for reducing complications include:

- Healthy lifestyle changes, such as regular exercise, heart-healthy diet, quitting smoking.

- Use of various drugs to control high blood pressure (such as ACE inhibitors and diuretics) and to lower cholesterol (statins and fibrates).

- Daily low-dose (75–162 mg) aspirin is recommended for men older than age 50 and women older than age 60 who have diabetes and at least one additional risk factor for heart disease (such as smoking, high blood pressure, unhealthy cholesterol levels, family history of heart disease, or albuminuria). Daily aspirin is not recommended for patients with diabetes who are younger than these ages and who do not have cardiovascular risk factors.

- Close follow-up with your doctor.

Treating Special Populations

Different goals may be necessary for specific individuals, including pregnant women, very old and very young people, and those with accompanying serious medical conditions. Treating children with type 2 diabetes depends on the severity of the condition at diagnosis. Metformin is approved for children. Formerly, only insulin was approved for treating children with diabetes.

The American Diabetes Association does not recommend tight blood glucose control for children because glucose is necessary for brain development. Elderly people should not generally be placed on tight control as low blood sugar can increase the risk of stroke or heart attack.

Medications

Many types of anti-hyperglycemic drugs are available to help patients with type 2 diabetes control their blood sugar levels. Most of these drugs are aimed at using or increasing sensitivity to the patient's own natural stores of insulin.

For the most part older oral hypoglycemic drugs—particularly metformin—are less expensive and work as well as newer diabetes drugs. Metformin is generally recommended as the first-line drug.

Adding a second oral hypoglycemic drug is usually recommended if adequate control is not achieved with the first medication. For the most part, doctors should add a second drug rather than trying to push the first drug dosage to the highest levels.

Insulin Replacement: Insulin replacement may be necessary when natural insulin reserves are depleted. It is typically started in combination with an oral drug (usually metformin).

Because type 2 diabetes is progressive, many patients eventually need insulin. However, when a single oral drug fails to control blood sugar it is not clear whether it is better to add insulin replacement or a second or third oral drug.

Some doctors advocate using insulin as early as possible for optimal control. However, in patients who still have insulin reserves, there is concern that extra natural insulin will have adverse effects. Low blood sugar (hypoglycemia) and weight gain are the main side effects of insulin therapy. It is still not clear if insulin replacement improves survival rates compared to oral drugs, notably metformin.

Finger-Prick Test

A typical blood sugar test includes the following: A drop of blood is obtained by pricking the finger. The blood is then applied to a chemically treated strip. Monitors read and provide results.

Home monitors are about 10–15% less accurate than laboratory monitors, and many do not meet the standards of the American Diabetes Association. Most doctors believe, however, that they are accurate enough to indicate when blood sugar is too low.

Source: © 2011 A.D.A.M., Inc. Reprinted with permission.

Monitoring Glucose (Blood Sugar) Levels

Both low blood sugar (hypoglycemia) and high blood sugar (hyperglycemia) are of concern, especially for patients who take insulin. Blood glucose levels are generally more stable in type 2 diabetes than in type 1, so doctors usually recommend measuring blood levels only once or twice a day. For patients who have become insulin-dependent, more intensive monitoring is necessary. Patients should aim for the following measurements:

- Pre-meal glucose levels of between 70–130 mg/dL

- Post-meal glucose levels of less than 180 mg/dL

Different goals may be required for specific individuals, including pregnant women, very old and very young people, and those with accompanying serious medical conditions.

Chapter 8

Double Diabetes

The incidences of both type 1 diabetes and type 2 diabetes are on the rise in children and teenagers. Indeed, type 1 diabetes is increasing particularly in the very young. Recent multi-country data from the EURODIAB study indicate that the overall prevalence of type 1 diabetes among young people under 15 years is growing by over 3% each year and by more than 6% a year in children aged up to four years.[1] Over the last decade and a half, there has been an increase in the incidence of obesity-driven type 2 diabetes in young people in countries around the world.

Before the 1990s, it was rare for U.S. pediatric diabetes centers to see young people with type 2 diabetes. But by 1994, in urban areas of the U.S., children with type 2 diabetes represented up to 16% of the new cases of diabetes in children, and by 1999, that figure was as high as 45% in some areas.[2,3] Similarly, there has been an approximate four-fold rise in the incidence of type 2 diabetes in six- to 15-year-olds in Japan.[4]

While, for the most part, it is easy to determine what type of diabetes a child or teenager has, in some instances it is not quite so clear. In my own practice at Children's Hospital Los Angeles in the U.S., I recently saw two cases that illustrated the potential difficulties in determining the type of diabetes.

Type 2 Diabetes?

The first was a 13-year-old girl with obesity, who had had symptoms of diabetes for about three months. Her blood glucose level was 17.8 mmol/L (322 mg/dL). Fortunately, she did not have ketones in her urine or blood, but her blood cholesterol levels were very high, and

About This Chapter: Text in this chapter is from "Double diabetes in young people and how to treat it," by Francine Kaufman, in *DiabetesVoice*, March 2006, Volume 51, Issue 1. © 2006 International Diabetes Federation (www.diabetesvoice.org); reprinted with permission. Text reviewed July 2011.

there was darkening of the skin around her neck (called acanthosis nigricans). The clinical picture was apparently typical of a person with type 2 diabetes.

However, she showed the distinctive feature of type 1 diabetes: very high levels of antibodies against the insulin-producing pancreatic beta cells. Therefore, she was treated with insulin injections rather than oral blood glucose-lowering medicines.

Type 1 Diabetes?

The other case was that of a 13-year-old girl who had been diagnosed with type 1 diabetes when she was four years old. When she went through puberty—having been on insulin for nine years—she gained excessive weight and her body developed insensitivity to insulin. She needed to take more than 150 units of insulin each day; she developed elevated levels of blood cholesterol and acanthosis nigricans. The oral medication, metformin, was added to her regimen, which improved her diabetes control on a significantly reduced dosage of insulin.

Double Diabetes

As mentioned earlier, the hallmark of type 1 diabetes is the presence of antibodies which attack the insulin-producing pancreatic beta cells—an indication that type 1 diabetes is an autoimmune disorder. The autoimmunity leads to the destruction of the beta-cell mass that results in profound insulin deficiency.

The hallmark of type 2 diabetes is the combination of insensitivity to insulin and the continuing ability to make the hormone—although not enough to overcome the body's insensitivity to the action of insulin.

What's It Mean?

Ketones: Ketones are chemicals that the body produces when there is not enough insulin in the blood and it must break down stored fat instead of glucose for its energy.

Ketoacidosis: Ketoacidosis occurs when excessive amounts of ketones build up in the blood. Ketoacidosis can lead to coma or even death.

C-peptide: C-peptide is a by-product of insulin made in the pancreas. A measurement of the levels of C-peptide (made up of amino acids) in the blood can indicate whether or not a person is producing insulin and roughly how much.

Table 8.1. Differential Diagnosis: Type 1 diabetes vs. type 2 diabetes in children and adolescents

	Type 1 diabetes	Type 2 diabetes
Typical clinical course	Usually rapid onset	Slow onset
Weight	Primarily lean	80%–90% obese
Diabetes ketoacidosis	35%–40%	5%–25%
Family history	5% have a relative with type 1 diabetes; Up to 20% may have a relative with type 2 diabetes	74%–100% have relative with type 2 diabetes
Co-morbid conditions	Thyroid and/or adrenal disorders; Vitiligo; Celiac disease	Polycystic ovary syndrome; Acanthosis nigricans
C-peptide	Usually reduced levels but can be preserved at diagnosis	Always present
Presence of islet auto-antibodies	85%	15%

Double diabetes suggests that elements of both type 1 diabetes and type 2 diabetes co-exist in the same person: people with type 1 diabetes have the insensitivity to insulin that is most often associated with obesity; people with type 2 diabetes have antibodies against the pancreatic beta cells. Blurring the issue further is the fact that people with type 1 diabetes have family members with type 2 diabetes and vice versa. This means that a considerable number of people may be at genetic risk for both kinds of diabetes.

In adults, latent autoimmune diabetes in adults (LADA) may be a form of double diabetes. Young adults with LADA have antibodies against the insulin-producing beta cells. At first, these young people can be treated with an oral diabetes medication; they then require insulin treatment earlier than most people with type 2 diabetes.

The SEARCH (Search for Diabetes in Youth) study in the U.S. identified a number of children with double diabetes.[5] This study—designed to determine the incidence and prevalence of childhood diabetes in the U.S.—has demonstrated that a relatively large proportion of the young people diagnosed with diabetes both continue to produce insulin and have antibodies against the beta cells.

The Accelerator Hypothesis

The accelerator hypothesis of diabetes development suggests that excessive weight gain—a significant and growing problem worldwide—results in insensitivity to insulin. This insensitivity to insulin puts the beta cells under stress by forcing them to manufacture more insulin.[6] The stressed beta cells are more susceptible to autoimmune injury, which can lead to their destruction.

The accelerator hypothesis predicts that heavier children will develop type 1 diabetes.[6] This is similar to type 2 diabetes: heavier children are also the ones who develop type 2 diabetes. The overall increase in insensitivity to insulin due to obesity is blurring the lines that differentiate between type 1 diabetes and type 2 diabetes.

Diagnostic Evaluation And Treatment

At the time of a diagnosis of diabetes in children and teenagers, the healthcare provider should of course attempt to determine which type of diabetes is present.

Table 8.1 shows the clinical features that can help to differentiate the type of diabetes. In lean, young children, it is probably correct to assume that the young person has type 1 diabetes. However, in overweight teenagers, it may be difficult to differentiate type 1 diabetes from type 2 diabetes.[7] Measuring antibodies that act against the pancreatic beta cells can be helpful; an assessment of insulin production by measuring C-peptide levels can also be used.

Everyone with type 1 diabetes requires insulin therapy. If it is determined that a person has type 2 diabetes, lifestyle interventions or oral blood glucose-lowering medication can be started—if blood glucose levels are not excessively elevated and there is no significant dehydration or acidosis. If the type of diabetes cannot be determined, the young person should be started on insulin therapy while waiting for test results that hopefully will clarify the situation.

For people with double diabetes, it is likely that they need both insulin and oral diabetes medicines to improve sensitivity to insulin. However, studies are required to evaluate the benefits of a dual approach to increasing sensitivity to insulin.

Conclusions

It is important to determine who has double diabetes since that will help to dictate which diagnostic and therapeutic approaches should be taken. However, we need to learn more about this relatively newly recognized condition. Since the emergence of double diabetes seems to be linked to the epidemic of obesity in young people, our focus should be on how to prevent childhood obesity as a primary means of reducing the emergence of this potentially devastating condition.

References

1. EURODIAB ACE Study Group. Variation and trends in incidence of childhood diabetes in Europe. *Lancet* 2000; 355: 873-6.

2. Pinhas-Hamiel O, Dolan LM, Daniels SR, et al. Increased incidence of non-insulin-dependent diabetes mellitus among adolescents. *J Pediatr* 1996; 128:608-15.

3. Fagot-Campagna A, Petit DJ, Engelgau MM. Type 2 diabetes among North American children and adolescents: An epidemiological review and a public health perspective. *J Pediatr* 2000; 136: 664-72.

4. Kitagawa T, Owada M, Urakami T, Yamauchi K. Increase incidence of non-insulin dependent diabetes mellitus among Japanese school children correlates with an increased intake of animal protein and fat. *Clin Pediatr* 1998; 37: 111-5.

5. www.niddk.nih.gov/patient/SEARCH/SEARCH.htm (Accessed 25 January 2006).

6. Wilkin TJ. The accelerator hypothesis: weight gain as the missing link between type I and type II diabetes. *Diabetologia* 2001; 44: 914-22.

7. Silverstein J, Klingensmith G, Copeland K, et al. Care of Children and Adolescents with Type 1 Diabetes Mellitus: A Statement of the American Diabetes Association. *Diabetes Care* 2005; 28: 186-212.

Chapter 9

Gestational Diabetes And Diabetes-Related Women's Concerns

Gestational Diabetes

Gestational (jes-TAY-shun-ul) diabetes is a type of diabetes that can happen during pregnancy. It means the woman has have never had diabetes before. Having gestational diabetes means she has a problem with high blood sugar while she is pregnant. The treatment is to control blood sugar. This can help prevent a difficult birth. It also helps keep her baby healthy.

What is gestational diabetes?

Gestational diabetes means that the body has a problem with insulin during pregnancy. When women are pregnant, their bodies need more insulin to keep blood sugar at the right level. Women's bodies make more insulin during pregnancy. When the extra insulin is not enough to keep blood sugar normal, women get high blood sugar. This is called gestational diabetes. Blood sugar usually returns to normal after delivery.

Who gets gestational diabetes?

About seven out of 100 pregnant women get gestational diabetes. Gestational diabetes is more likely for women who are overweight, women with family members who have had gestational diabetes, women with family members who have type 2 diabetes, and African American, American Indian, and Hispanic/Latina American women.

About This Chapter: Excerpted and adapted from "Gestational Diabetes: A Guide for Pregnant Women," Agency for Healthcare Research and Quality, August 5, 2009. Text under the heading "How are women especially affected by diabetes?" is excerpted from "Groups Especially Affected," Centers for Disease Control and Prevention, August 9, 2010. Text under the heading "What is PCOS?" is excerpted from "Polycystic Ovary Syndrome (PCOS)," National Institute of Child Health and Human Development, May 27, 2007.

Fast Facts On Gestational Diabetes

- Gestational diabetes is a kind of diabetes that can happen during pregnancy. It usually goes away after delivery.

- Gestational diabetes is treated by controlling blood sugar. Some women can do this with a special diet for diabetes and staying active. Other women will need insulin shots or diabetes pills.

- Insulin and two kinds of diabetes pills can lower blood sugar for women with gestational diabetes.

- Many women who have gestational diabetes get type 2 diabetes later in life. Controlling weight gain during pregnancy may prevent type 2 diabetes later on.

- It is important to keep being tested for type 2 diabetes regularly after pregnancy.

Source: Agency for Healthcare Research and Quality, August 5, 2009.

Why is it important to treat gestational diabetes?

High blood sugar can cause the baby to get too big—nine pounds or more. This is the most common problem with gestational diabetes. It is called macrosomia (mak-ruh-SO-me-uh). A baby that is too big can cause problems during delivery. At birth, the baby can also have breathing problems or blood sugar that is too low.

Women with gestational diabetes can give birth to healthy babies. Keeping blood sugar under control may help prevent problems.

If a woman has gestational diabetes, her doctor or midwife may discuss different delivery options. The goal is to have a safe delivery and a healthy baby.

Many times doctors or midwives induce (or start) a woman's labor before her due date if she has gestational diabetes. Sometimes this is done so the baby does not get so big. Research can't tell us if inducing labor early is better for the mom and baby than waiting for labor to start on its own.

Sometimes doctors or midwives suggest cesarean section, or c-section. It is another option to prevent problems with delivery from a big baby. A c-section is an operation done to deliver the baby from the mom's belly. Research also can't tell us if a c-section is better for the mom and baby than inducing labor or waiting for labor to start on its own.

How is gestational diabetes treated?

Eating healthy and staying active are two of the most important ways to control blood sugar and treat gestational diabetes. Activities like walking and swimming are helpful. The activity does not have to be hard. The goal is to get up and move.

All women with gestational diabetes need to follow a special diabetes meal plan. A woman's doctor or midwife may ask her to meet with a diabetes educator or dietitian. Diabetes educators or dietitians can help create a plan just for her.

The diabetes meal plan follows simple guidelines like watching portion size and eating a variety of foods, including fresh fruits, vegetables, and whole grains. It may also limit fat calories to 30 percent or less each day. Being careful about weight gain during pregnancy is also very important to control gestational diabetes.

Is medicine used to treat gestational diabetes?

Most women can control their gestational diabetes by following a diabetes meal plan and being more active. Some will also need insulin or diabetes pills to control their blood sugar. Insulin and two kinds of diabetes pills are used to treat gestational diabetes. They all work to lower blood sugar. So far, research shows that they all seem safe to use while pregnant.

Insulin: Insulin needs to be injected (given by a shot). The insulin injected is like the insulin the body makes, but it is made in a lab. There are many kinds of insulin.

Diabetes Pills: Two kinds of diabetes pills have been used to treat gestational diabetes. Glyburide (DiaBeta®, Glynase PresTab®, Micronase®) is a pill that helps raise the amount of insulin in the body. Metformin (Glucophage®) blocks the liver from making glucose (sugar). The two pills used to treat gestational diabetes are also used for type 2 diabetes.

How often is blood sugar tested?

Some women will need to check their blood sugar several times a day. This is usually done in the morning before breakfast and after each meal.

The Risk For Type 2 Diabetes

About 60 out of 100 women who have gestational diabetes will have type 2 diabetes by 10 years after their pregnancy. The good news is this risk can be reduced by staying at a healthy weight, eating a healthy diet, getting active, and being tested regularly.

Source: Agency for Healthcare Research and Quality, August 5, 2009.

How is blood sugar tested?

Blood sugar is tested by a finger stick done at home. This test uses a glucose meter that shows blood sugar level. Following instructions from their physicians or midwives, most women with gestational diabetes check their blood sugar at different times of the day. Typical blood sugar targets for pregnant women are as follows (but they may be different in individual circumstances, so women should ask their healthcare providers about the right targets):

- Before eating: Less than 95

- One hour after eating: Less than 130

- Two hours after eating: Less than 120

It is important for women with gestational diabetes to keep track of blood sugar test results. Their healthcare providers will use the results to decide about the need to start medicine for blood sugar control or adjust doses.

What is hypoglycemia?

Blood sugar that is too low is called hypoglycemia (high-po-gly-SEE-mee-ah). It can make a person feel dizzy, sweaty, confused, shaky, hungry, and weak.

Insulin and pills for gestational diabetes can cause blood sugar to drop too low, but more women using insulin develop very low blood sugar than women taking metformin (Glucophage®).

A pregnant woman with low blood sugar should eat or drink something with sugar in it right away. Her healthcare provider may suggest something like hard candy, juice, or glucose tablets.

What happens after delivery?

After birth, gestational diabetes usually goes away. Blood sugar returns to normal after delivery. Most women won't need to keep checking blood sugar at home with the finger sticks. But there are important things to keep in mind.

Women who have had gestational diabetes are more likely to get type 2 diabetes later in life. They have a higher chance than women who have not had gestational diabetes. Women who gain more weight than normal during pregnancy also have a higher chance of getting type 2 diabetes later.

There are ways a woman can help lower her risk of getting diabetes later on. Staying at a healthy weight, following a healthy diet, and being active can help. These small steps are important during and after pregnancy.

It is very important for women who have had gestational diabetes to have their blood sugar checked at their doctor's office from time to time. The test will make sure that that have not developed type 2 diabetes. A doctor or nurse can give advice about how often blood sugar should be tested.

Women And Diabetes: Other Issues

How are women especially affected by diabetes?

Of the 20.8 million people with diabetes in the United States, 9.7 million are women. The risk of heart disease, the most common complication of diabetes, is more serious among women than men. Among people with diabetes who have had a heart attack, women have lower survival rates and a poorer quality of life than men. Women with diabetes have a shorter life expectancy than women without diabetes, and women are at greater risk of blindness from diabetes than men. Death rates for women aged 25–44 years with diabetes are more than three times the rate for women without diabetes.

Women with diabetes must also plan childbearing carefully. It is especially important to keep blood glucose levels as near to normal as possible before and during pregnancy, to protect both mother and baby. Pregnancy itself may affect insulin levels, as well as diabetes-related eye and kidney problems.

What is PCOS?

Polycystic ovary syndrome (PCOS) is a condition in which a woman's ovaries and, in some cases the adrenal glands, produce more androgens (a type of hormone) than normal. High levels of these hormones interfere with the development and release of eggs as part of ovulation. As a result, fluid-filled sacs or cysts can develop on the ovaries.

Because women with PCOS do not release eggs during ovulation, PCOS is the most common cause of female infertility. In addition to infertility, women with PCOS may also have pelvic pain; hirsutism (excess hair growth on the face, chest, stomach, thumbs, or toes); male-pattern baldness or thinning hair; acne, oily skin, or dandruff; or patches of thickened and dark brown or black skin. Also, women who are obese are more likely to have PCOS.

Although it is hard for women with PCOS to get pregnant, some do get pregnant, naturally or using assistive reproductive technology. Women with PCOS are at higher risk for miscarriage if they do become pregnant.

Women with PCOS are also at higher risk for associated conditions, such as diabetes or metabolic syndrome. Sometimes called a precursor to diabetes, metabolic syndrome indicates that the body has trouble regulating its insulin. In addition, women with PCOS are at higher risk for cardiovascular disease—including heart disease and high blood pressure.

Chapter 10

Monogenic Forms Of Diabetes

Neonatal Diabetes Mellitus And Maturity-Onset Diabetes Of The Young

The most common forms of diabetes, type 1 and type 2, are polygenic, meaning the risk of developing these forms of diabetes is related to multiple genes. Environmental factors, such as obesity in the case of type 2 diabetes, also play a part in the development of polygenic forms of diabetes. Polygenic forms of diabetes often run in families. Doctors diagnose polygenic forms of diabetes by testing blood glucose in individuals with risk factors or symptoms of diabetes.

Genes provide the instructions for making proteins within the cell. If a gene has a mutation, the protein may not function properly. Genetic mutations that cause diabetes affect proteins that play a role in the ability of the body to produce insulin or in the ability of insulin to lower blood glucose. People have two copies of most genes; one gene is inherited from each parent.

What are monogenic forms of diabetes?

Some rare forms of diabetes result from mutations in a single gene and are called monogenic. Monogenic forms of diabetes account for about one to five percent of all cases of diabetes in young people. In most cases of monogenic diabetes, the gene mutation is inherited; in the remaining cases the gene mutation develops spontaneously. Most mutations in monogenic diabetes reduce the body's ability to produce insulin, a protein produced in the pancreas that helps

About This Chapter: This chapter begins with excerpts from "Monogenic Forms of Diabetes: Neonatal Diabetes Mellitus and Maturity-onset Diabetes of the Young," National Institute of Diabetes and Digestive and Kidney Diseases (NIDDK), March 2007. Text under the heading "Other Types of Diabetes," is from "Diagnosis of Diabetes," NIDDK, October 2008.

the body use glucose for energy. Neonatal diabetes mellitus (NDM) and maturity-onset diabetes of the young (MODY) are the two main forms of monogenic diabetes. MODY is much more common than NDM. NDM first occurs in newborns and young infants; MODY usually first occurs in children or adolescents but may be mild and not detected until adulthood.

Genetic testing can diagnose most forms of monogenic diabetes. If genetic testing is not performed, people with monogenic diabetes may appear to have one of the polygenic forms of diabetes. When hyperglycemia is first detected in adulthood, type 2 is often diagnosed instead of monogenic diabetes. Some monogenic forms of diabetes can be treated with oral diabetes medications while other forms require insulin injections. A correct diagnosis that allows the proper treatment to be selected should lead to better glucose control and improved health in the long term. Testing of other family members may also be indicated to determine whether they are at risk for diabetes.

What is neonatal diabetes mellitus (NDM)?

NDM is a monogenic form of diabetes that occurs in the first six months of life. It is a rare condition occurring in only one in 100,000 to 500,000 live births. Infants with NDM do not produce enough insulin, leading to an increase in blood glucose. NDM can be mistaken for the much more common type 1 diabetes, but type 1 diabetes usually occurs later than the first six months of life. In about half of those with NDM, the condition is lifelong and is called permanent neonatal diabetes mellitus (PNDM). In the rest of those with NDM, the condition is transient and disappears during infancy but can reappear later in life; this type of NDM is called transient neonatal diabetes mellitus (TNDM). Specific genes that can cause NDM have been identified. See Table 10.1 for more information.

Symptoms of NDM include thirst, frequent urination, and dehydration. NDM can be diagnosed by finding elevated levels of glucose in blood or urine. In severe cases, the deficiency of insulin may cause the body to produce an excess of acid, resulting in a potentially life-threatening condition called ketoacidosis. Most fetuses with NDM do not grow well in the womb and newborns are much smaller than those of the same gestational age, a condition called intrauterine growth restriction. After birth, some infants fail to gain weight and grow as rapidly as other infants of the same age and sex. Appropriate therapy improves and may normalize growth and development.

What is maturity-onset diabetes of the young (MODY)?

MODY is a monogenic form of diabetes that usually first occurs during adolescence or early adulthood. However, MODY sometimes remains undiagnosed until later in life. A number of different gene mutations have been shown to cause MODY, all of which limit the ability of the pancreas to produce insulin. This process leads to the high blood glucose levels characteristic of diabetes and, in time, may damage body tissues, particularly the eyes, kidneys, nerves, and blood vessels. MODY accounts for about one to five percent of all cases of diabetes in the United States. Family members of people with MODY are at greatly increased risk for the condition.

People with MODY may have only mild or no symptoms of diabetes and their hyperglycemia may only be discovered during routine blood tests. MODY may be confused with type 1 or type 2 diabetes. People with MODY are generally not overweight and do not have other risk factors for type 2 diabetes, such as high blood pressure or abnormal blood fat levels. While both type 2 diabetes and MODY can run in families, people with MODY typically have a family history of diabetes in multiple successive generations, meaning that MODY is present in a grandparent, a parent, and a child. Unlike people with type 1 diabetes who always require insulin, people with MODY can often be treated with oral diabetes medications. Treatment varies depending on the genetic mutation that has caused the MODY.

Table 10.1. Neonatal Diabetes Mellitus (NDM)

Permanent Neonatal Diabetes Mellitus (PNDM)

Gene	How Common	Usual Age of Onset
KCNJ11	Most common type of PNDM	3 to 6 months
ABCC8	Rare	1 to 3 months
GCK	Rare	1 week
IPF1 (PDX1)	Rare	1 week
PTF1A	Rare	At birth
FOXP3, IPEX syndrome	Rare	Sometimes present at birth
EIF2AK3, Wolcott-Rallison syndrome	Rare	3 months

Transient Neonatal Diabetes Mellitus (TNDM)

Gene	How Common	Usual Age of Onset
ZAC/HYMAI	Most common form of NDM	Birth to 3 months
ABCC8	Rare	Birth to 6 months
KCNJ11	Uncommon cause of TNDM but most common cause of PNDM	Birth to 6 months
HNF1-beta (HNF1B)	rare	Birth to 6 months

What do I need to know about genetic testing and counseling?

Testing for monogenic diabetes involves providing a blood sample from which DNA is isolated. The DNA is analyzed for changes in the genes that cause monogenic diabetes. Abnormal results can determine the gene responsible for diabetes in a particular individual or show whether someone is likely to develop a monogenic form of diabetes in the future. Genetic testing can also be helpful in selecting the most appropriate treatment for individuals with monogenic diabetes. Prenatal testing can diagnose these conditions in unborn children.

Most forms of monogenic diabetes are caused by dominant mutations, meaning that the condition can be passed on to children when only one parent is affected. In contrast, if the mutation is a recessive mutation, a disease gene must be inherited from both parents for diabetes to occur. For recessive forms of monogenic diabetes, testing can indicate whether parents or siblings without disease are carriers for recessive genetic conditions that could be inherited by their children.

If you suspect that you or a member of your family may have a monogenic form of diabetes, you should seek help from health care professionals—physicians and genetic counselors—who have specialized knowledge and experience in this area. They can determine whether genetic testing is appropriate, select the genetic tests that should be performed, and provide information about the basic principles of genetics, genetic testing options, and confidentiality issues. They also can review the test results with the patient or parent after testing, make recommendations about how to proceed, and discuss testing options for other family members.

> ## Points To Remember
>
> - Mutations in single genes can cause rare forms of diabetes.
> - Genetic testing can identify many forms of monogenic diabetes.
> - A physician evaluates whether genetic testing is appropriate.
> - A correct diagnosis aided by genetic testing can lead to optimal treatment.
> - Recent research results show that people with certain forms of monogenic diabetes can be treated with oral diabetes medications instead of insulin injections.
>
> Source: National Institute of Diabetes and Digestive and Kidney Diseases (NIDDK), March 2007

What research is underway?

Researchers are studying the genetic causes of and metabolic processes related to diabetes. Discoveries about monogenic forms of diabetes may contribute to the search for the causes of and treatments for type 1 and type 2 diabetes. For information about clinical trials related to diabetes and genetics, see http://www.clinicaltrials.gov.

Other Types Of Diabetes

A number of other types of diabetes exist. A person may exhibit characteristics of more than one type. For example, in latent autoimmune diabetes in adults (LADA), also called type 1.5 diabetes or double diabetes, people show signs of both type 1 and type 2 diabetes. Diagnosis usually occurs after age 30.

Most people with LADA still produce their own insulin when first diagnosed, like those with type 2 diabetes, but within a few years, they must take insulin to control blood glucose levels. In LADA, as in type 1 diabetes, the beta cells of the pancreas stop making insulin because the body's immune system attacks and destroys them. Some experts believe that LADA is a slowly developing kind of type 1 diabetes.

Other types of diabetes include those caused by other factors:

- Genetic defects in insulin action, resulting in the body's inability to control blood glucose levels, as seen in leprechaunism and the Rabson-Mendenhall syndrome

- Diseases of the pancreas or conditions that damage the pancreas, such as pancreatitis and cystic fibrosis

- Excess amounts of certain hormones resulting from some medical conditions—such as cortisol in Cushing syndrome—that work against the action of insulin

- Medications that reduce insulin action, such as glucocorticoids, or chemicals that destroy beta cells

- Infections, such as congenital rubella and cytomegalovirus

- Rare autoimmune disorders, such as stiff-man syndrome, an autoimmune disease of the central nervous system

- Genetic syndromes associated with diabetes, such as Down syndrome and Prader-Willi syndrome

Chapter 11

Diabetes Research

Diabetes, Type 1

Yesterday

In the 1950s, about one in five people died within 20 years after a diagnosis of type 1 diabetes. One in three people died within 25 years of diagnosis.

About one in four people developed kidney failure within 25 years of a type 1 diabetes diagnosis. Doctors could not detect early kidney disease and had no tools for slowing its progression to kidney failure. Survival after kidney failure was poor, with one of ten patients dying each year.

About 90 percent of people with type 1 diabetes developed diabetic retinopathy within 25 years of diagnosis. Blindness from diabetic retinopathy was responsible for about 12 percent of new cases of blindness between the ages of 45 and 74. Studies had not proven the value of laser surgery in reducing blindness.

Major birth defects in the offspring of mothers with type 1 diabetes were three times higher than in the general population.

Patients relied on injections of animal-derived insulin. The insulin pump would soon be introduced but would not become widely used for years.

Studies had not yet shown the need for intensive glucose control to delay or prevent the debilitating eye, nerve, kidney, heart, and blood vessel complications of diabetes. Also, the importance of blood pressure control in preventing complications had not been established yet.

About This Chapter: This chapter includes "Diabetes, Type 1," National Institutes of Health (NIH), November 22, 2010; "Diabetes, Type 2," NIH, November 22, 2010; and "Pancreatic Islet Transplantation," National Institute of Diabetes and Digestive and Kidney Diseases, March 2007.

Patients monitored their glucose levels with urine tests, which recognized high but not dangerously low glucose levels and reflected past, not current, glucose levels. More reliable methods for testing glucose levels in the blood had not been developed yet.

Researchers had just discovered autoimmunity as the underlying cause of type 1 diabetes. However, they couldn't assess an individual's level of risk for developing type 1 diabetes, and they didn't know enough to even consider ways to prevent type 1 diabetes.

Today

The long-term survival of those with type 1 diabetes has dramatically improved in the last 30 years. For people born between 1975 and 1980, about 3.5 percent die within 20 years of diagnosis, and 7 percent die within 25 years of diagnosis. These death rates are much lower than those of patients born in the 1950s, but are still significantly increased compared to the general population.

After 20 years of annual increases from 5 to 10 percent, rates for new kidney failure cases have leveled off. The most encouraging trend is in diabetes, where rates for new cases in whites under age 40 are the lowest in 20 years. Improved control of glucose and blood pressure and the use of specific antihypertensive drugs prevent or delay the progression of kidney disease to kidney failure.

Annual eye exams are recommended because, with timely laser surgery and appropriate follow-up care, people with advanced diabetic retinopathy can reduce their risk of blindness by 90 percent. A new study shows that vision loss that is often associated with laser therapy can be reduced when the drug ranibizumab is used in combination with laser.

For expectant mothers with type 1 diabetes, tight control of glucose that begins before conception lowers the risk of birth defects, miscarriage, and newborn death to a range that is close to that of the general population.

Patients use genetically engineered human insulin in a variety of formulations, for example, rapid-acting, intermediate acting, and long-acting insulin, to control their blood glucose. Insulin pumps are widely used.

A major clinical trial, the Diabetes Control and Complications Trial (DCCT; http://diabetes.niddk.nih.gov/dm/pubs/control), showed that intensive glucose control dramatically delays or prevents the eye, nerve, and kidney complications of type 1 diabetes. A paradigm shift in the way type 1 diabetes is controlled was based on this finding. As researchers continued to follow study participants, they found that tight glucose control also reduces cardiovascular complications, such as heart attack and stroke. This research has contributed to greatly improved health outcomes for patients.

Patients can regularly monitor their blood glucose with precise, less painful methods, including a continuous glucose monitor (CGM). Technology pairing a CGM with an insulin pump is also available and was found to help patients achieve better blood glucose control with fewer episodes of dangerously low blood glucose compared to standard insulin injection therapy.

The widely used HbA1c test shows average blood glucose over the past three months. The HbA1c Standardization Program enabled the translation of tight blood glucose control into common practice.

Scientists have identified a key gene region that contributes nearly half the increased risk of developing type 1 diabetes and have also learned a great deal about the underlying biology of autoimmune diabetes. They have used this knowledge to develop accurate genetic and antibody tests to predict who is at high, moderate, and low risk for developing type 1 diabetes. This knowledge and recent advances in immunology have enabled researchers to design and conduct studies that seek to prevent type 1 diabetes and to preserve insulin production in newly diagnosed patients. This new understanding has prevented life-threatening complications in clinical trial participants at risk for developing diabetes.

Scientists have identified nearly 50 genes or gene regions associated with type 1 diabetes.

Many people who received islet transplants for poorly controlled type 1 diabetes are free of the need for insulin administration a year later, and episodes of dangerously low blood glucose are greatly reduced for as long as five years after transplant. But, the function of transplanted islets is lost over time, and patients have side effects from immunosuppressive drugs.

The SEARCH for Diabetes in Youth Study (www.searchfordiabetes.org) provided the first national data on prevalence of diabetes in youth: One of every 523 youth had physician diagnosed diabetes in 2001 (this number included both type 1 and type 2 diabetes). SEARCH also found that about 15,000 youth are diagnosed with type 1 diabetes each year.

Tomorrow

By finding the environmental factors (for example, viruses, toxins, dietary factors) that trigger type 1 diabetes through the National Institutes of Health (NIH)'s TEDDY study (www.teddystudy.org), researchers will identify ways to safely prevent the autoimmune destruction of insulin-producing cells.

Approaches to prevent or slow progression of type 1 diabetes will be identified through research conducted by NIH's Type 1 Diabetes TrialNet (www.diabetestrialnet.org). TrialNet will also be poised to test new therapies emerging from research on environmental and genetic contributors to disease.

Research by the NIH's Clinical Islet Transplantation Consortium (www.citisletstudy.org) will improve methods for islet transplantation, allowing more people to benefit from this treatment strategy.

Methods for safely imaging the insulin-producing beta cells will help scientists better understand the disease process and assess the benefits of treatments and preventions that are under study.

Knowledge from the NIH's Beta Cell Biology Consortium (www.betacell.org) about biological pathways regulating development and growth of insulin-producing beta cells will help scientists generate beta cells in the lab. This progress may relieve the shortage of beta cells for transplantation and lead to ways to promote beta cell regeneration in people with type 1 diabetes.

New technologies, such as a closed loop system that automatically senses blood glucose and adjusts insulin dosage precisely, will become available—allowing patients to more easily control their blood glucose levels and develop fewer complications.

As molecular pathways by which blood glucose causes cell injury are better understood, scientists will develop medicines to prevent and repair the damage.

Tracking the number of children with diabetes through SEARCH will allow scientists to see how rates are changing over time and inform research and public health efforts to combat the disease.

Diabetes, Type 2

Yesterday

No proven strategies existed to prevent the disease or its complications.

The only ways to treat diabetes were the now-obsolete forms of insulin from cows and pigs, and drugs that stimulate insulin release from the beta cells of the pancreas (sulfonylureas). Both of these therapies cause dangerous low blood sugar reactions and weight gain. Patients monitored their glucose levels with urine tests, which recognized high but not dangerously low glucose levels and reflected past, not current, glucose levels. More reliable methods for testing glucose levels in the blood had not been developed yet.

While scientists knew that genes played a role (that is, the disease often runs in families), they had not identified any specific culprit genes.

National efforts were not being made to combat obesity—a serious risk factor for the disease. Fewer people developed type 2 diabetes compared to today because overweight, obesity, and physical inactivity were not pervasive.

Patients were almost exclusively adults—the reason that the disease was formerly called "adult onset diabetes." It was rare in children or young adults.

Today

Type 2 diabetes can be prevented or delayed. The NIH-funded Diabetes Prevention Program (DPP) clinical trial (http://diabetes.niddk.nih.gov/dm/pubs/preventionprogram/) found a lifestyle intervention (modest weight loss of five to seven percent of body weight and 30 minutes of exercise five times weekly) reduced the risk of getting type 2 diabetes by 58 percent in a diverse population of more than 3,000 adults at high risk for diabetes. In another arm of the study, the drug metformin reduced development of diabetes by 31 percent.

Based on the DPP findings, the National Diabetes Education Program developed the education campaign, "Small Steps. Big Rewards. Prevent Type 2 Diabetes" to help people at high risk take the necessary steps to prevent the disease (www.ndep.nih.gov).

Ongoing NIH translational research efforts are testing cost effective ways to deliver the DPP-proven lifestyle change in real-world settings. This vigorous effort is needed to address the escalating prevalence of type 2 diabetes which now affects 7.8 percent of Americans, disproportionate affects minorities, and is conservatively estimated to be the seventh leading cause of death in the U.S.

Type 2 diabetes is increasing in children, in tandem with rising obesity rates. This trend is alarming because, as younger people develop the disease, the complications, morbidity, and mortality associated with diabetes are all likely to occur earlier. Also, offspring of women with type 2 diabetes are more likely to develop the disease. Thus, the burgeoning of diabetes in younger populations could lead to a vicious cycle of ever-growing rates of diabetes.

The SEARCH for Diabetes in Youth Study (www.searchfordiabetes.org) has provided the first national data on incidence and prevalence of diabetes in youth. About 3,700 youth under 20 years old are diagnosed with type 2 diabetes each year, and the disease is particularly prevalent in minority youth.

Research has vastly expanded understanding of the molecular underpinnings of diabetes and its complications. Recent work has boosted to nearly 40 the number of gene regions associated with increased risk of type 2 diabetes, laying the foundation for new approaches to prevention and therapy.

NIH-supported clinical trials validated a marker called hemoglobin A1C (A1C). This marker reflects average blood sugar control over a three month period. This technology, along with tests that allow patients to monitor their own blood glucose throughout the day, helps make better blood glucose control achievable for many people with type 2 diabetes.

Because lower A1C levels have been shown to be predictive of longer life and fewer complications, the test has helped speed development and approval of better forms of insulin and new diabetes medicines that work though a variety of mechanisms. New drugs are available that lower glucose without weight gain or even with modest weight loss. Several agents targeting the specific metabolic abnormalities of type 2 diabetes are now available and can be combined, thus delaying the need for insulin.

Tight blood sugar control has become a standard of treatment for most diabetes patients based on results from NIH clinical trials demonstrating that keeping A1C below 7 can prevent or delay devastating disease complications.

A large clinical trial showed that older patients with longstanding type 2 diabetes at high risk of heart disease do not benefit from more intensive blood glucose control than is currently recommended. These findings spare patients from unneeded therapy and provide important data to help individualize therapy, with less stringent A1C targets suggested for some people such as those with advanced diabetes complications.

Clinical trials have shown that blood pressure and lipid control reduce diabetes complications by up to 50 percent. Physicians are now much better equipped to prevent and control heart disease, which often accompanies diabetes, and is the leading cause of death in people with diabetes.

Nationwide improvements in risk factor control show research-proven strategies are being translated into practice. Improvements in control of cholesterol, blood glucose, and blood pressure have added an estimated one year to the expected lifespan of a person with type 2 diabetes since 1992, and improved quality of life by reducing the incidence of burdensome complications like blindness, lower limb amputations, kidney failure, and coronary heart disease.

As a result of research proving their benefits, Medicare now covers blood glucose self-monitoring materials and diabetes education services, helping people to better control their diabetes.

Kidney disease can be detected earlier via urine tests. Therefore, patients can be treated earlier to slow the rate of kidney damage. Improved control of glucose and blood pressure prevents or delays progression of kidney disease to kidney failure. With good care, less than ten percent of patients develop kidney failure.

With timely laser surgery and appropriate follow-up care, people with advanced diabetic retinopathy can reduce their risk of blindness by 90 percent. A recent study showed a drug which limits blood vessel growth can be an important supplement to laser therapy for diabetic macular edema.

The NIH spent over $1.1 billion on diabetes research in fiscal year 2009. In 2007, total costs attributable to diabetes for Americans was estimated at $174 billion—an increase of 32 percent since 2002.

Tomorrow

Research will find better ways to bring proven diabetes prevention strategies to more people at lower cost.

Earlier and more aggressive treatment approaches may help better prevent diabetes complications.

New understanding of the biology of obesity and insulin resistance is informing the development of new therapeutics to prevent and treat type 2 diabetes.

Identification of susceptibility genes for diabetes and its complications will enable earlier implementation of prevention measures targeted to those at highest risk.

Research on the effect of maternal diabetes on offspring may help to break the vicious diabetes cycle.

Continued research on the mechanisms underlying the development and progression of disease complications will result in the ability to predict who is likely to develop them. Personalized treatments could then be developed to preempt complications. This strategy would dramatically improve the health and well-being of patients.

NIH clinical trials will identify new approaches to prevent and treat the emerging problem of type 2 diabetes in children.

Pancreatic Islet Transplantation

The pancreas, an organ about the size of a hand, is located behind the lower part of the stomach. It makes insulin and enzymes that help the body digest and use food. Throughout the pancreas are clusters of cells called the islets of Langerhans. Islets are made up of several types of cells, including beta cells that make insulin.

The pancreas is located in the abdomen behind the stomach. Islets within the pancreas contain beta cells, which produce insulin.

In an experimental procedure called islet transplantation, islets are taken from the pancreas of a deceased organ donor. The islets are purified, processed, and transferred into another person. Once implanted, the beta cells in these islets begin to make and release insulin. Researchers hope that islet transplantation will help people with type 1 diabetes live without daily injections of insulin.

Research Developments

Scientists have made many advances in islet transplantation in recent years. Since reporting their findings in the June 2000 issue of the *New England Journal of Medicine*, researchers at the University of Alberta in Edmonton, Canada, have continued to use and refine a procedure called the Edmonton protocol to transplant pancreatic islets into selected patients with type 1

Researchers Identify Genetic Elements Influencing The Risk Of Type 2 Diabetes

A team led by researchers at the National Human Genome Research Institute (NHGRI), part of the National Institutes of Health, has captured the most comprehensive snapshot to date of DNA regions that regulate genes in human pancreatic islet cells, a subset of which produces insulin. The study highlights the importance of genome regulatory sequences in human health and disease, particularly type 2 diabetes.

Epigenomic research focuses on the mechanisms that regulate the expression of genes in the human genome. Genetic information is written in the chemical language of DNA, a long molecule of nucleic acid wound around specialized proteins called histones. Together, they constitute chromatin, the DNA-protein complex that forms chromosomes during cell division. The researchers used DNA sequencing technology to search the chromatin of islet cells for specific histone modifications and other signals marking regulatory DNA. Computational analysis of the large amounts of DNA sequence data generated in this study identified different classes of regulatory DNA.

Among the results, the researchers detected about 18,000 promoters, which are regulatory sequences immediately adjacent to the start of genes. Promoters are like molecular on-off switches and more than one switch can control a gene. Several hundred of these were previously unknown and found to be highly active in the islet cells.

The researchers also identified at least 34,000 distal regulatory elements, so called because they are farther away from the genes. Many of these were bunched together, suggesting they may cooperate to form regulatory modules. These modules may be unique to islets and play an important role in the maintenance of blood glucose levels.

The researchers also found that 50 single nucleotide polymorphisms, or genetic variants, associated with islet-related traits or diseases are located within or very close to non-promoter regulatory elements. Variants associated with type 2 diabetes are present in six such elements that function to boost gene activity. These results suggest that regulatory elements may be a key component to understanding the molecular defects that contribute to type 2 diabetes.

Source: Excerpted from "NIH Researchers Identify Genetic Elements Influencing the Risk of Type 2 Diabetes," *NIH News*, National Institutes of Health, November 2, 2010.

diabetes that is difficult to control. In 2005, the researchers published five-year follow-up results for 65 patients who received transplants at their center and reported that about 10 percent of the patients remained free of the need for insulin injections at five-year follow-up. Most recipients returned to using insulin because the transplanted islets lost their ability to function over time. The researchers noted, however, that many transplant recipients were able to reduce their need for insulin, achieve better glucose stability, and reduce problems with hypoglycemia.

In its 2006 annual report, the Collaborative Islet Transplant Registry, which is funded by the National Institute of Diabetes and Digestive and Kidney Diseases, presented data from 23 islet transplant programs on 225 patients who received islet transplants between 1999 and 2005. According to the report, nearly two-thirds of recipients achieved "insulin independence"—defined as being able to stop insulin injections for at least 14 days—during the year following transplantation. However, other data from the report showed that insulin independence is difficult to maintain over time. Six months after their last infusion of islets, more than half of recipients were free of the need for insulin injections, but at two-year follow-up, the proportion dropped to about one-third of recipients. The report described other benefits of islet transplantation, including reduced need for insulin among recipients who still needed insulin, improved blood glucose control, and greatly reduced risk of episodes of severe hypoglycemia.

In a 2006 report of the Immune Tolerance Network's international islet transplantation study, researchers emphasized the value of transplantation in reversing a condition known as hypoglycemia unawareness. People with hypoglycemia unawareness are vulnerable to dangerous episodes of severe hypoglycemia because they are not able to recognize that their blood glucose levels are too low. The study showed that even partial islet function after transplant can eliminate hypoglycemia unawareness.

Transplant Procedure

Researchers use specialized enzymes to remove islets from the pancreas of a deceased donor. Because the islets are fragile, transplantation occurs soon after they are removed. Typically a patient receives at least 10,000 islet "equivalents" per kilogram of body weight, extracted from two donor pancreases. Patients often require two transplants to achieve insulin independence. Some transplants have used fewer islet equivalents taken from a single donated pancreas.

Transplants are often performed by a radiologist, who uses x-rays and ultrasound to guide placement of a catheter—a small plastic tube—through the upper abdomen and into the portal vein of the liver. The islets are then infused slowly through the catheter into the liver. The patient receives a local anesthetic and a sedative. In some cases, a surgeon may perform the transplant through a small incision, using general anesthesia.

Islets extracted from a donor pancreas are infused into the liver. Once implanted, the beta cells in the islets begin to make and release insulin.

Islets begin to release insulin soon after transplantation. However, full islet function and new blood vessel growth associated with the islets take time. The doctor will order many tests to check blood glucose levels after the transplant, and insulin is usually given until the islets are fully functional.

The Benefits And Risks

The goal of islet transplantation is to infuse enough islets to control the blood glucose level without insulin injections. Other benefits may include improved glucose control and prevention of potentially dangerous episodes of hypoglycemia. Because good control of blood glucose can slow or prevent the progression of complications associated with diabetes, such as heart disease, kidney disease, and nerve or eye damage, a successful transplant may reduce the risk of these complications.

Risks of islet transplantation include the risks associated with the transplant procedure—particularly bleeding and blood clots—and side effects from the immunosuppressive drugs that transplant recipients must take to stop the immune system from rejecting the transplanted islets.

Part Two
Medical Management
Of Diabetes

Chapter 12

You And Your Diabetes Care Team

Visiting The Health Care Team

Because most newly diagnosed cases of type 1 diabetes occur in individuals younger than 18 years of age, and more children and teens are now getting type 2 diabetes, care of this group requires integration of diabetes management with the complicated physical and emotional growth needs of children, adolescents, and their families, as well as consideration of teens' emerging autonomy and independence.

Diabetes care for children and teens should be provided by a team that can deal with these special medical, educational, nutritional, and behavioral issues. The team usually consists of a physician, diabetes educator, dietitian, and social worker or psychologist, along with the patient and family. Children should be seen by the team at diagnosis and in follow-up, as agreed upon by the primary care provider and the diabetes team. The following schedule of care is based on the American Diabetes Association's Standards of Medical Care.

At Diagnosis

- Establish the goals of care and required treatment.

- Begin diabetes self-management education about healthy eating habits, daily physical activity, and insulin/medication administration, and self-monitoring of blood glucose levels if appropriate. A solid educational base is needed so that the individual and family can become increasingly independent in self-management of diabetes. Diabetes educators play an important role in this aspect of management.

About This Chapter: Text in this chapter begins with an excerpt from "Overview of Diabetes in Children and Adolescents," National Diabetes Education Program (http://ndep.nih.gov), August 2008. The chapter continues with "Staying Healthy with Diabetes," Centers for Disease Control and Prevention, June 4, 2010.

- Provide nutritional therapy by an individual experienced with the nutritional needs of the growing child and the behavioral issues that have an impact on adolescent diets.

- Conduct a psychosocial assessment to identify emotional and behavioral disorders.

- Check lipids in children with a significant family history. In children with no significant family history, check lipids at puberty after glucose control has been established and if normal, repeat profile every five years.

- Check for microalbumin in type 2 diabetes.

- Provide ophthalmologic examination shortly after diagnosis in type 2 diabetes.

Each Quarterly Visit

Most young people with diabetes are seen by the health care team every three months. At each visit, the following should be monitored or examined:

- A1C, an indicator of average blood glucose control
- Growth (height and weight)
- Body mass index (BMI)
- Blood pressure
- Injection sites
- Self-testing blood glucose records
- Psychosocial assessment

Annually

- Evaluate nutrition therapy
- Provide ophthalmologic examination (less often on the advice of an eye care professional). The first ophthalmologic examination should be obtained once the child is age 10 or older and has had type 1 diabetes for three to five years. For children with type 2 diabetes, the first examination should be shortly after diagnosis.
- Check for microalbuminuria (once the child is 10 years old and has had diabetes for five years)
- Perform thyroid function test (for children with type 1 diabetes)
- Administer influenza vaccination
- Examine feet

Questions About Staying Healthy With Diabetes

What routine medical examinations and tests are needed for people with diabetes?

Your doctors should take these steps:

- Measure your blood pressure at every visit

- Check your feet for sores at every visit, and give a thorough foot exam at least once a year

- Give you a hemoglobin A1C test at least twice a year, to determine what your average blood glucose level was for the past two to three months

- Test your urine and blood to check your kidney function at least once a year

- Test your blood lipids (fats)—total cholesterol; LDL, or low-density lipoprotein ("bad" cholesterol); HDL, or high-density lipoprotein ("good" cholesterol); and triglycerides at least once a year

You should also get a dental checkup twice a year, a dilated eye exam once a year, an annual flu shot, and a pneumonia shot.

How does maintaining healthy blood glucose levels help people with diabetes stay healthy?

Research studies in the United States and other countries have shown that controlling blood glucose benefits people with either type 1 or type 2 diabetes. In general, for every 1% reduction in results of A1C blood tests (for example, from 8.0% to 7.0%), the risk of developing eye, kidney, and nerve disease is reduced by 40%.

You Need A Health Care Team

Diabetes is a serious disease. It affects almost every part of your body. That is why a health care team may help you take care of your diabetes:

- Doctor
- Dentist
- Diabetes educator
- Dietitian
- Eye doctor
- Foot doctor
- Mental health counselor
- Nurse
- Nurse practitioner
- Pharmacist
- Social worker
- Friends and family

You are the most important member of the team.

Source: From "4 Steps to Control Your Diabetes. For Life." National Diabetes Education Program, November, 2009.

How does maintaining a healthy body weight help people with diabetes stay healthy?

Most people newly diagnosed with type 2 diabetes are overweight. Excess weight, particularly in the abdomen, makes it difficult for cells to respond to insulin, resulting in high blood glucose. Often, people with type 2 diabetes are able to lower their blood glucose by losing weight and increasing physical activity. Losing weight also helps lower the risk for other health problems which especially affect people with diabetes, such as cardiovascular disease.

How does maintaining a healthy blood pressure level help people with diabetes stay healthy?

About 73% of adults with diabetes have high blood pressure or use prescription medications to reduce high blood pressure. Maintaining normal blood pressure—less than 130/80 millimeters of mercury (mm Hg) helps to prevent damage to the eyes, kidneys, heart, and blood vessels. Blood pressure measurements are written like a fraction, with the two numbers separated by a slash. The first number represents the pressure in your blood vessels when your heart beats (systolic pressure); the second number represents the pressure in the vessels when your heart is at rest (diastolic pressure).

In general, for every 10 mm Hg reduction in systolic blood pressure (the first number in the fraction), the risk for any complication related to diabetes is reduced by 12%. Maintaining normal blood pressure control can reduce the risk of eye, kidney, and nerve disease (microvascular disease) by approximately 33%, and the risk of heart disease and stroke (cardiovascular disease) by approximately 33% to 50%. Healthy eating, medications, and physical activity can help you bring high blood pressure down.

How does maintaining healthy cholesterol levels help people with diabetes stay healthy?

Several things, including having diabetes, can make your blood cholesterol level too high. When cholesterol is too high, the insides of large blood vessels become narrowed, even clogged, which can lead to heart disease and stroke, the biggest health problems for people with diabetes. Maintaining normal cholesterol levels will help prevent these diseases, and can help prevent circulation problems, also an issue for people with diabetes. Have your cholesterol checked at least once a year. Total cholesterol should be under 200; LDL ("bad" cholesterol) should be under 100; HDL ("good" cholesterol) should be above 40 in men and above 50 in women; and triglycerides should be under 150. Healthy eating, medications, and physical activity can help you reach your cholesterol targets. Keeping cholesterol levels under control can reduce the risk of cardiovascular complications of diabetes by 20% to 50%.

How does exercise help people with diabetes stay healthy?

Physical activity can help you control your blood glucose, weight, and blood pressure, as well as raise your "good" cholesterol and lower your "bad" cholesterol. It can also help prevent heart and blood flow problems.

Experts recommend moderate-intensity physical activity for at least 30 minutes on five or more days of the week. Talk to your health care provider about a safe exercise plan. He or she may check your heart and your feet to be sure you have no special problems. If you have high blood pressure, eye, or foot problems, you may need to avoid some kinds of exercise.

How does quitting smoking help people with diabetes stay healthy?

Smoking puts people with diabetes at particular risk. Smoking raises your blood glucose, cholesterol, and blood pressure, all of which people with diabetes need to be especially concerned about. When you have diabetes and use tobacco, the risk of heart and blood vessel problems is even greater. If you quit smoking, you'll lower your risk for heart attack, stroke, nerve disease, kidney disease, and oral disease.

Why is it important for people with diabetes to get an annual flu shot?

Diabetes can make the immune system more vulnerable to severe cases of the flu. People with diabetes who come down with the flu may become very sick and may die. You can help keep yourself from getting the flu by getting a flu shot every year. Everyone with diabetes—even pregnant women—should get a yearly flu shot. The best time to get one is between October and mid-November, before the flu season begins.

Work With Your Health Care Team

Work with your health care team to create a plan to help you reach your self-care goals:

- Make a list of all your reasons to manage your diabetes for life.
- Set goals you can reach. Break a big goal into small steps.
- Engage your whole family in being more physically active.
- Stay at a healthy weight by using your meal plan and being physically active.
- Learn what causes you to slip up in reaching your goals. Plan how to do better next time.
- Reach out to friends or family for support or when you feel down.
- Give yourself a healthy reward for doing well.

Source: Excerpted from "Tips to Help You Stay Healthy," National Diabetes Education Program, November 2007.

Chapter 13

Improving Self-Care In Young People With Diabetes

Young people with diabetes face a range of challenges in managing their condition. Reasons for inadequate self-care include the nature of the many tasks involved; the nature of the skills and supports needed to identify and resolve barriers to following a therapeutic regimen; and the need for ongoing motivation and self-efficacy. Self-care tasks can be quite challenging for a young person due to their frequency and relationship to food, and the need to apply skills, such as self-control, insight, and planning. Some of the most significant barriers reported during adolescence are related to prioritizing diabetes in social situations. Solving social problems that impact on diabetes involves applying skills related to personal insight, communication with others, and situational decision-making.

Self-Efficacy And Self-Care

Regardless of developmental stage or specific self-care goals, consistent, independent self-care is the result of many repeated lessons related to identifying and solving barriers to diabetes care. In many instances, young people know what they are supposed to do, but psychosocial barriers, such as embarrassment, get in the way. One of the most critical aspects of successfully developing and applying problem-solving to diabetes-related barriers over a lifespan is known as "self-efficacy"—a person's belief in his or her own ability to successfully perform the tasks involved in diabetes self-management.[1]

About This Chapter: Text in this chapter is from "Improving self-care in young people with diabetes—the importance of self-efficacy," by Shelagh Mulvaney, in *DiabetesVoice*, October 2009, Volume 54, Special Issue. © 2009 International Diabetes Federation (www.diabetesvoice.org); reprinted with permission.

When young people believe that they are capable of carrying out self-care tasks, they are more likely to be successful in those tasks.[2,3] Across many studies involving children, adolescents, and adults, self-efficacy has been consistently identified as an important facilitator of self-care.

In younger children with type 1 diabetes, self-efficacy is first needed in order to learn about self-care tasks, such as checking blood glucose, carbohydrate counting, and insulin dosing. At this stage of development, parental self-efficacy also plays a critical role. As a child matures, efforts to develop self-efficacy should be focused on implementing diabetes knowledge in day-to-day living, solving barriers to self-management, and applying related skills, such as communication.

The effects of high self-efficacy in young people with diabetes may be evident when we observe them becoming more confident in their diabetes-related decisions—not shying away from difficult tasks (like talking to friends about how to deal with hypoglycemia), or experiencing a determination for, and an enjoyment of, solving diabetes problems. In the context of high self-efficacy, a failure to solve a diabetes problem or attain a desired outcome is not interpreted as a personal failing, and there is increased motivation for solving barriers to self-care.

Ways To Improve Self-Efficacy

Alfred Bandura, the social scientist who first described self-efficacy, identified four sources through which we obtain self-efficacy information about ourselves. Self-efficacy for diabetes self-care may be influenced through successfully performing self-care tasks (mastery experiences), watching others learn to perform a task or solve a problem (modeling), being persuaded that one is capable of carrying out a task (social persuasion), and individually interpreting subjective emotional or physiological experiences (such as interpreting a rapid heart beat as excitement versus fear).[1]

Before young people are able to estimate their own ability to carry out a task, they need to understand the nature of the task and any potential barriers, and have a clear definition of success. One of the most challenging aspects of diabetes goal-setting and problem-solving for young people is that they may attempt goals that are unrealistic or beyond their skill level. Mastery experiences are typically labelled as "guided mastery" because they involve planned appropriate behavioral challenges with appropriate guidance and support. Through guided mastery-learning cycles (setting small goals and attaining those goals through practice), people develop a sense of self-efficacy.[4]

If goals are set too high, failure is more likely to occur. If failure occurs too often and self-efficacy has not yet been developed, those failures will have an even greater negative impact on

Caring For Your Diabetes Supplies

Be kind to your glucose meter. Since your glucose meter plays a vital role in your diabetes management, be sure to take good care of it. That means you should never expose it to extreme temperatures, whether that may be freezing cold or intense heat. If you have more than one glucose meter, or if you store one in your car, make sure you remove it if extreme conditions are forecasted.

Get organized. Whether you have type 1 or type 2 diabetes, storing your medication neatly will not only help you find your supplies easier, but they'll also make your diabetes management a bit more predictable. If you can, designate a drawer in your kitchen (or another safe spot in your home) for neatly storing syringes, alcohol swabs, lancets, and other supplies. Drawer organizers sold at office or craft supply stores can be used to conveniently separate these items, and make them easily accessible.

Keep your insulin cool—but not frozen. Exposing your insulin to extreme heat will most certainly ruin it, so be sure to keep insulin pens and vials refrigerated. It is perfectly fine to carry these supplies with you during the day unrefrigerated, just as long as you're careful to keep them out of direct sunlight and in a cool environment. On the other hand, never store insulin next to a frozen ice pack—freezing insulin will also destroy its efficacy.

Protect your pump. Pump housing provides some insulation from the heat. If you are concerned about heat, you can use a protective pouch with a small, cold (but not freezing) gel pack placed inside the pouch as a way to protect your insulin from the effects of heat, advises Catherine Carver, M.S., A.N.P., C.D.E, and Vice President for Clinical Services at Joslin Diabetes Center. If you are spending an extended amount of time in the sun, cover the pump with a towel to protect it from prolonged direct sunlight, and limit the exposure to direct light. Disconnecting your pump for up to an hour is another option, but if it is disconnected for a longer time, you will need to adjust your insulin infusion rate accordingly to allow for the missed doses.

Keep testing strips safe. As anyone with diabetes will tell you, testing strips are a very costly but very helpful supply for managing diabetes. You should protect your investment accordingly—never leave your strips exposed to extreme temperatures, and always close the cap on a canister of testing strips. Keeping the lid closed at all times will protect the integrity of the strips and also keep out moisture and debris.

motivation. Key to this process is that young people are applying themselves and not having a parent or clinician complete a task, so that they may accurately attribute success to themselves. Diabetes-related stress may be related to feelings of not being in control. So guided mastery may be used to reduce stress as well as to build diabetes self-management skills.

Modeling

Another method that has been used to improve self-efficacy in diabetes is vicarious learning or modeling. This involves watching or experiencing others successfully perform a task. Several interventions designed to improve pediatric diabetes education and self-care have successfully used this approach. An important factor in the effectiveness of this method is that the person demonstrating the task, or "actor," is perceived as being similar to the young person who is watching. For example, if a clinic wants to teach young people how to resolve barriers to making healthy food choices at restaurants, they should use people to model that behavior who most closely match that population in terms of age, gender, race, and socioeconomic status. This will facilitate engagement in the learning experience.

Peer Interactions

Peer interactions often build on modeling and are a promising means to enhance diabetes education. Peers are generally perceived as similar to ourselves and, in theory, can provide positive modeling of critical diabetes attitudes, beliefs, and behaviors. However, peer interactions, such as online forums and social networking sites, cannot be controlled by diabetes healthcare providers and researchers, and have the potential to reduce self-efficacy in some young people. Although adolescents report enjoying online social interactions about diabetes, and knowing that others have the same experiences, the specific ways that these peer interactions may be used to enhance self-care have not yet been well studied.

Family Interactions

Interactions with family members represent another potential source for enhancing diabetes self-efficacy. For example, young people with type 2 diabetes often have one or more family members with the same condition. In the best situations, family members who are in good control of their diabetes share their successes with the young person, and provide guided mastery support for goal-setting and to help build self-efficacy.

However, similar to peers, family members may act as positive or negative role models.[5] Regardless of the quality of their own self-care, adults need to be aware of the influence that their own behavior can have on the self-efficacy of young people around them. In contrast, children and adolescents with type 1 diabetes may be isolated in dealing with diabetes, and are likely to have no one in their immediate family with the condition. Adolescents with type 1 diabetes report benefits from using technologies, such as the internet, that bring them into contact with other young people with diabetes. Mobile phones are also being used as a means to improve diabetes problem-solving support through the provision of "just-in-time" information, guidance, and prompts.

The "Silver Bullet"

There is no single solution to developing and maintaining adequate self-care practices in young people. However, regardless of the specific learning or behavioral goal, the relevance of self-efficacy in facilitating behavioral change is a consistent finding across studies involving people with type 1 diabetes or type 2 diabetes in a variety of populations and in a variety of cultures. Self-efficacy has an important role in facilitating health behaviors, and has implications for the way diabetes professionals create and structure learning experiences for young people.

A first step towards promoting behavior change is to incorporate a proven method to promote and enhance the belief that a young person can and will be successful in taking care of him- or herself. If they believe that they are capable of self-care, young people will be more motivated to apply themselves to solving their diabetes problems and will benefit in terms of overall health and quality of life throughout adulthood.

References

1. Bandura A. Self-efficacy: the exercise of control. WH Freeman. New York, 1997.

2. Holmes CS, Chen R, Streisand R, et al. Predictors of youth diabetes care behaviors and metabolic control: a structural equation modeling approach. *J Pediatr Psychol* 2006; 31: 770-84.

3. Stewart SM, Lee PWH, Waller D, et al. A follow-up study of adherence and glycemic control among Hong Kong youths with diabetes. *J Pediatr Psychol* 2003; 28: 67-79.

4. Ott J, Greening L, Palardy N, et al. Self-efficacy as a mediator variable for adolescents' adherence to treatment for insulin-dependent diabetes mellitus. *Child Health Care* 2000; 29: 47-63.

5. Mulvaney SA, Mudasiru E, Schlundt DG, et al. Self-management in type 2 diabetes: the adolescent perspective. *Diabetes Educ* 2008; 34: 674-82.

Chapter 14

Know Your Blood Sugar Numbers

If you have diabetes, keeping your blood glucose (sugar) numbers in your target range can help you feel good today and stay healthy in the future.

There are two ways to measure blood glucose.

1. The A1C is a lab test that measures your average blood glucose level over the last two to three months. It shows whether your blood glucose stayed close to your target range most of the time, or was too high or too low.

2. Self-tests are the blood glucose checks you do yourself. They show what your blood glucose is at the time you test. Both ways help you and your health care team to get a picture of how your diabetes care plan is working.

About The A1C Test

Why should I have an A1C test?

The A1C tells you and your health care team how well your diabetes care plan worked over the last two to three months. It also helps decide the type and amount of diabetes medicine you need.

What is a good A1C target for me?

For many people with diabetes, the A1C target is below 7. You and your health care team will decide on an A1C target that is right for you.

About This Chapter: "Know Your Blood Sugar Numbers," National Diabetes Education Program, February 2011.

If your A1C stays too high, it may increase your chances of having eye, kidney, nerve, and heart problems.

How often do I need an A1C?

You need an A1C at least twice a year. You need it more often if it is too high, if your diabetes treatment changes, or if you become pregnant. (Women who plan to become pregnant should talk to their doctors before becoming pregnant.)

Self-Tests For Blood Glucose

Why should I do self-tests?

Self-tests can help you learn how being active, having stress, taking medicine, and eating food can make your blood glucose go up or down. They give you the facts you need to make wise choices as you go through the day.

Hemoglobin Variants Can Affect A1C Test Results

If you are of African, Mediterranean, or Southeast Asian heritage, you could have a variant form of hemoglobin in your red blood cells that affects your diabetes care. Hemoglobin in red blood cells gives blood its red color and carries oxygen from your lungs to all parts of your body. Some forms of hemoglobin can cause false results for a diabetes blood test called the A1C test. If the A1C test gives a false result, your doctor may think your blood glucose level is higher or lower than it really is.

Most people have only one kind of hemoglobin called hemoglobin A. Some people have both hemoglobin A and another kind such as hemoglobin S, C, or E. These less common forms of hemoglobin are called hemoglobin variants. You can have a hemoglobin variant but not know it because you might not have any symptoms of blood disease. Having a variant without symptoms of the disease is also called having the trait or being a carrier.

Many people have heard of sickle cell trait, which occurs most often in people of African heritage. Again, having the trait means you inherited a gene for a hemoglobin variant from one parent. Genes carry information about which characteristics are passed down from parents to children. People with sickle cell trait usually have no symptoms. (Inheriting genes from both parents for the variant hemoglobin "S," however, results in sickle cell disease, which is painful. You would know if you had sickle cell disease.)

People of Mediterranean or Southeast Asian heritage also can inherit hemoglobin variants. Some of these variants cause no symptoms; others cause some health problems.

Variant hemoglobin does not increase your risk for diabetes, but your doctor needs accurate results from your A1C test in order to plan how best to control your diabetes.

Source: Excerpted from "For People of African, Mediterranean, or Southeast Asian Heritage: Important Information about Diabetes Blood Tests," National Institute of Diabetes and Digestive and Kidney Diseases, November 2007.

Keep a record of your results. Look for times when your blood glucose is often too high or too low. Talk about your results with your health care team at each visit. Ask what you can do when your glucose is out of your target range.

How do I check my blood glucose?

Blood glucose meters use a small drop of blood to tell you how much glucose is in your blood at that moment. Ask your health care team how to get the supplies you need. They will also show you how to use them.

What is a good target range for my self-tests?

Many people with diabetes aim to keep their blood glucose between 70 and 130 before meals. About two hours after a meal starts, they aim for less than 180. Talk with your health care team about the best target range for you.

Can my blood glucose get too low?

Yes it can. If you feel shaky, sweaty, or hungry, do a check to see if it is below your target range. Carry something sweet with you at all times, such as four hard candies or glucose tablets. If your blood glucose is too low, eat the candy or glucose tablets right away. Let your health care team know if this happens often. Ask how you can prevent it.

How often should I check my blood glucose?

Self-tests are often done before meals, after meals, and at bedtime. People who take insulin need to check more than those who do not take insulin. Test whenever you want to know your blood glucose.

Other Information

Are there other numbers I need to know?

Yes, you need tests of your blood pressure and cholesterol (a blood fat). You and your health care team need to decide the best targets for these too. Keeping them in your target range can help lower your chances for having a heart attack or stroke.

Are these tests expensive?

Medicare and most insurance plans pay for the A1C, cholesterol, and some self blood test supplies. Check with your insurance plan or ask your health care team for help.

What is in it for me?

Finding the time to check your blood glucose can be a struggle. It is also hard when your glucose levels do not seem to match your efforts to manage your diabetes. Keep in mind that your self-test and A1C results are numbers to help you, not to judge you.

Many people find that self-testing and using the results to manage their diabetes pays off. They are more able to take charge of their diabetes so that they can feel good today and stay healthy in the future.

Chapter 15

Blood Glucose Monitoring

Keeping Track Of Your Blood Glucose

It's important to your health to control your blood glucose (also called blood sugar). Keeping your glucose level close to normal helps prevent or delay some diabetes problems, such as eye disease, kidney disease, and nerve damage. One thing that can help you control your glucose level is to keep track of it. You can do this by taking these steps:

- Checking your own glucose a number of times each day (self-monitoring blood glucose). Many people with diabetes check their glucose two to four times a day.

- Getting an A1C test from your health care provider about every three months.

These tests can help you and the rest of your diabetes health care team—doctor, diabetes educator, and others—work together to help you control your blood glucose.

Checking Your Blood Glucose Each Day

You can do a test to find out what your blood glucose is at any moment. Your health care team can show you how to do the test yourself. Using a finger prick, you place a drop of blood on a special coated strip, which "reads" your blood glucose. Many people use an electronic meter to get this reading.

Blood glucose testing can help you understand how food, physical activity, and diabetes medicine affect your glucose levels. Testing can help you make day-to-day choices about how

About This Chapter: This chapter begins with "Keeping Track of Your Blood Glucose," excerpted from *Take Charge of Your Diabetes,* Centers for Disease Control and Prevention, 2007. It continues with "Medical Devices: Glucose Testing Devices," U.S. Food and Drug Administration, December 23, 2010.

Daily Log   Week Starting _____

Insulin type	Breakfast		Lunch		Dinner		Bedtime		Other		Notes
	Dose	Blood Sugar	Dose	Blood Sugar	Dose	Blood Sugar	Dose	Blood Sugar	Dose	Blood Sugar	
Mon											
Tues											
Wed											
Thurs											
Fri											
Sat											
Sun											

Figure 15.1. Glucose Log Sheet For People Who Use Insulin. Use this log sheet—or one like it that your health care provider may give you—to keep a record of your daily blood glucose levels.

Daily Log

Week Starting _____

	Breakfast Blood Sugar	Lunch Blood Sugar	Dinner Blood Sugar	Bedtime Blood Sugar	Other Blood Sugar	Notes
Mon						
Tues						
Wed						
Thurs						
Fri						
Sat						
Sun						

Figure 15.2. Glucose Log Sheet For People Who Do Not Use Insulin. Use this log sheet—or one like it that your health care provider may give you—to keep a record of your daily blood glucose levels.

to balance these things. It can also tell you when your glucose is too low or too high so that you can treat these problems.

Ask your health care team to help you set a goal for your glucose range and show you how to record your glucose readings in a logbook or record sheet. If you need a daily logbook, ask your health care provider for one. Or you can make copies the log sheets shown in Figures 15.1 and 15.2.

Be sure to write down each glucose reading and the date and time you took it. When you review your records, you can see a pattern of your recent glucose control. Keeping track of your glucose on a day-to-day basis is one of the best ways you can take charge of your diabetes.

Getting A Summary Lab Test (A1C)

By performing an A1C test, health providers can sum up your diabetes control for the past few months. An A1C test measures how much glucose has been sticking to your red blood cells. Since each red blood cell is replaced by a new one every three to four months, this test tells you how high the glucose levels have been during the life of the cells.

If most of your recent blood glucose readings have been near normal (70 to 140 milligrams per deciliter or mg/dL, with the higher reading mainly after meals), the A1C test will be near normal (usually about 6%–7%). If you've had many readings above normal, the extra glucose sticking to your red blood cells will make your A1C test read higher.

You should get an A1C test every three months if your test results are not yet at goal. You should get an A1C test at least twice times a year if your A1C results are at goal. Ask your team to tell you the normal range of values and help you set a goal for yourself.

If your A1C test results are high, work with your team to adjust your balance of food, physical activity, and diabetes medicine. When your A1C test result is near your goal, you'll know you've balanced things well.

Having Problems With Low Blood Glucose

In general, a blood glucose reading lower than 70 mg/dL is too low. If you take insulin or diabetes pills, you can have low blood glucose (also called hypoglycemia). Low blood glucose is usually caused by eating less or later than usual, being more active than usual, or taking too much diabetes medicine. Drinking beer, wine, or liquor may also cause low blood glucose or make it worse.

Low blood glucose happens more often when you're trying to keep your glucose level near normal. This is no reason to stop trying to control your diabetes. It just means you have to watch more carefully for low levels. Talk this over with your health care team.

Some possible signs of low blood glucose are feeling nervous, shaky, or sweaty. Sometimes people just feel tired.

The signs may be mild at first. But a low glucose level can quickly drop much lower if you don't treat it. When your glucose level is very low, you may get confused, pass out, or have seizures. If you have any signs that your glucose may be low, test it right away. If it's less than 60 to 70 mg/dL, you need to treat it right away.

If you feel like your blood glucose is getting too low but you can't test it right then, play it safe—go ahead and treat it. Eat 10 to 15 grams of carbohydrate right away. Here are some examples of foods and liquids with this amount of carbohydrate; each item has 15 grams of carbohydrate:

- Sugar packets: 3 to 4
- Fruit juice: 1/2 cup (4 ounces)
- Soda pop (not diet): 1/2 cup (4 ounces)
- Hard candy: 3 to 5 pieces
- Sugar or honey: 4 teaspoons
- Glucose tablets: 3 to 4

Check your blood glucose again in 15 minutes. Eat another 10 to 15 grams of carbohydrate every 15 minutes until your blood glucose is above 70 mg/dL. Eating or drinking an item from this list will keep your glucose up for only about 30 minutes. So if your next planned meal or snack is more than 30 minutes away, you should go ahead and eat a small snack, something like crackers and a tablespoon of peanut butter.

In your glucose logbook or record sheet, write down the numbers and the times when low levels happen. Think about what may be causing them. If you think you know the reason, write it beside the numbers you recorded. You may need to call your health care provider to talk about changing your diet, activity, or diabetes medicine.

Tell family members, close friends, teachers, and people at work that you have diabetes. Tell them how to know when your blood glucose is low. Show them what to do if you can't treat yourself. Someone will need to give you fruit juice, soda pop (not diet), or sugar.

If you can't swallow, someone will need to give you a shot of glucagon and call for help. Glucagon is a prescription medicine that raises the blood glucose and is injected like insulin. If you take insulin, you should have a glucagon kit handy. Teach family members, roommates, and friends when and how to use it.

Waiting to treat low blood glucose is not safe. You may be in danger of passing out. If you get confused, pass out, or have a seizure, you need emergency help. Don't try to drive yourself to get help.

Having Problems With High Blood Glucose

For most people, blood glucose levels that stay higher than 140 mg/dL (before meals) are too high. Talk with your health care team about the glucose range that is best for you. Eating too much food, being less active than usual, or taking too little diabetes medicine are some common reasons for high blood glucose (or hyperglycemia). Your blood glucose can also go up when you're sick or under stress. Over time, high blood glucose can damage body organs. For this reason, many people with diabetes try to keep their blood glucose in balance as much as they can.

Some people with type 2 diabetes may not feel the signs of high blood glucose until their blood glucose is higher than 300. People with blood glucose higher than 300 are more likely to have dehydration. Dehydration can become a serious problem if not treated right away.

Your blood glucose is more likely to go up when you're sick—for example, when you have the flu or an infection. You'll need to take special care of yourself during these times.

Some common signs of high blood glucose are having a dry mouth, being thirsty, and urinating often. Other signs include feeling tired, having blurred vision, and losing weight without trying. If your glucose is very high, you may have stomach pain, feel sick to your stomach, or even throw up. This is an emergency and you need to go to the hospital right away.

If you have any signs that your blood glucose is high, check your blood. In your logbook or on your record sheet, write down your glucose reading and the time you did the test. If your glucose is high, think about what could have caused it to go up. If you think you know of something, write this down beside your glucose reading.

Emergency Identification

Always wear something (like an identification bracelet) that says you have diabetes. Carry a card in your wallet that says you have diabetes and tells if you use medicine to treat it. Wear something that lets others know you have diabetes, in case of an emergency.

Source: Centers for Disease Control and Prevention, 2007.

Try to stay with your food and activity plan as much as you can. Drink water. Take your diabetes medicine about the same time each day. Work with your health care team to set goals for weight, blood glucose level, and activity.

Keep track of your blood glucose and go over your records often. You'll learn how certain foods or activities affect your glucose. Show your records to your health care team. Ask how you can change your food, activity, and medicine to avoid or treat high blood glucose. Ask when you should call for help. Balance is the key to taking charge of your diabetes.

What's It Mean?

Continuous Glucose Monitoring: Continuous glucose monitoring (CGM) systems use a tiny sensor inserted under the skin to check glucose levels in tissue fluid. The sensor stays in place for several days to a week and then must be replaced. A transmitter sends information about glucose levels via radio waves from the sensor to a pager-like wireless monitor. The user must check blood samples with a glucose meter to program the devices. Because currently approved CGM devices are not as accurate and reliable as standard blood glucose meters, users should confirm glucose levels with a meter before making a change in treatment.

CGM systems are more expensive than conventional glucose monitoring, but they may enable better glucose control. CGM devices produced by Abbott, DexCom, and Medtronic have been approved by the U.S. Food and Drug Administration (FDA) and are available by prescription. These devices provide real-time measurements of glucose levels, with glucose levels displayed at five-minute or one-minute intervals. Users can set alarms to alert them when glucose levels are too low or too high. Special software is available to download data from the devices to a computer for tracking and analysis of patterns and trends, and the systems can display trend graphs on the monitor screen.

Additional CGM devices are being developed and tested. To learn more about such monitors and new products after approval, call the FDA at 888-INFO-FDA (463-6332) or check the FDA's website section titled "Glucose Meters and Diabetes Management" at www.fda.gov/diabetes/glucose.html.

Source: Excerpted from "Continuous Glucose Monitoring," U.S. Food and Drug Administration, October 2008.

Glucose Testing Devices

A glucose testing device is home-use test kit to measure blood sugar (glucose) in your blood. This is a quantitative test—you find out the amount of glucose present in your sample. You can use the results to help you determine your daily adjustments in treatment, know if you have dangerously high or low levels of glucose, and understand how your diet and exercise change your glucose levels.

Follow your doctor's recommendations about how often you test your glucose. You may need to test yourself several times each day to determine adjustments in your treatment.

The accuracy of this test depends on many factors including the quality of your meter, the quality of your test strips, and how well you do the test. Other factors can also affect the test's accuracy:

- Your hematocrit (the amount of red blood cells in the blood). If you have a high hematocrit, you may test low for blood glucose. Or, if you have a low hematocrit, you may test high for glucose. If you know your hematocrit is low or high, discuss with your health care provider how it may affect your glucose testing.

- Interfering substances (some substances, such as Vitamin C and uric acid, may interfere with your glucose testing). Check the package insert for your meter and test strips to find out what substances may affect the testing accuracy.

- Altitude, temperature, and humidity (high altitude, low and high temperatures, and humidity can cause unpredictable effects on glucose results). Check the meter and test strip package inserts for more information. Store and handle the meter and strips according to instructions.

How The Test Is Done

Before you self-monitor your blood glucose, you must read and understand the instructions for your meter. In general, you prick your finger with a lancet to get a drop of blood. Place the blood on a disposable "test strip" that is coated with chemicals that react with glucose. Then place the test strip in your meter. Some meters measure the amount of electricity that passes through the test strip. Others measure how much light reflects from it. In the U.S., meters report results in milligrams of glucose per deciliter of blood or mg/dl.

You can get information about your meter and test strips from several different sources including the toll-free number in the user manual or the manufacturer's web site. If you have an urgent problem, always contact your healthcare provider or a local emergency room for advice.

Choosing A Glucose Meter

You can purchase more than 25 different types of meters. They differ in several ways including the following:

- Amount of blood needed for each test

- How easy it is to use

- Pain associated with using the product

- Accuracy

- Testing speed

- Overall size

- Ability to store test results in memory

- Cost of the meter

- Cost of the test strips used

- Doctor's recommendation

- Technical support provided by the manufacturer

- Special features such as automatic timing, error codes, large display screen, or spoken instructions or results

Talk to your health care practitioner about glucose meters and how to use them.

Comparing Home Test Glucose Values With Laboratory Values

Most home blood glucose meters in the U.S. measure glucose in whole blood. Most lab tests, in contrast, measure glucose in plasma. Plasma is blood without the cells. A lab test of your blood glucose will be about 10–15% higher than the value given by your meter. Look at the instructions for your meter to find out if it gives its results as "whole blood" or "plasma equivalent." Many meters now sold give values that are "plasma equivalent," which means they can be compared more directly to lab test values.

Generic Test Strips

You may choose test strips that are made by a different company than the one that made meter. Sometimes, generic test strips are cheaper. If you choose generic test strips make sure the generic strips will work with your meter. Check the label of the test strips to make sure they will work with the make and model of your meter. Just because the generic test strip looks like it will work does not mean that it will work. Watch for inconsistent results. If you get poor results, try strips made or recommended by the maker of your meter until you again get consistent results.

Check Your Meter's Performance

There are three ways to make sure your meter works properly:

1. Use liquid control solution: every time you open a new container of test strips; occasionally as you use the container of test strips; whenever you get unusual results. You test a

drop of these solutions just like you test a drop of your blood. The value you get should match that written on the liquid control solution bottle.

2. Use electronic checks. Every time you turn on your meter, it does an electronic check. If it detects a problem it will give you an error code. Look in your owner's manual to see what the error codes mean and how to fix the problem.

3. Compare your meter with a laboratory meter. Take your meter with you to your next appointment with your health care provider. Ask your provider to watch your technique to make sure you are using the meter correctly. Ask your healthcare provider have your blood tested with a routine laboratory method. If the values you obtain on your glucose meter match the laboratory values, then your meter is working well and you are using good technique.

If your meter malfunctions, you should tell your health care professional and the company that made your meter and strips.

Alternate Testing Sites

Some new meters allow you to test blood from the base of your thumb, upper arm, forearm, thigh, or calf. If your glucose changes rapidly, these other sites may not give you accurate results. You should probably use your fingers to get your blood for testing if any of the following applies:

- You have just taken insulin
- You think your blood sugar is low
- You are not aware of symptoms when you become hypoglycemic
- The site results do not agree with the way you feel
- You have just eaten
- You have just exercised
- You are ill
- You are under stress

Chapter 16

Alternate Site Testing

Fingerstick Test And Alternate Site Test Techniques

Fingerstick

Wash hands with soap and water. Stick the finger on the side of the fingertip (you can do it on the fingertip, but, since we use our fingertips to write, grab, work... it will make it more sensitive). Don't squeeze the finger, but, you can use your other hand to gently squeeze the hand in a downward motion all the way to the fingertip. Place the blood drop on the strip and wait for your results. If you have a difficult time getting enough blood, use warm wet towels to soak your hand for a couple of minutes before you perform your test or adjust your lancet device to have a deeper penetration.

Alternate Site Testing

Alternative site refers to testing blood glucose on parts of the body other than the fingertip: most commonly the forearm, palm, or thigh. Testing somewhere other than the finger may bring a sigh of relief to many people with diabetes.

However, alternative test sites are not all the same. With all meters, routine testing on an unrubbed forearm, upper arm, thigh, or calf gives a test result that is 20 to 30 minutes old. We will call these sites 'lagging' alternative test sites.

The fingertips and the palm hold the most recent 'memories' of your blood glucose. Fingertip and palm testing tell you what your blood glucose level is right now.

About This Chapter: "Alternate Blood Glucose Testing on Arm, Palm, and Thigh," reprinted courtesy of and © Becton, Dickinson and Company, 2011. For additional information, visit www.bd.com.

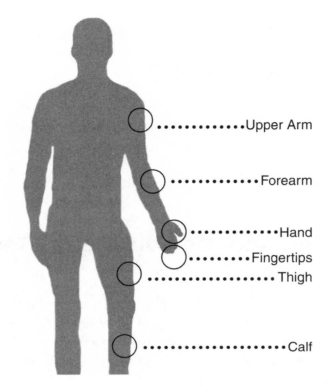

Figure 16.1. Alternate Site Testing (AST) now available.

On the other hand, lagging test sites, such as the forearm or thigh, tell you what your blood glucose was around 20 to 35 minutes ago—not what it is right now. That difference can be crucial if your blood glucose is dropping fast—a forearm test might tell you that the level is fine, because the forearm is a lagging test site, while a fingertip test correctly alerts you to a low number. Because of this, lagging test sites cannot replace the fingertip or palm completely for any person.

Several monitoring companies give people the choice to test their blood glucose using alternative sites. However, lagging test sites such as the forearm or thigh are only reliable when your blood glucose levels are relatively stable, such as fasting blood glucose.

So when is alternative site testing not recommended? The U.S. Food and Drug Administration gives these guidelines:

1. People with hypoglycemia unawareness should not use alternative site testing at all.

2. Don't use alternative sites when a seriously low blood glucose might go undetected:

- When you have just taken insulin, or any time during or after exercise.

- When there are unknown variables occurring in your day, such as illness.

- Any time you just feel "low."

- Whenever you are about to drive.

Talk to your doctor to see if alternative site testing (AST) is right for you. With a little bit of education, you can give your fingertips a rest and maybe test more often than you do now. For people with diabetes, more frequent testing is a good thing. Just remember: any time you want to be sure of an accurate, up-to-date blood glucose reading, test on your fingertip or palm.

You may find that getting an adequate sample from another site other than the fingertip a little more difficult, so here are some tips to help with successful AST testing:

- Only use a meter recommended for AST (check the instruction manual to be sure).

- Use a lancet device suited to AST (such as Accu-Chek Softclix with AST cap).

- Dial up the highest number on your lancet device for the first try (remember it won't hurt nearly as much as a fingerprick).

- Vigorously rub the site to stimulate blood flow.

- Lance the site but keep some pressure on it with the device until you see a drop of blood start to form.

It may take a few tests to get the technique right and you may want to do an AST and a fingerprick test at the same time just to compare results.

If you decide to use AST you should regularly make sure that your AST results match your fingerprick test results AND be sure the AST results confirm how you are feeling.

Until you discuss the suitability of AST with your healthcare professional, please continue to use only fingerprick test results.

Chapter 17

Diabetes Medicines

Different Medicines For Different Forms Of Diabetes

Diabetes medicines help keep your blood glucose in your target range. The target range is suggested by diabetes experts and your doctor or diabetes educator.

Type 1 diabetes, once called juvenile diabetes or insulin-dependent diabetes, is usually first found in children, teenagers, or young adults. If you have type 1 diabetes, you must take insulin because your body no longer makes it. You also might need to take other types of diabetes medicines that work with insulin. [For more information about insulin, see Chapter 18.]

Type 2 diabetes, once called adult-onset diabetes or noninsulin-dependent diabetes, is the most common form of diabetes. It can start when the body doesn't use insulin as it should, a condition called insulin resistance. If the body can't keep up with the need for insulin, you may need diabetes medicines. Many choices are available. Your doctor might prescribe two or more medicines. The American Diabetes Association (ADA) recommends that most people start with metformin, a kind of diabetes pill.

Gestational diabetes is diabetes that occurs for the first time during pregnancy. The hormones of pregnancy or a shortage of insulin can cause gestational diabetes. Most women with gestational diabetes control it with meal planning and physical activity. But some women need insulin to reach their target blood glucose levels.

If you have one of the rare forms of diabetes, such as diabetes caused by other medicines or monogenic diabetes, talk with your doctor about what kind of diabetes medicine would be best for you.

About This Chapter: This chapter includes excerpts from "What I Need to Know about Diabetes Medicines," National Institute of Diabetes and Digestive and Kidney Diseases, October 2010.

Diabetes Pills

Along with meal planning and physical activity, diabetes pills help people with type 2 diabetes or gestational diabetes keep their blood glucose levels on target. Several kinds of pills are available. Each works in a different way. Many people take two or three kinds of pills. Some people take combination pills. Combination pills contain two kinds of diabetes medicine in one tablet. Some people take pills and insulin.

Diabetes pills help people with type 2 diabetes or gestational diabetes keep their blood glucose levels on target.

Your doctor may ask you to try one kind of pill. If it doesn't help you reach your blood glucose targets, your doctor may ask you to take more of the same pill, add another kind of pill, change to another type of pill, start taking insulin, or start taking another injected medicine.

If your doctor suggests that you take insulin or another injected medicine, it doesn't mean your diabetes is getting worse. Instead, it means you need insulin or another type of medicine to reach your blood glucose targets. Everyone is different. What works best for you depends on your usual daily routine, eating habits, and activities, and your other health conditions.

The information below explains some of the most commonly used non-insulin diabetes medicines:

Alpha-Glucosidase Inhibitor

This is pronounced alpha (AL-fuh)-glucosidase (-gloo-KOH-sih-dayss) inhibitor (in-HIB-ih-tur). Brand and generic names are Glyset (pronounced GLY-set)—the generic name is miglitol (pronounced MIG-lih-tol) and Precose (pronounced PREE-kohss)—the generic name is acarbose (pronounced A-kahr-bohss)

What does this type of pill do?

This type of pill helps keep your blood glucose from going too high after you eat, a common problem in people with diabetes. It works by slowing down the digestion of foods high in carbohydrate, such as rice, potatoes, bread, milk, and fruit.

Who should not take Glyset or Precose?

Talk with your doctor about whether to take this type of pill if you have bowel disease or other intestinal conditions, you have advanced kidney or liver disease, or you are pregnant, planning to get pregnant, or breastfeeding.

Table 17.1. Kinds Of Diabetes Pills And How They Work

Generic Name	Brand Name	How They Work
Biguanides		
Metformin	Glucophage	Block the liver from making sugar
Sulfonylureas (second-generation)		
Glimepiride	Amaryl	Raise the amount of insulin in the body
Glipizide	Glucotrol	
Glyburide	DiaBeta	
	Glynase PresTab	
	Micronase	
Meglitinides		
Repaglinide	Prandin	Raise the amount of insulin in the body
Nateglinide	Starlix	
Thiazolidinediones		
Pioglitazone	Actos	Help the body use insulin better
Rosiglitazone	Avandia	
Alpha-glucosidase inhibitors		
Acarbose	Precose	Slow the digestion of sugar
Miglitol	Glyset	

Source: Excerpted from "Pills for Type 2 Diabetes: A Guide for Adults," Agency for Healthcare Research and Quality, December 5, 2007.

What are the possible side effects?

This type of pill doesn't cause low blood glucose by itself. But your risk of having low blood glucose goes up if you also take diabetes pills that cause low blood glucose or insulin.

Your doctor may ask you to take a lower dose of your other diabetes medicines while you take this type of pill.

Taking Glyset or Precose may cause stomach pain, gas, bloating, or diarrhea. These symptoms usually go away after you have taken these pills for a while.

What do I need to know about low blood glucose?

If you take Glyset or Precose, only glucose tablets or glucose gel will bring your blood glucose level back to normal quickly. Other quick-fix foods and drinks won't raise your blood glucose as quickly because Glyset and Precose slow the digestion of other quick-fix foods and drinks.

Biguanide

This is pronounced biguanide (by-GWAH-nyd). Brand and generic names are Glucophage (GLOO-coh-fahj)—the generic is metformin (met-FOR-min); Glucophage XR—the generic is metformin long-acting; and Riomet (RY-oh-met)—the generic is metformin liquid.

What does this type of medicine do?

This type of medicine, which comes in pill or liquid form, lowers the amount of glucose made by your liver. Then your blood glucose levels don't go too high. This type of medicine also helps treat insulin resistance. With insulin resistance, your body doesn't use insulin the way it should. When your insulin works properly, your blood glucose levels stay on target and your cells get the energy they need. This type of medicine improves your cholesterol levels. It also may help you lose weight.

Who should not take Glucophage, Glucophage XR, or Riomet?

Talk with your doctor about whether to take this type of medicine if you have advanced kidney or liver disease, you drink excessive amounts of alcoholic beverages, or you are pregnant, planning to get pregnant, or breastfeeding.

What are the possible side effects?

This type of pill doesn't cause low blood glucose by itself. But your risk of having low blood glucose goes up if you also take diabetes pills that cause low blood glucose or insulin. Your doctor may ask you to take a lower dose of your other diabetes medicines while you take this type of pill.

You may have nausea, diarrhea, or an upset stomach when you first start taking this type of medicine. These side effects are likely to go away after a while.

Rarely, a serious condition called lactic acidosis occurs as a side effect of taking this medicine. Call your doctor right away if you become weak and tired, become dizzy, feel very cold, have trouble breathing, have unusual muscle pain and stomach problems, or have a sudden change in the speed or steadiness of your heartbeat.

Sometimes you'll need to stop taking this type of medicine for a short time so you can avoid developing lactic acidosis. If you have severe vomiting, diarrhea, or a fever, or if you can't keep fluids down, call your doctor right away. You should also talk with your doctor well ahead of time about stopping this type of medicine if you'll be having special x-rays that require an injection of dye or if you'll be having surgery. Your doctor will tell you when it's safe to start taking your medicine again.

D-Phenylalanine Derivative

This is pronounced d-phenylalanine (dee-FEN-il-AL-uh-neen) derivative (duh-RIV-uh-tiv). The brand name is Starlix (STAR-liks)—the generic name is nateglinide (nuh-TEG-lih-nyd).

What does this type of pill do?

This type of pill helps your body make more insulin for a short period of time right after meals. The insulin helps keep your blood glucose from going too high after you eat, a common problem in people with diabetes.

Who should not take Starlix?

Talk with your doctor about whether to take this type of pill if you are pregnant, planning to get pregnant, or breastfeeding or if you have liver disease.

What are the possible side effects?

Possible side effects are low blood glucose, also called hypoglycemia, weight gain, and dizziness.

DPP-4 Inhibitor

DPP4 stands for dipeptidyl (dy-PEP-tih-dil) peptidase-4 (PEP-tih-dayss-FOR). The brand name is Januvia (juh-NOO-vee-uh)—the generic name is sitagliptin (sih-tuh-GLIP-tin) phosphate (FOSS-fayt).

What does this type of pill do?

This type of pill lowers your blood glucose by helping your body make more insulin when it's needed, especially right after meals. It also helps keep your liver from putting stored glucose into your blood.

Who should not take Januvia?

Talk with your doctor about whether to take this type of pill if you are pregnant, planning to get pregnant, or breastfeeding, if you have kidney disease, or if you have type 1 diabetes and if you have a condition called diabetic ketoacidosis.

What are the possible side effects?

This type of pill doesn't cause low blood glucose by itself. But your risk of having low blood glucose goes up if you also take diabetes pills that cause low blood glucose or insulin. Your doctor may ask you to take a lower dose of your other diabetes medicines while you take this type of pill.

Possible side effects are a cold, runny nose, sore throat, and headache. If you take Januvia and have kidney problems, your health care provider might order blood tests to see how well your kidneys are working.

Meglitinide

This is pronounced meglitinide (meh-GLIH-tih-nyde). The brand name is Prandin (PRAN-din), and the generic name is repaglinide (ruh-PAG-luh-nyd).

What does this type of pill do?

This type of pill helps your body make more insulin for a short period of time right after meals. The insulin helps keep your blood glucose from going too high after you eat, a common problem in people with diabetes.

Who should not take Prandin?

Talk with your doctor about whether to take this type of pill if you are pregnant, planning to get pregnant, or if you are breastfeeding or if you have liver disease.

What are the possible side effects?

Prandin can cause low blood glucose (also called hypoglycemia), weight gain, upset stomach, back pain, or a headache.

Sulfonylurea

This is pronounced sulfonylurea (SUHL-foh-nil-yoo-REE-uh). There are several brand names for this type of medication (Brand name; generic name):

- Amaryl (AM-uh-ril); glimepiride (gly-MEP-ih-ryd)
- DiaBeta (dy-uh-BAY-tuh); glyburide (GLY-buh-ryd)
- Diabinese (dy-AB-ih-neez); chlorpropamide (klor-PROH-puh-myd)
- Glucotrol (GLOO-kuh-trohl); glipizide (GLIP-ih-zyd)
- Glucotrol XL (GLOO-kuh-trohl)(EKS-EL); glipizide (GLIP-ih-zyd) (long-acting)

- Glynase (GLY-nayz) PresTab; glyburide (GLY-buh-ryd)

- Micronase (MY-kroh-nayz); glyburide (GLY-buh-ryd)

Two others are available only in generic form: tolazamide (tahl-AZ-uh-myd) and tolbutamide (tahl-BYOO-tuh-myd).

What does this type of pill do?

This type of pill helps your body make more insulin. The insulin helps lower your blood glucose.

Who should not take sulfonylureas?

Talk with your doctor about whether to take this type of pill if you are allergic to sulfa drugs or if you are pregnant, planning to get pregnant, or breastfeeding.

What are the possible side effects?

Possible side effects include low blood glucose (hypoglycemia), upset stomach, skin rash, and weight gain.

Diabetes Pills Use Up—Insulin Use Down

The proportion of Americans reporting treatment for diabetes who took oral medications to treat their condition increased from 60 percent in 1997 to 77 percent in 2007—a 28 percent increase—according to the Agency for Healthcare Research and Quality (AHRQ). During the same period, the proportion taking insulin to control their diabetes fell from 38 percent to 24 percent.

The federal agency's analysis also revealed a shift in the three most commonly prescribed oral medications between 1997 and 2007. The proportion of Americans using sulfonylureas—which stimulate the pancreas to produce more insulin—declined from 1997 to 2007. The proportions using biguanides—which reduces the liver's excess glucose production—and thiazolidinediones—which increases insulin sensitivity—rose during the period.

Specifically the proportions of people who were treated for diabetes who used the three most commonly prescribed oral medications were as follows:

- Sulfonylureas declined from 51 percent to 40 percent.
- Biguanides rose from 21 percent to 55 percent.
- Thiazolidinediones increased from 5 percent to 25 percent.

Source: From "Diabetes Pills Use Up—Insulin Use Down," *AHRQ News and Numbers*, Agency for Healthcare Research and Quality, September 20, 2010.

Thiazolidinedione

This is pronounced thiazolidinedione (THY-uh-ZOHL-ih-deen-DY-ohn). Brand and generic names are Actos (AK-tohss)—the generic names is pioglitazone (py-oh-GLIH-tuh-zohn), and Avandia (uh-VAN-dee-uh)—the generic name is rosiglitazone (rohss-ih-GLIH-tuh-zohn).

In September 2010, the U.S. Food and Drug Administration (FDA) restricted access to Avandia. The FDA based this decision on studies linking Avandia to an increased risk of cardiovascular events, such as heart attacks and strokes.

If you are currently taking Avandia discuss treatment options with your doctor before stopping your diabetes medicines. Stopping your diabetes medicines without talking with your doctor can cause serious short-term health problems and could increase the risk of long-term diabetes-related complications.

For more information about FDA's restrictions on the use of Avandia, visit www.fda.gov/Drugs/DrugSafety/PostmarketDrugSafetyInformationforPatientsandProviders/ucm226976.htm or call the FDA at 888-INFO-FDA (888-463-6332).

What does this type of pill do?

This type of pill helps treat insulin resistance. With insulin resistance, your body doesn't use insulin the way it should. Thiazolidinediones help your insulin work properly. Then your blood glucose levels stay on target and your cells get the energy they need.

Who should not take this type of pill?

People with heart failure, also called congestive heart failure, should not take this type of pill. This type of pill can cause heart failure or make it worse.

Heart failure is a condition in which your heart no longer pumps properly. Then your body keeps too much fluid in your legs, ankles, and lungs.

Call your doctor right away if you have signs of heart failure. Warning signs include having swelling in your legs or ankles, gaining a lot of weight in a short time, having trouble breathing, having a cough, or being very tired.

You should also talk with your doctor about whether to take this type of pill if you are pregnant, planning to get pregnant, or breastfeeding or if you have liver disease.

What are the possible side effects?

Heart failure is a serious side effect. Avandia is also linked to an increased risk of cardiovascular events, such as heart attacks and strokes.

This type of pill doesn't cause low blood glucose by itself. But your risk of having low blood glucose goes up if you also take diabetes pills that cause low blood glucose or insulin. Your doctor may ask you to take a lower dose of your other diabetes medicines while you take this type of pill.

Possible side effects, in addition to the side effects related to heart failure, are anemia, a condition that can make you feel very tired, and an increased risk of getting pregnant even if you're taking birth control pills.

Women who take Actos, Avandia, or combination diabetes pills containing pioglitazone or rosiglitazone may have an increased risk of bone fractures.

If you take Actos or Avandia, your health care provider should make sure your liver is working properly. Call your doctor right away if you have any signs of liver disease: nausea, vomiting, stomach pain, tiredness, dark-colored urine, or loss of appetite.

Combination Diabetes Pills

Combination pills contain two different types of diabetes pills. Several combination pills are available.

Actoplus Met: The brand name is Actoplus Met (AK-toh-pluhss)(met); the generic name is pioglitazone (py-oh-GLIH-tuh-zohn) + metformin (met-FOR-min). Actoplus Met is a combination of two types of pills. One pill lowers the amount of glucose made by your liver. Both types help your insulin work the way it should.

Avandamet: The brand name is Avandamet (uh-VAN-duh-met); the generic name is rosiglitazone (rohss-ih-GLIH-tuh-zohn) + metformin (met-FOR-min). Avandamet is a combination of two types of pills. One pill lowers the amount of glucose made by your liver. Both types help your insulin work the way it should.

Avandaryl: The brand name is Avandaryl (uh-VAN-duh-ril); the generic name is rosiglitazone (rohss-ih-GLIH-tuh-zohn) + glimepiride (gly-MEP-ih-ryd). Avandaryl is a combination of two types of pills. One pill helps your insulin work the way it should. The other pill helps your body make more insulin.

Duetact: The brand name is Duetact (DOO-uh-tak); the generic name is pioglitazone (py-oh-GLIH-tuh-zohn) + glimepiride (gly-MEP-ih-ryd). Duetact is a combination of two types of pills. One pill helps your insulin work the way it should. The other pill helps your body make more insulin.

Glucovance: The brand name is Glucovance (GLOO-koh-vanss); the generic name is glyburide (GLY-buh-ryd) + metformin (met-FOR-min). Glucovance is a combination of two types of pills. One pill helps your body make more insulin. The other pill lowers the amount of glucose made by your liver and helps your insulin work the way it should.

Janumet: The brand name is Janumet (JAN-yoo-met); the generic name is sitagliptin (sih-tuh-GLIP-tin) + metformin (met-FOR-min). Janumet is a combination of two types of pills. One pill helps your body make more insulin when it's needed, especially right after meals. It also helps keep your liver from putting stored glucose into your blood. The other pill lowers the amount of glucose made by your liver and helps your insulin work the way it should.

Metaglip: The brand name is Metaglip (MET-uh-glip); the generic name is glipizide (GLIP-ih-zyd) + metformin (met-FOR-min). Metaglip is a combination of two types of pills. One pill helps your body make more insulin. The other pill lowers the amount of glucose made by your liver and helps your insulin work the way it should.

Amylin Mimetic

This is pronounced amylin (AM-ih-lin) mimetic (mih-MET-ik). The brand name is Symlin (SIM-lin), and the generic name is pramlintide (PRAM-lin-tyd) acetate (ASS-ih-tayt).

What does this medicine do?

Symlin helps keep your blood glucose from going too high after you eat, a common problem in people with diabetes. It works by helping food move more slowly through your stomach. Symlin helps keep your liver from putting stored glucose into your blood. It also may prevent hunger, helping you eat less and maybe lose weight.

Symlin is for people who already take insulin. However, you should always use a separate syringe to inject Symlin. Symlin is not used in place of insulin. But taking Symlin may change the amount of insulin you take.

Who should not take Symlin?

Talk with your doctor about whether you should take this type of medicine if you can't tell when you are having low blood glucose (a condition called hypoglycemia unawareness), if you have recently had severe low blood glucose, if you have stomach problems caused by diabetes-related nerve damage, or if you are pregnant, planning to get pregnant, or breastfeeding. Symlin has not been studied for use in children.

There may be times when you should not take your usual dose of Symlin. If you're having surgery or you're sick and can't eat, you should not take your Symlin. Ask your doctor about other times to not take it.

Evaluating Diabetes Claims? Be Smart. Be Skeptical.

Evaluating online claims for diabetes products is a two-step process. First, be smart. Then, be skeptical. The Federal Trade Commission, the nation's consumer protection agency, says it's best to check any product out with your health care provider before you buy it. That's because some fraudulent marketers try to make money by peddling products that sound great, but just don't—and can't—work as promised.

Here are some tips on how to spot scams before you get stung.

- A promise that a product can cure diabetes is a tip-off to a rip-off. There's no pill, patch, tea, herb, or other "miracle" treatment you can buy on the internet that can make your diabetes go away forever.
- Ads that promise too much generally deliver nothing. Don't buy any product that claims it can do it all—stabilize your blood sugar, end your need for insulin, regenerate your pancreas, reduce your cholesterol, and cause easy weight loss.
- A product that claims to be a "scientific breakthrough" may be a bust. Researchers around the world are racing to find better treatments for diabetes, so genuine scientific discoveries make front-page news. If the first you hear about a new treatment is an ad on the internet, be suspicious.
- Ads that try hard to sound scientific are suspect. Technical terms don't necessarily mean medical proof. And the presence of a doctor in an ad is no guarantee the product works. Scam artists have been known to dress models to look like experts.
- Don't be swayed by a questionable "success" story. Despite what a company claims, there's no guarantee that "A.B. of Hometown, USA" had the advertised results—or is even a real person.
- A money-back guarantee does not prove that a product works. Scam artists who offer a guarantee have been known to take your money and run.

If an ad for a product makes you curious, ask your healthcare provider about it before you try it—or buy it. If you're thinking about trying a new product, run it past a doctor, nurse, dietician, or other health professional who knows your case well.

Source: From "Evaluating Diabetes Claims? Be Smart. Be Skeptical." Federal Trade Commission (www.ftc.gov), October 2008.

What are the possible side effects?

Symlin can cause nausea and vomiting—most often when you first start taking Symlin, swelling, redness, or itching of the skin where Symlin is injected, headache, decreased appetite, stomach pain and indigestion, tiredness, and dizziness. This type of medicine doesn't cause low blood glucose by itself. But your risk of having low blood glucose is higher because Symlin is always taken along with insulin.

Incretin Mimetic

This is pronounced incretin (in-KREE-tin) mimetic (mih-MET-ik). The brand name is Byetta (by-YAY-tuh) and the generic name is exenatide (eks-EN-uh-tyd).

What does this medicine do?

Byetta helps your body make more insulin when it's needed. It helps keep your blood glucose from going too high after you eat, a common problem in people with diabetes. It works by helping food move more slowly through your stomach. Byetta helps keep your liver from putting stored glucose into your blood. It also may prevent hunger, helping you eat less and maybe lose weight.

Byetta is not used in place of insulin.

Who should not take Byetta?

Talk with your doctor about whether you should take this type of medicine if you have severe stomach or digestive problems, if you have any symptoms of kidney disease or are on dialysis, if you are pregnant, planning to get pregnant, or breastfeeding, or if you have type 1 diabetes. Byetta has not been studied for use in children.

What are the possible side effects?

Byetta can cause nausea and vomiting—most often when you first start taking Byetta, headache, diarrhea, and dizziness. Byetta also can cause an acid stomach or make you feel nervous.

If you take Byetta, you need to know about possible problems with your kidneys. Talk with your doctor right away if you notice any of the following:

- Changes in the color of your urine, how often you urinate, or the amount you urinate
- Swelling of your hands or feet
- Tiredness
- Changes in your appetite or digestion
- A dull ache in your mid to lower back

This type of medicine doesn't cause low blood glucose by itself. But your risk of having low blood glucose goes up if you also take diabetes pills that cause low blood glucose or insulin. Your doctor may ask you to take a lower dose of your other diabetes medicines while you take this type of medicine.

Chapter 18

Facts About Insulin

Taking Insulin

If your body no longer makes enough insulin, you'll need to take it. Insulin is used for all types of diabetes. Your doctor can help you decide which way of taking insulin is best for you.

- **Taking Injections:** You'll give yourself shots using a needle and syringe. The syringe is a hollow tube with a plunger. You will put your dose of insulin into the tube. Some people use an insulin pen, which looks like a pen but has a needle for its point.

- **Using An Insulin Pump:** An insulin pump is a small machine about the size of a cell phone, worn outside of your body on a belt or in a pocket or pouch. The pump connects to a small plastic tube and a very small needle. The needle is inserted under the skin and stays in for several days. Insulin is pumped from the machine through the tube into your body.

- **Using An Insulin Jet Injector:** The jet injector, which looks like a large pen, sends a fine spray of insulin through the skin with high-pressure air instead of a needle.

Insulin helps keep blood glucose levels on target by moving glucose from the blood into your body's cells. Your cells then use glucose for energy. In people who don't have diabetes, the body makes the right amount of insulin on its own. But when you have diabetes, you and your doctor must decide how much insulin you need throughout the day and night.

Possible side effects include low blood glucose and weight gain.

About This Chapter: This chapter begins with excerpts from "What I Need to Know about Diabetes Medicines," National Institute of Diabetes and Digestive and Kidney Diseases (NIDDK), October 2010. It continues with excerpts from "Alternative Devices for Taking Insulin," NIDDK, May 2009.

Your plan for taking insulin will depend on your daily routine and your type of insulin. Some people with diabetes who use insulin need to take it two, three, or four times a day to reach their blood glucose targets. Others can take a single shot. Your doctor or diabetes educator will help you learn how and when to give yourself insulin.

Insulin Injections: What You Should Know

Insulin cannot be taken orally because the body's digestive juices destroy it. Injections of insulin under the skin ensure that it is absorbed slowly by the body for a long-lasting effect. The timing and frequency of insulin injections depend upon a number of factors:

- The duration of insulin action. Insulin is available in several forms, including: standard, intermediate, long-acting, and rapid-acting.
- Amount and type of food eaten. Ingestion of food makes the blood glucose level rise. Alcohol lowers levels.
- The person's level of physical activity. Exercise lowers glucose levels.

Fast-Acting Insulin: Insulin lispro (Humalog) and insulin aspart (Novo Rapid, NovoLog) lower blood sugar very quickly, usually within five minutes after injection. Insulin peaks in about four hours and continues to work for about four more hours. This rapid action reduces the risk for hypoglycemic events after eating (postprandial hypoglycemia). Optimal timing for administering this insulin is about 15 minutes before a meal, but it can also be taken immediately after a meal (but within 30 minutes). Fast-acting insulins may be especially useful for meals with high carbohydrates.

Regular Insulin: Regular insulin begins to act 30 minutes after injection, reaches its peak at two to four hours, and lasts about six hours. Regular insulin may be administered before a meal and may be better for high-fat meals.

Intermediate Insulin: NPH (neutral protamine hagedorn) insulin has been the standard intermediate form. It works within two to four hours, peaks four to twelve hours later, and lasts up to 18 hours. Lente (insulin zinc) is another intermediate insulin that peaks four to twelve hours and lasts up to 18 hours.

Long-Acting (Ultralente) Insulin: Long-acting insulins, such as insulin glargine (Lantus), are released slowly. Long-acting insulin peaks at 10 hours and lasts up to 20 hours. Researchers are studying new types of long-acting insulins including one called degludec that requires injections only three times a week.

Combinations: Regimens generally include combinations of short and longer-acting insulins to help match the natural cycle. For example, one approach in patients who are intensively controlling their glucose levels uses three injections of insulin, which includes a mixture of regular insulin and NPH at dinner. Another approach uses four injections, including a separate short-acting form at dinner and NPH at bedtime, which may pose a lower risk for nighttime hypoglycemia than the three-injection regimen.

Source: Excerpted from "Diabetes, Type 1," 2011 A.D.A.M., Inc. Reprinted with permission.

Types Of Insulin

Each type of insulin works at a different speed. For example, rapid-acting insulin starts to work right after you take it. Long-acting insulin works for many hours. Most people need two or more types of insulin to reach their blood glucose targets.

Each type of insulin has an onset, a peak, and a duration time. The onset is how soon the insulin starts to lower your blood glucose after you take it. The peak is the time the insulin is working the hardest to lower your blood glucose. The duration is how long the insulin lasts—the length of time it keeps lowering your blood glucose.

The times shown in below are estimates. Your onset, peak, and duration times may be different. You'll work with your health care team to come up with an insulin plan that works best for you.

Rapid-Acting

- NovoLog (insulin aspart). Onset: 15 minutes; Peak: 30 to 90 minutes; Duration: 3 to 5 hours
- Apidra (insulin glulisine). Onset: 15 minutes; Peak: 30 to 90 minutes; Duration: 3 to 5 hours
- Humalog (insulin lispro). Onset: 15 minutes; Peak: 30 to 90 minutes; Duration: 3 to 5 hours

Short-Acting

- Humulin R; Novolin R (Regular [R]). Onset: 30 to 60 minutes; Peak: 2 to 4 hours; Duration: 5 to 8 hours

Intermediate-Acting

- Humulin N; Novolin N (NPH [N]). Onset: 1 to 3 hours; Peak: 8 hours; Duration: 12 to 16 hours

Long-Acting

- Levemir (insulin detemir). Onset: 1 hour; Peakless; Duration: 20 to 26 hours
- Lantus (insulin glargine). Onset: 1 hour; Peakless; Duration: 20 to 26 hours

Pre-Mixed NPH (Intermediate-Acting) And Regular (Short-Acting)

- Humulin 70/30; Novolin 70/30 (70% NPH and 30% regular). Onset: 30 to 60 minutes: Peak: varies; Duration 10 to 16 hours
- Humulin 50/50 (50% NPH and 50% regular). Onset: 30 to 60 minutes: Peak: varies; Onset: 10 to 16 hours

Pre-Mixed Insulin Lispro Protamine Suspension (Intermediate-Acting) And Insulin Lispro (Rapid-Acting)

- Humalog Mix 75/25 (75% insulin lispro protamine and 25% insulin lispro). Onset: 10 to 15 minutes; Peak: varies; Duration: 10 to 16 hours

- Humalog Mix 50/50 (50% insulin lispro protamine and 50% insulin lispro). Onset: 10 to 15 minutes; Peak: varies; Duration: 10 to 16 hours

Pre-Mixed Insulin Aspart Protamine Suspension (Intermediate-Acting) And Insulin Aspart (Rapid-Acting)

- NovoLog Mix 70/30 (70% insulin aspart protamine and 30% insulin aspart). Onset: 5 to 15 minutes; Peak: varies; Duration: 10 to 16 hours

Alternative Devices For Taking Insulin

Most people who take insulin use a needle and syringe to inject insulin just under the skin. Several other devices for taking insulin are available and new approaches are under development. No matter which approach a person uses for taking insulin, consistent monitoring of blood glucose levels is important. Good blood glucose control can prevent complications of diabetes.

What alternative devices for taking insulin are available?

Insulin Pens: Insulin pens provide a convenient, easy-to-use way of injecting insulin and may be less painful than a standard needle and syringe. An insulin pen looks like a pen with a cartridge. Some of these devices use replaceable cartridges of insulin. Other pens are prefilled with insulin and are totally disposable after the insulin is injected. Insulin pen users screw a short, fine, disposable needle on the tip of the pen before an injection. Then users turn a dial to select the desired dose of insulin, inject the needle, and press a plunger on the end to deliver the insulin just under the skin. Insulin pens are less widely used in the United States than in many other countries.

Insulin Pumps: External insulin pumps are typically about the size of a deck of cards or cell phone, weigh about 3 ounces, and can be worn on a belt or carried in a pocket. Most pumps use a disposable plastic cartridge as an insulin reservoir. A needle and plunger are temporarily attached to the cartridge to allow the user to fill the cartridge with insulin from a vial. The user then removes the needle and plunger and loads the filled cartridge into the pump.

Why Did I Gain Weight When I Started Taking Insulin?

There are several factors at work to lead you to believe that insulin is "to blame" for your weight gain.

People who have poorly controlled diabetes also sometimes experience weight loss because their bodies are unable to properly convert food into energy. This is because they either are not producing enough insulin or their bodies are unable to use the insulin they produce properly. This food winds up as excess glucose circulating in the blood (resulting in high blood glucose!). Ultimately the body can't use all that extra glucose circulating in the blood and so it is eliminated in the urine.

When your blood glucose runs high, you can become dehydrated as your body works to clear itself of all that excess glucose—which makes you think you've lost weight, but you've only lost water. Then, when you start taking insulin and get your blood glucose under better control, you start over-retaining fluids initially to make up for your dehydration, which makes you think you've rapidly gained a lot of weight. You associate it with taking insulin, but really what is happening is taking your insulin properly is just enabling your body to better use food and maintain a proper water balance.

Also, once you start taking insulin injections and start getting your blood glucose under control, you now have enough insulin circulating in your blood to help the glucose get into the body's cells where it can be used as energy. So the glucose produced by the food you eat is no longer spending time in your bloodstream and being excreted out as urine. You gain weight.

Your high blood glucose may have also made you feel more hungry because not all the food you were eating was able to get into the cells as energy to nourish the cells. Then, you started taking insulin—and continued to eat the same amount of food. Only this time, because your body has enough insulin to process the food you're eating, you gain weight. Before, you were getting away with eating more food because your body couldn't use it properly. But once your blood glucose is in a more normal range, you're just using the food properly—and you gain weight.

Some people quickly come to associate taking insulin with weight gain. They will sometimes cut back on their insulin and let their blood glucose run high once they discover they can lose a few pounds in a few days times by doing so. Unfortunately, when they go back to using the right amount of insulin to maintain good control, they are dismayed to discover that they gain the weight back—and perhaps more—in equally rapid fashion. Manipulating insulin to lose weight is an unhealthy pattern to get into. Letting your blood glucose run high can lead to long-term complications—and up and down weight problems when you try to bring your blood glucose back to a normal range.

When you begin taking insulin, discuss with your health team how to address your weight concerns. It may mean making adjustments in how much you eat. You will need to eat enough to make sure you don't have a low blood glucose reaction, but perhaps not as much as you have been eating to offset the problems caused by having had high blood glucose for a while.

Insulin pumps contain enough insulin for several days. An infusion set carries insulin from the pump to the body through flexible plastic tubing and a soft tube or needle inserted under the skin.

Disposable infusion sets are used with insulin pumps to deliver insulin to an infusion site on the body, such as the abdomen. Infusion sets include a cannula—a needle or a small, soft tube—that the user inserts into the tissue beneath the skin. Devices are available to help insert the cannula. Narrow, flexible plastic tubing carries insulin from the pump to the infusion site. On the skin's surface, an adhesive patch or dressing holds the infusion set in place until the user replaces it after a few days.

Users set the pumps to give a steady trickle or "basal" amount of insulin continuously throughout the day. Pumps can also give "bolus" doses—one-time larger doses—of insulin at meals and at times when blood glucose is too high based on the programming set by the user. Frequent blood glucose monitoring is essential to determine insulin dosages and to ensure that insulin is delivered.

Injection Ports: Injection ports provide an alternative to daily injections. Injection ports look like infusion sets without the long tubing. Like infusion sets, injection ports have a cannula that is inserted into the tissue beneath the skin. On the skin's surface, an adhesive patch or dressing holds the port in place. The user injects insulin through the port with a needle and syringe or an insulin pen. The port remains in place for several days and is then replaced. Use of an injection port allows a person to reduce the number of skin punctures to one every few days to apply a new port.

Injection Aids: Injection aids are devices that help users give injections with needles and syringes through the use of spring-loaded syringe holders or stabilizing guides. Many injection aids have a button the user pushes to inject the insulin.

Jet Injectors: Insulin jet injectors send a fine spray of insulin into the skin at high pressure instead of using a needle to deliver the insulin.

What are the prospects for an artificial pancreas?

To overcome the limitations of current insulin therapy, researchers have long sought to link glucose monitoring and insulin delivery by developing an artificial pancreas. An artificial pancreas is a system that will mimic, as closely as possible, the way a healthy pancreas detects changes in blood glucose levels and responds automatically to secrete appropriate amounts of insulin. Although not a cure, an artificial pancreas has the potential to significantly improve diabetes care and management and to reduce the burden of monitoring and managing blood glucose.

An artificial pancreas based on mechanical devices requires at least three components a continuous glucose monitoring (CGM) system, an insulin delivery system, and a computer program that adjusts insulin delivery based on changes in glucose levels.

CGM systems approved by the U.S. Food and Drug Administration (FDA) include those made by Abbott, DexCom, and Medtronic. A CGM system paired with an insulin pump is available from Medtronic. This integrated system, called the MiniMed Paradigm REAL-Time System, is not an artificial pancreas, but it does represent the first step in joining glucose monitoring and insulin delivery systems using the most advanced technology available.

Chapter 19

Insulin Pumps

- Insulin pumps replace the need for periodic injections by delivering rapid-acting insulin continuously throughout the day using a catheter.
- They offer many advantages that can simplify diabetes management.
- There are some downsides, but most pump users agree that the benefits are worth it.
- Switching to a pump requires some adjustment, so discuss the options with your health care team before making a decision.

By using an insulin pump, you can match your insulin to your lifestyle rather than adjusting your lifestyle to your body's response to insulin injections. With help from your health care team, insulin pumps can help you keep your blood glucose levels within your target ranges both day and night. People of all ages with type 1 diabetes use insulin pumps, and people with type 2 diabetes have started to use them as well.

How Do Insulin Pumps Work

If you have been diagnosed with diabetes, you may feel overwhelmed by all the new information you have learned and will continue to learn about managing your diabetes. You already know your main goal should be to get your blood glucose (sugar) levels under control in order to increase your chances of a complication-free life. Many people know this, but need to know how to achieve good diabetes management, while balancing the day-to-day demands of diabetes with other life demands.

An insulin pump can help you manage your diabetes. By using an insulin pump, you can match your insulin to your lifestyle, rather than getting an insulin injection and matching your life to how the insulin is working. When you work closely with your diabetes care team, insulin pumps can help you keep your blood glucose levels within your target ranges. People of all ages with type 1 diabetes use insulin pumps and people with type 2 diabetes have started to use them as well.

Insulin pumps deliver rapid- or short-acting insulin 24 hours a day through a catheter placed under the skin. Your insulin doses are separated into:

- Basal rates
- Bolus doses to cover carbohydrate in meals
- Correction or supplemental doses

Basal insulin is delivered continuously over 24 hours, and keeps your blood glucose levels in range between meals and overnight. Often, you program different amounts of insulin at different times of the day and night.

When you eat, you use buttons on the insulin pump to give additional insulin called a bolus. You take a bolus to cover the carbohydrate in each meal or snack. If you eat more than you planned, you can simply program a larger bolus of insulin to cover it.

You also take a bolus to treat high blood glucose levels. If you have high blood glucose levels before you eat, you give a correction or supplemental bolus of insulin to bring it back to your target range.

Knowing how an insulin pump works is one thing. But you may be wondering where you are supposed to put it. You can buy a pump case or it can be attached to a waistband, pocket, bra, garter belt, sock, or underwear. You can also tuck any excess tubing into the waistband of your underwear or pants.

When you sleep, you could try laying the pump next to you on the bed. You could even try wearing it on a waistband, armband, legband, or clip it to the blanket, sheet, pajamas, stuffed toy, or pillow with a belt clip.

Showering and bathing are other instances when you should know where to put your insulin pump. Although insulin pumps are water resistant, they should not be set directly in the water. Instead, you can disconnect it. All insulin pumps have a disconnect port for activities, such as swimming, bathing, or showering. Some pumps can be placed on the side of the tub, in a shower caddy, or in a soap tray. There are also special cases you can buy. You can hang these cases from your neck or from a shower curtain hook.

No matter what you may think, you can still have fun when you are using an insulin pump. When you exercise or play sports, you can wear a strong elastic waist band with a pump case. You can also wear it on an armband where it is visible. Women can tape the insulin pump to the front of their sports bra. Some coaches do not allow any devices to be worn because getting the pump knocked into you or falling on it can be painful. In this case, you may just need to take the insulin pump off.

When you disconnect your pump, you are stopping all delivery (basal and bolus) by the pump. Here are some important tips to remember when disconnecting your pump.

1. It is important for you to remember that if you stop your pump while it is in the middle of delivering any bolus—it will NOT be resumed. You may need to program a new one.

2. Be sure to bolus to cover the basal rate you will miss. If your blood glucose level is under 150, you can wait an hour to bolus.

3. Do not go longer than one to two hours without any insulin.

4. Monitor your blood glucose every three to four hours.

Now that you know how the insulin pump works and how to wear it, take a look at some of the facts to see if this is right for you.

Advantages Of Using An Insulin Pump

Some advantages of using an insulin pump instead of insulin injections are:

- Using an insulin pump means eliminating individual insulin injections.
- Insulin pumps deliver insulin more accurately than injections.
- Insulin pumps often improve A1C.
- Using an insulin pump usually results in fewer large swings in your blood glucose levels.
- Using an insulin pump makes diabetes management easier—if your glucose level is high or you feel like eating, figure out how much insulin you need and push the little button on the pump.
- Insulin pumps allow you to be flexible about when and what you eat.
- Using an insulin pump can improve your quality of life.
- Using an insulin pump reduces severe low blood glucose episodes.
- Using an insulin pump eliminates unpredictable effects of intermediate- or long-acting insulin.

• Insulin pumps allow you to exercise without having to eat large amounts of carbohydrate.

Disadvantages Of Using An Insulin Pump

Although there are many good reasons as to why using an insulin pump can be an advantage, there are some disadvantages.

The disadvantages of using a pump are that it:

• Can cause weight gain.

• Can cause diabetic ketoacidosis (DKA) if your catheter comes out and you don't get insulin for hours.

• Can be expensive.

• Can be bothersome since you are attached to the pump most of the time.

• Can require a hospital stay or maybe a full day in the outpatient center to be trained.

There are pluses and minuses to using a pump. Even though using an insulin pump has disadvantages, most pump users agree the advantages outweigh the disadvantages.

Getting Started With An Insulin Pump

Once you have talked with your diabetes care team and have become comfortable with all of the options on your insulin pump, you and your team will need to do the following in order to get you started.

1. Determine how much insulin to use in the insulin pump by averaging the total units of insulin you use per day for several days. (You may start with about 20% less if you are switching to rapid-acting insulin.)

2. Divide the total dosage into 40–50% for basal and 50–60% for bolus insulin.

3. Divide the basal portion by 24 to determine a beginning hourly basal rate.

4. Then, adjust the hourly basal rate up or down for patterns of highs and lows, such as more insulin for dawn phenomenon and less for daily activity.

5. Determine a beginning carbohydrate dose (insulin:carb ratio) using the 450 (or 500) rule. Divide by the total units of insulin/day to get the number of grams of carbohydrate covered by one unit of insulin. This dose may be raised or lowered based on your history and how much fast-acting insulin you took in the past.

Insulin Injections vs. Insulin Pump

Are you considering switching from insulin injections to insulin pump therapy? Stacy O'Donnell, RN, BS, CDE, and Andrea Penney, RN, CDE, at Joslin Diabetes Center, give the pros and cons of each method.

Insulin Injections

Pros

- Injections require less education and training than pump therapy. "Many people don't realize the amount of work involved with pumps," Penney says. "Using a pump requires professional training and close diabetes management."
- Injection therapy is cheaper than pump therapy.

Cons

- Low blood glucose levels can occur because you may be using different types of insulin.
- Frequent injections mean you may develop resistant areas of the body where insulin will not absorb properly.

Insulin Pump

Pros

- The pump delivers insulin continuously throughout the day, causing fewer sudden highs and lows in blood glucose levels.
- Insulin delivery is more accurate and precise.
- There will be less needle sticks. You may have one injection (hook up) every three days versus 15–18 injections in a three-day period with injection therapy, according to O'Donnell.
- Adjusting your own insulin allows a more flexible lifestyle.

Cons

- There is a greater risk of developing diabetic ketoacidosis (DKA), however, O'Donnell believes this can be prevented. "Patients are testing blood glucose levels frequently and are also well-educated on what to do if this occurs."
- It is attached to your body all day, reminding you and others that you have diabetes.
- Pump supplies are expensive.

6. Determine the dose of insulin to correct high blood glucose with the 1800 (or 1500) rule. Divide 1800 by the total units of insulin/day to see how much one unit of insulin lowers your blood glucose. This dose must be evaluated by your health care team. It is often too high for children or for people who have not had diabetes very long.

It may take several months to get comfortable with the pump. During those first months is the time to adopt some good habits. Here are some tips to help you adjust:

- Take your insulin at a specific time, such as five minutes before you eat, so you don't forget boluses.

- When traveling anywhere, bring extra supplies or at least an insulin pen, in case you are unable to use your pump for some reason.

- With an insulin pump, when you eat, what you eat, and how much you eat is up to you. You can eat more carbohydrate and still manage your blood glucose, but weight gain can happen. Talk to a dietitian about this when you start on the pump. It's a lot easier to not to gain weight, than it is to lose it after you have already gained it.

- When you take the insulin pump off or turn it off, figure out a system to remember to turn it back on. Listen to the alarms on the pump or set a timer.

- Make a habit of recording blood glucose checks, carbohydrate amounts, carbohydrate doses, correction doses, and exercise when you do them. It really helps to sit down and look over your blood glucose record at the end of every week (or even every day) to see if you have any problem areas. Reviewing your records is the key to improving blood glucose control.

- Your diabetes provider and insulin pump company have record forms, or you can make your own. Just be sure that you have enough room to record everything you need. Keeping daily records is best, but some people find keeping records for two weekdays and one weekend day gives enough information to see the patterns.

This is a lot of information. Fortunately, you don't need to be an expert on insulin pumps overnight. If you are uncertain about anything, you can go to your diabetes care team for help. Everyone learns at a different pace and it is okay if it takes you a while to get the hang of it. In addition, the American Diabetes Association also has resources to help you. [Contact and website information can be found in Chapter 52.]

Chapter 20

Managing Hypoglycemia

What is hypoglycemia?

Hypoglycemia, also called low blood glucose or low blood sugar, occurs when blood glucose drops below normal levels. Glucose, an important source of energy for the body, comes from food. Carbohydrates are the main dietary source of glucose. Rice, potatoes, bread, tortillas, cereal, milk, fruit, and sweets are all carbohydrate-rich foods.

After a meal, glucose is absorbed into the bloodstream and carried to the body's cells. Insulin, a hormone made by the pancreas, helps the cells use glucose for energy. If a person takes in more glucose than the body needs at the time, the body stores the extra glucose in the liver and muscles in a form called glycogen. The body can use glycogen for energy between meals. Extra glucose can also be changed to fat and stored in fat cells. Fat can also be used for energy.

When blood glucose begins to fall, glucagon—another hormone made by the pancreas—signals the liver to break down glycogen and release glucose into the bloodstream. Blood glucose will then rise toward a normal level. In some people with diabetes, this glucagon response to hypoglycemia is impaired and other hormones such as epinephrine, also called adrenaline, may raise the blood glucose level. But with diabetes treated with insulin or pills that increase insulin production, glucose levels can't easily return to the normal range.

Hypoglycemia can happen suddenly. It is usually mild and can be treated quickly and easily by eating or drinking a small amount of glucose-rich food. If left untreated, hypoglycemia can get worse and cause confusion, clumsiness, or fainting. Severe hypoglycemia can lead to seizures, coma, and even death.

About This Chapter: From "Hypoglycemia," National Institute of Diabetes and Digestive and Kidney Diseases (www.niddk.nih.gov), October 2008.

In adults and children older than ten years, hypoglycemia is uncommon except as a side effect of diabetes treatment. Hypoglycemia can also result, however, from other medications or diseases, hormone or enzyme deficiencies, or tumors.

What are the symptoms of hypoglycemia?

Hypoglycemia causes symptoms such as the following:

- Hunger
- Shakiness
- Nervousness
- Sweating
- Dizziness or light-headedness

- Sleepiness
- Confusion
- Difficulty speaking
- Anxiety
- Weakness

Hypoglycemia can also happen during sleep. Some signs of hypoglycemia during sleep include crying out or having nightmares, finding pajamas or sheets damp from perspiration, and feeling tired, irritable, or confused after waking up.

What causes hypoglycemia in people with diabetes?

Hypoglycemia can occur as a side effect of some diabetes medications, including insulin and oral diabetes medications—pills—that increase insulin production. Here are some examples of medications that may cause hypoglycemia:

- Chlorpropamide (Diabinese)
- Glimepiride (Amaryl)
- Glipizide (Glucotrol, Glucotrol XL)
- Glyburide (DiaBeta, Glynase, Micronase)

- Nateglinide (Starlix)
- Repaglinide (Prandin)
- Sitagliptin (Januvia)
- Tolazamide
- Tolbutamide

Certain combination pills can also cause hypoglycemia:

- Glipizide + metformin (Metaglip)
- Glyburide + metformin (Glucovance)
- Pioglitazone + glimepiride (Duetact)

- Rosiglitazone + glimepiride (Avandaryl)
- Sitagliptin + metformin (Janumet)

What's It Mean?

Hyper/hypoglycemia: Diabetes causes high blood sugar, also known as hyperglycemia (hi-per-gly-SEE-me-uh). Because we now know a lot about the disease, and since there are lots of different medicines to treat it, most people with diabetes can keep their blood sugar pretty well controlled. But, sometimes a diabetics' blood sugar gets too low—and that can be really scary, and sometimes it can be really serious.

Low blood sugar is called hypoglycemia (hi-poe-gly-SEE-me-uh). This can happen when someone with diabetes doesn't eat enough, takes too much medicine, or gets too much exercise. Symptoms of low blood sugar include sweating, shakiness, and confusion, and in extreme cases, a person can faint or have a seizure. A person with diabetes who has low blood sugar needs to eat sugar—and fast—to get it under control. In fact, many people with diabetes keep glucose pills with them in case they get low blood sugar. But, if you are around someone who has diabetes and starts to feel this way, you can also help him or her out by knowing what else he or she can eat. Good options include a couple of hard candies or gumdrops, orange juice, soda or pop (not diet!), a spoonful of honey, or some cake icing. Low blood sugar isn't an excuse to gorge on sweets, though—most people with diabetes only need a little sugar to get themselves back on track.

Source: From "Under the Microscope: Hyper/Hypo Glycemia," BAM! Body and Mind, Centers for Disease Control and Prevention, 2005. Reviewed by David A. Cooke, MD, FACP, August 2011.

Other types of diabetes pills, when taken alone, do not cause hypoglycemia. Examples of these medications are acarbose (Precose), metformin (Glucophage), miglitol (Glyset), pioglitazone (Actos), and rosiglitazone (Avandia). However, taking these pills along with other diabetes medications (insulin, pills that increase insulin production, or both) increases the risk of hypoglycemia.

In addition, use of the following injectable medications can cause hypoglycemia:

- Pramlintide (Symlin), which is used along with insulin
- Exenatide (Byetta), which can cause hypoglycemia when used in combination with chlorpropamide, glimepiride, glipizide, glyburide, tolazamide, and tolbutamide.

In people on insulin or pills that increase insulin production, low blood glucose can be due to meals or snacks that are too small, delayed, or skipped; increased physical activity; and alcoholic beverages.

How can hypoglycemia be prevented?

Diabetes treatment plans are designed to match the dose and timing of medication to a person's usual schedule of meals and activities. Mismatches could result in hypoglycemia. For example, taking a dose of insulin—or other medication that increases insulin levels—but then skipping a meal could result in hypoglycemia.

To help prevent hypoglycemia, people with diabetes should always consider the following:

- **Diabetes Medications:** A health care provider can explain which diabetes medications can cause hypoglycemia and explain how and when to take medications. For good diabetes management, people with diabetes should take diabetes medications in the recommended doses at the recommended times. In some cases, health care providers may suggest that patients learn how to adjust medications to match changes in their schedule or routine.

- **Meal Plan:** A registered dietitian can help design a meal plan that fits one's personal preferences and lifestyle. Following one's meal plan is important for managing diabetes. People with diabetes should eat regular meals, have enough food at each meal, and try not to skip meals or snacks. Snacks are particularly important for some people before going to sleep or exercising. Some snacks may be more effective than others in preventing hypoglycemia overnight. The dietitian can make recommendations for snacks.

- **Daily Activity:** To help prevent hypoglycemia caused by physical activity, health care providers may advise checking blood glucose before sports, exercise, or other physical activity and having a snack if the level is below 100 milligrams per deciliter (mg/dL); adjusting medication before physical activity; checking blood glucose at regular intervals during extended periods of physical activity and having snacks as needed; and checking blood glucose periodically after physical activity.

- **Alcoholic Beverages:** Although teens should not drink alcohol, it is important for them to know that drinking alcoholic beverages, especially on an empty stomach, can cause hypoglycemia, even a day or two later. Heavy drinking can be particularly dangerous for people taking insulin or medications that increase insulin production. Adults with diabetes who choose to drink should consume alcoholic beverages with a snack or meal at the same time.

- **Diabetes Management Plan:** Intensive diabetes management—keeping blood glucose as close to the normal range as possible to prevent long-term complications—can increase the risk of hypoglycemia. Those whose goal is tight control should talk with a health care provider about ways to prevent hypoglycemia and how best to treat it if it occurs.

People who take diabetes medications should ask their doctor or health care provider whether their diabetes medications could cause hypoglycemia, when they should take their diabetes medications, how much medication they should take, whether they should keep taking their diabetes medications when they are sick, whether they should adjust their medications before physical activity, and whether they should adjust their medications if they skip a meal.

How is hypoglycemia treated?

Signs and symptoms of hypoglycemia vary from person to person. People with diabetes should get to know their signs and symptoms and describe them to their friends and family so they can help if needed. School staff should be told how to recognize a child's signs and symptoms of hypoglycemia and how to treat it.

People who experience hypoglycemia several times in a week should call their health care provider. They may need a change in their treatment plan: less medication or a different medication, a new schedule for insulin or medication, a different meal plan, or a new physical activity plan.

When people think their blood glucose is too low, they should check the blood glucose level of a blood sample using a meter. If the level is below 70 mg/dL, one of these quick-fix foods should be consumed right away to raise blood glucose (recommended amounts may be less for small children):

- 3 or 4 glucose tablets
- 1 serving of glucose gel—the amount equal to 15 grams of carbohydrate
- 1/2 cup, or 4 ounces, of any fruit juice
- 1/2 cup, or 4 ounces, of a regular—not diet—soft drink
- 1 cup, or 8 ounces, of milk
- 5 or 6 pieces of hard candy
- 1 tablespoon of sugar or honey

Table 20.1. Normal And Target Blood Glucose Ranges

Normal Blood Glucose Levels in People Who Do Not Have Diabetes	
Upon waking—fasting	70 to 99 mg/dL
After meals	70 to 140 mg/dL
Target Blood Glucose Levels In People Who Have Diabetes	
Before meals	70 to 130 mg/dL
1 to 2 hours after the start of a meal	below 180 mg/dL

Source: American Diabetes Association. Standards of Medical Care in Diabetes—2008. *Diabetes Care.* 2008;31:S12–S54.

The next step is to recheck blood glucose in 15 minutes to make sure it is 70 mg/dL or above. If it's still too low, another serving of a quick-fix food should be eaten. These steps should be repeated until the blood glucose level is 70 mg/dL or above. If the next meal is an hour or more away, a snack should be eaten once the quick-fix foods have raised the blood glucose level to 70 mg/dL or above.

People who take either acarbose (Precose) or miglitol (Glyset) should know that only pure glucose, also called dextrose—available in tablet or gel form—will raise their blood glucose level during a low blood glucose episode. Other quick-fix foods and drinks won't raise the level quickly enough because acarbose and miglitol slow the digestion of other forms of carbohydrate.

What is hypoglycemia unawareness?

Some people with diabetes do not have early warning signs of low blood glucose, a condition called hypoglycemia unawareness. This condition occurs most often in people with type 1 diabetes, but it can also occur in people with type 2 diabetes. People with hypoglycemia unawareness may need to check their blood glucose level more often so they know when hypoglycemia is about to occur. They also may need a change in their medications, meal plan, or physical activity routine.

Hypoglycemia unawareness develops when frequent episodes of hypoglycemia lead to changes in how the body reacts to low blood glucose levels. The body stops releasing the hormone epinephrine and other stress hormones when blood glucose drops too low. The loss of the body's ability to release stress hormones after repeated episodes of hypoglycemia is called hypoglycemia-associated autonomic failure, or HAAF.

Epinephrine causes early warning symptoms of hypoglycemia such as shakiness, sweating, anxiety, and hunger. Without the release of epinephrine and the symptoms it causes, a person may not realize that hypoglycemia is occurring and may not take action to treat it. A vicious cycle can occur in which frequent hypoglycemia leads to hypoglycemia unawareness and HAAF, which in turn leads to even more severe and dangerous hypoglycemia. Studies have shown that preventing hypoglycemia for a period as short as several weeks can sometimes break this cycle and restore awareness of symptoms. Health care providers may therefore advise people who have had severe hypoglycemia to aim for higher-than-usual blood glucose targets for short-term periods.

How should people be prepared for hypoglycemia?

People who use insulin or take an oral diabetes medication that can cause low blood glucose should always be prepared to prevent and treat low blood glucose by taking these steps:

Hypoglycemia-Related Concerns

Severe Hypoglycemia: Severe hypoglycemia—very low blood glucose—can cause a person to pass out and can even be life threatening. Severe hypoglycemia is more likely to occur in people with type 1 diabetes. People should ask a health care provider what to do about severe hypoglycemia. Another person can help someone who has passed out by giving an injection of glucagon. Glucagon will rapidly bring the blood glucose level back to normal and help the person regain consciousness. A health care provider can prescribe a glucagon emergency kit. Family, friends, or coworkers—the people who will be around the person at risk of hypoglycemia—can learn how to give a glucagon injection and when to call 911 or get medical help.

Physical Activity: Physical activity has many benefits for people with diabetes, including lowering blood glucose levels. However, physical activity can make levels too low and can cause hypoglycemia up to 24 hours afterward. A health care provider can advise about checking the blood glucose level before exercise. For those who take insulin or one of the oral medications that increase insulin production, the health care provider may suggest having a snack if the glucose level is below 100 mg/dL or adjusting medication doses before physical activity to help avoid hypoglycemia. A snack can prevent hypoglycemia. The health care provider may suggest extra blood glucose checks, especially after strenuous exercise.

Hypoglycemia When Driving: Hypoglycemia is particularly dangerous if it happens to someone who is driving. People with hypoglycemia may have trouble concentrating or seeing clearly behind the wheel and may not be able to react quickly to road hazards or to the actions of other drivers. To prevent problems, people at risk for hypoglycemia should check their blood glucose level before driving. During longer trips, they should check their blood glucose level frequently and eat snacks as needed to keep the level at 70 mg/dL or above. If necessary, they should stop for treatment and then make sure their blood glucose level is 70 mg/dL or above before starting to drive again.

Source: National Institute of Diabetes and Digestive and Kidney Diseases (www.niddk.nih.gov), October 2008.

- Learning what can trigger low blood glucose levels

- Having their blood glucose meter available to test glucose levels; frequent testing may be critical for those with hypoglycemia unawareness, particularly before driving a car or engaging in any hazardous activity

- Always having several servings of quick-fix foods or drinks handy

- Wearing a medical identification bracelet or necklace

- Planning what to do if they develop severe hypoglycemia

- Telling their family, friends, and co-workers about the symptoms of hypoglycemia and how they can help if needed

For people with diabetes, a blood glucose level below 70 mg/dL is considered hypoglycemia.

Can hypoglycemia occur in people who do not have diabetes?

Two types of hypoglycemia can occur in people who do not have diabetes:

- Reactive hypoglycemia, also called postprandial hypoglycemia, occurs within four hours after meals.

- Fasting hypoglycemia, also called postabsorptive hypoglycemia, is often related to an underlying disease.

Symptoms of both reactive and fasting hypoglycemia are similar to diabetes-related hypoglycemia. Symptoms may include hunger, sweating, shakiness, dizziness, light-headedness, sleepiness, confusion, difficulty speaking, anxiety, and weakness.

To find the cause of a patient's hypoglycemia, the doctor will use laboratory tests to measure blood glucose, insulin, and other chemicals that play a part in the body's use of energy.

Reactive Hypoglycemia: To diagnose reactive hypoglycemia, the doctor may ask about signs and symptoms, test blood glucose while the patient is having symptoms by taking a blood sample from the arm (a personal blood glucose monitor cannot be used to diagnose reactive hypoglycemia) and sending it to a laboratory for analysis, and check to see whether the symptoms ease after the patient's blood glucose returns to 70 mg/dL or above after eating or drinking.

A blood glucose level below 70 mg/dL at the time of symptoms and relief after eating will confirm the diagnosis. The oral glucose tolerance test is no longer used to diagnose reactive hypoglycemia because experts now know the test can actually trigger hypoglycemic symptoms.

The causes of most cases of reactive hypoglycemia are still open to debate. Some researchers suggest that certain people may be more sensitive to the body's normal release of the hormone epinephrine, which causes many of the symptoms of hypoglycemia. Others believe deficiencies in glucagon secretion might lead to reactive hypoglycemia.

A few causes of reactive hypoglycemia are certain, but they are uncommon. Gastric—or stomach—surgery can cause reactive hypoglycemia because of the rapid passage of food into the small intestine. Rare enzyme deficiencies diagnosed early in life, such as hereditary fructose intolerance, also may cause reactive hypoglycemia.

To relieve reactive hypoglycemia, some health professionals recommend eating small meals and snacks about every three hours, being physically active, and eating a variety of foods, including meat, poultry, fish, or nonmeat sources of protein; starchy foods such as whole-grain bread, rice, and potatoes; fruits; vegetables; and dairy products, as well as eating foods high in fiber and avoiding or limiting foods high in sugar, especially on an empty stomach.

The doctor can refer patients to a registered dietitian for personalized meal planning advice. Although some health professionals recommend a diet high in protein and low in carbohydrates, studies have not proven the effectiveness of this kind of diet to treat reactive hypoglycemia.

Fasting Hypoglycemia: Fasting hypoglycemia is diagnosed from a blood sample that shows a blood glucose level below 50 mg/dL after an overnight fast, between meals, or after physical activity.

Causes of fasting hypoglycemia include certain medications, alcoholic beverages, critical illnesses, hormonal deficiencies, some kinds of tumors, and certain conditions occurring in infancy and childhood.

Medications, including some used to treat diabetes, are the most common cause of hypoglycemia. Other medications that can cause hypoglycemia include salicylates, including aspirin, when taken in large doses; sulfa medications, which are used to treat bacterial infections; pentamidine, which treats a serious kind of pneumonia; and quinine, which is used to treat malaria. If using any of these medications causes a person's blood glucose level to fall, the doctor may advise stopping the medication or changing the dose.

Drinking alcoholic beverages, especially binge drinking, can cause hypoglycemia. The body's breakdown of alcohol interferes with the liver's efforts to raise blood glucose. Hypoglycemia caused by excessive drinking can be serious and even fatal.

Some illnesses that affect the liver, heart, or kidneys can cause hypoglycemia. Sepsis, which is an overwhelming infection, and starvation are other causes of hypoglycemia. In these cases, treating the illness or other underlying cause will correct the hypoglycemia.

Hormonal deficiencies may cause hypoglycemia in very young children, but rarely in adults. Shortages of cortisol, growth hormone, glucagon, or epinephrine can lead to fasting hypoglycemia. Laboratory tests for hormone levels will determine a diagnosis and treatment. Hormone replacement therapy may be advised.

Insulinomas are insulin-producing tumors in the pancreas. Insulinomas can cause hypoglycemia by raising insulin levels too high in relation to the blood glucose level. These tumors are rare and do not normally spread to other parts of the body. Laboratory tests can pinpoint the exact cause. Treatment involves both short-term steps to correct the hypoglycemia and medical or surgical measures to remove the tumor.

Children rarely develop hypoglycemia. If they do, causes may include the following:

- Brief intolerance to fasting, often during an illness that disturbs regular eating patterns. Children usually outgrow this tendency by age 10.

- Hyperinsulinism, which is the overproduction of insulin. This condition can result in temporary hypoglycemia in newborns, which is common in infants of mothers with diabetes. Persistent hyperinsulinism in infants or children is a complex disorder that requires prompt evaluation and treatment by a specialist.

- Enzyme deficiencies that affect carbohydrate metabolism. These deficiencies can interfere with the body's ability to process natural sugars, such as fructose and galactose, glycogen, or other metabolites.

- Hormonal deficiencies such as lack of pituitary or adrenal hormones.

Points To Remember

- When people with diabetes think their blood glucose level is low, they should check it and treat the problem right away.
- To treat hypoglycemia, people should have a serving of a quick-fix food, wait 15 minutes, and check their blood glucose again. They should repeat the treatment until their blood glucose is 70 mg/dL or above.
- People at risk for hypoglycemia should keep quick-fix foods in the car, at work—anywhere they spend time.
- People at risk for hypoglycemia should be careful when driving. They should check their blood glucose frequently and snack as needed to keep their level 70 mg/dL or above.

Source: National Institute of Diabetes and Digestive and Kidney Diseases (www.niddk.nih.gov), October 2008.

Chapter 21

Managing Hyperglycemia

What is high blood glucose?

People who do not have diabetes typically have fasting plasma blood glucose levels that run under 126 mg/dl.

Your physician will define for you what your target blood glucose should be—identifying a blood glucose target that is as close to normal as possible that you can safely achieve given your overall medical health. In general, high blood glucose, also called 'hyperglycemia', is considered "high" when it is 160 mg/dl or above your individual blood glucose target. Be sure to ask your healthcare provider what he or she thinks is a safe target for you for blood glucose before and after meals.

If your blood glucose runs high for long periods of time, this can pose significant problems for you long-term—increased risk of complications, such as eye disease, kidney disease, heart attacks, and strokes and more. High blood glucose can pose health problems in the short-term as well. Your treatment plan may need adjustment if the blood glucose stays over 180 mg/dl for three days in a row. It is important to aim to keep your blood glucose under control, and treat hyperglycemia when it occurs.

What are the symptoms of high blood glucose?

- Increased thirst
- Increased urination
- Dry mouth or skin

- Tiredness or fatigue

- Blurred vision

- More frequent infections

- Slow healing cuts and sores

- Unexplained weight loss

What causes high blood glucose?

- Too much food

- Too little exercise or physical activity

- Skipped or not enough diabetes pills or insulin

- Insulin that has spoiled after being exposed to extreme heat or freezing cold

- Stress, illness, infection, injury or surgery

- A blood glucose meter that is not reading accurately

What should you do for high blood glucose?

- Be sure to drink plenty of water. It is recommended to drink a minimum of eight glasses each day.

- If your blood glucose is 250 or greater and you are on insulin, check your urine for ketones. If you have ketones, follow your sick day rules or call your healthcare team if you are not sure what to do.

- Ask yourself what may have caused the high blood sugar, and take action to correct it. Ask your healthcare team if you are not sure what to do.

- Try to determine if there is a pattern to your blood glucose levels. Check your blood glucose before meals three days in a row. If greater than your target level for three days, a change in medication may be needed. Call your healthcare team or adjust your insulin dose following well day rules. Call your healthcare team if you are currently using diabetes pills.

Determine why your blood glucose is high.

Ask yourself the questions outlined below. The answers will give you the information you need to determine what to do about the hyperglycemia.

Cause: Food

- Have you increased your portion sizes?
- Have you changed your eating habits or food choices?
- Have you eaten too many high-fat foods?

If your answers to the questions are yes, follow these suggestions: You may need to measure food more accurately to check portion control. If you think your eating pattern is changing, your medication or exercise plan may need to change.

Cause: Activity

- Have you decreased or eliminated your usual activity?
- Are you doing too little physical activity?

If your answers to the questions are yes, follow these suggestions: Physical activity is a key to blood glucose control. Ask your healthcare team about starting a program.

Cause: Medication

- Have you been taking the prescribed doses?
- Have you been taking the medication at the right time?

If your answers to the questions are yes, follow these suggestions: Take the right dose at the right time. If you have any questions ask a diabetes educator.

- Do you have "spoiled" insulin?

If your answer is yes, throw away the bottle and open a new bottle.

- Does your insulin look different?
- Was your insulin exposed to very hot or cold temperatures?
- Has your insulin expired?

If your answers to the questions are yes, follow this suggestion: Check the expiration date on bottle.

Cause: Monitoring

- Is the drop of blood too small?
- Are you using the correct technique?

- Could your meter be dirty?

If your answers to the questions are yes, follow these suggestions: See a nurse educator to be sure your technique is correct and your meter is functioning the right way. Learn how to clean the meter.

- Have your strips expired?
- Have your strips been exposed to very hot or cold temperatures or not been kept in an airtight, dry, container?
- Is your meter calibrated to the current bottle of strips?

If your answers to the questions are yes, follow these suggestions: Throw away the strips and get a new bottle. Check the code on the strip bottle.

Cause: Illness, Infection, Injury And Surgery

- Are you feeling well?
- Do you have any infections?

If your answers to the questions are yes, follow these suggestions: Follow sick day rules. Contact your healthcare team for questions or help.

Chapter 22

Diabetic Ketoacidosis

Ketoacidosis (key-toe-ass-i-DOE-sis) is a serious condition that can lead to diabetic coma (passing out for a long time) or even death. When your cells don't get the glucose they need for energy, your body begins to burn fat for energy, which produces ketones. Ketones are acids that build up in the blood and appear in the urine when your body doesn't have enough insulin. They are a warning sign that your diabetes is out of control or that you are getting sick. High levels of ketones can poison the body. When levels get too high, you can develop diabetic ketoacidosis, or DKA.

Ketoacidosis may happen to anyone with diabetes, though it is rare in people with type 2. Some older people with type 2 diabetes may experience a different serious condition called hyperosmolar nonketotic coma (hi-per-oz-MOE-lar non-key-TOT-ick KO-ma) in which the body tries to get rid of excess sugar by passing it into the urine.

Treatment for ketoacidosis usually takes place in the hospital. But you can help prevent ketoacidosis by learning the warning signs and checking your urine and blood regularly.

What are the warning signs of ketoacidosis?

Ketoacidosis usually develops slowly. But when vomiting occurs, this life-threatening condition can develop in a few hours. Early symptoms include the following:

- Thirst or a very dry mouth
- Frequent urination

- High blood glucose (sugar) levels

- High levels of ketones in the urine

Then, other symptoms appear:

- Constantly feeling tired

- Dry or flushed skin

- Nausea, vomiting, or abdominal pain (Vomiting can be caused by many illnesses, not just ketoacidosis. If vomiting continues for more than two hours, contact your health care provider.)

- A hard time breathing (short, deep breaths)

- Fruity odor on breath

- A hard time paying attention, or confusion

Ketoacidosis is dangerous and serious. If you have any of the above symptoms, contact your health care provider IMMEDIATELY, or go to the nearest emergency room of your local hospital.

How do I check for ketones?

You can detect ketones with a simple urine test using a test strip, similar to a blood testing strip. Ask your health care provider when and how you should test for ketones. Many experts advise to check your urine for ketones when your blood glucose is more than 240 mg/dl.

When you are ill (when you have a cold or the flu, for example), check for ketones every four to six hours. And check every four to six hours when your blood glucose is more than 240 mg/dl.

Also, check for ketones when you have any symptoms of ketoacidosis.

Remember
- Ketones are produced when your body starts burning fat for energy instead of glucose.
- Dangerously high levels of ketones can lead to diabetic coma or death.
- Know the warning signs and check urine for ketones, especially when sick.

What if I find higher-than-normal levels of ketones?

If your health care provider has not told you what levels of ketones are dangerous, then call when you find moderate amounts after more than one test. Often, your health care provider can tell you what to do over the phone.

Call your health care provider at once if you experience the following conditions:

- Your urine tests show high levels of ketones.

- Your urine tests show high levels of ketones and your blood glucose level is high.

- Your urine tests show high levels of ketones and you have vomited more than twice in four hours.

Do NOT exercise when your urine tests show ketones and your blood glucose is high. High levels of ketones and high blood glucose levels can mean your diabetes is out of control. Check with your health care provider about how to handle this situation.

What causes ketoacidosis?

Here are three basic reasons for moderate or large amounts of ketones:

- **Not Enough Insulin:** Maybe you did not inject enough insulin. Or your body could need more insulin than usual because of illness.

- **Not Enough Food:** When you're sick, you often don't feel like eating, sometimes resulting in high ketone levels. High levels may also occur when you miss a meal.

- **Insulin Reaction (Low Blood Glucose):** If testing shows high ketone levels in the morning, you may have had an insulin reaction while asleep.

Part Three
Nutrition, Physical Activity, And Weight Management

Chapter 23

The Truth About The Diabetes Diet

The So-Called "Diabetes Diet"

Despite all the publicity surrounding new research and new nutrition guidelines, some people with diabetes still believe that there is something called a "diabetic diet." For some, this so-called diet consists of avoiding sugar, while others believe it to be a strict way of eating that controls glucose. Unfortunately, neither are quite right.

The "diabetes diet" is not something that people with type 1 or type 2 diabetes should be following. "That just simply isn't how meal planning works today for patients with diabetes," says Amy Campbell, MS, RD, LDN, CDE, a nutritionist at Joslin and co-author of *16 Myths of a Diabetic Diet*.

"The important message is that with proper education and within the context of healthy eating, a person with diabetes can eat anything a person without diabetes eats," Campbell states.

What's The Truth About Diabetes And Diet?

We know now that it is okay for people with diabetes to substitute sugar-containing food for other carbohydrates as part of a balanced meal plan. Prevailing beliefs up to the mid-1990s were that people with diabetes should avoid foods that contain so-called "simple" sugars and replace them with "complex" carbohydrates, such as those found in potatoes and cereals. A

About This Chapter: This chapter includes "The Truth About the So-Called 'Diabetes Diet,'" "The Best Kinds of Low-Carb Snacks," "Healthy Alternatives to Your Favorite Foods," "Tips on Vegetarian Eating and Diabetes," and "Dining Out with Diabetes," all Copyright 2011 by Joslin Diabetes Center. All rights reserved. Excerpted with permission from Joslin Diabetes Center's website (www.joslin.org). Please refer to the website for updates to this information.

review of the research at that time revealed that there was relatively little scientific evidence to support the theory that simple sugars are more rapidly digested and absorbed than starches, and therefore more apt to produce high blood glucose levels.

Now many patients are being taught to focus on how many total grams of carbohydrate they can eat throughout the day at each meal and snack, and still keep their blood glucose under good control. Well-controlled blood glucose is a top priority because other research studies have concluded that all people with diabetes can cut their risk of developing diabetes complications such as heart disease, stroke, kidney and eye disease, nerve damage, and more, by keeping their blood glucose as closely controlled as possible.

What Does This Mean For People With Diabetes?

This means that a person who has worked with a dietitian and a diabetes treatment team to figure out how many grams of carbohydrate they can eat throughout the day can decide at any given meal what they will eat. Those with diabetes who are not on insulin need to focus on keeping the amount of carbohydrate they eat consistent throughout the day. Those on insulin can decide both what and how much to eat at a given meal (as long as it doesn't exceed their daily allotment), and can then adjust their insulin accordingly. "There aren't any foods that are 'off-limits,'" says Campbell. "Rather, one just needs to learn how to spend his or her grams of carbohydrate wisely over the course of the day."

Frequent home blood glucose monitoring is then used to keep track of the effects of meals and activity levels on their blood glucose. They work with their healthcare team to make adjustments in their food intake, physical activity, and medication to keep their blood glucose as close to normal as possible.

How Does Carbohydrate Counting Work?

Most foods—except meat and fat—contain some carbohydrate, and carbohydrate increases blood glucose faster than any other food. The number of grams of carbohydrate that a person can eat each day or at each meal is determined by:

- Weight and weight loss goals
- How physically active an individual is (because physical activity will lower their blood glucose)
- What diabetes medication or insulin they are taking, and when
- Other factors such as age or the presence of high blood fats (or any other medical issue, for that matter)

For example, a 6'2" tall man with diabetes who weighs 180 pounds and wants to maintain his current weight might be told he could eat 350 grams of carbohydrate spread out over the day. His goal would be to spread those grams out over the course of the day so that he doesn't send his blood glucose too high at any one time. If he is taking insulin or oral diabetes medication, he might also have to manage when he eats his carbohydrate in such a way that there is enough sugar from his meals in his bloodstream when his medication is working its hardest.

"We now know that in general, a sugar-containing food like a brownie may have 30 grams of carbohydrate in it, but that brownie will have the same effect on your blood glucose as 2/3 cup of rice or one cup of applesauce, both of which have 30 grams of carbohydrate in them," says Campbell. "So, if this man's meal plan developed with a dietitian states that he can eat 60 grams of carbohydrate at a meal, he can decide how he 'spends' those 60 grams. One time he may have 2/3 cup of rice and one cup of peas. Another time he may decide, for his carb choices, to eat a small baked potato, a cup of milk, and have the brownie for dessert."

People who develop diabetes when they are over 40 frequently develop diabetes in part because they are overweight. Being overweight makes it more difficult for their bodies to use insulin to convert food into energy. For this reason, many patients with diabetes also have weight loss as a goal. Because each gram of fat contains nine calories (while a gram of protein or carbohydrate contains only four calories), fat gram counting as a means of losing weight becomes an additional nutritional tool for many patients.

Frequently people with diabetes also have problems with high blood fats and/or cholesterol levels, and will be prescribed a meal plan that is low in fat as well. So even if they aren't overweight, some patients may be counting grams of fat eaten at each meal or over the course of the day, as well as how many grams of carbohydrate.

There are many food lists available that show how many grams of carbohydrate and fat are in most foods. Also, most any food you purchase in a grocery story lists carbohydrate and fat content as part of the food label requirements mandated by the federal government.

Not A Do-It-Yourself Project

"Obviously using nutrition as part of an overall diabetes treatment plan is not an entirely do-it-yourself project," notes Campbell. It's best, she states, if you work with a dietitian to determine which type of meal planning approach will work best for you.

"But then the rest of it is pretty much up to you," she adds. "You get your meal plan 'budget,' and then you decide how to spend it at each meal. And just like people without diabetes, you need to eat a variety of foods in order to be healthy.

The Best Kinds Of Low-Carb Snacks

Low/no-carb snacks can be an excellent choice for people with diabetes to satisfy cravings between meals, while still keeping blood glucose levels under control, according to Elizabeth Staum, MS, RD, LDN, Nutrition Educator at Joslin Diabetes Center.

Tips On Vegetarian Eating And Diabetes

What is a vegetarian?

A vegetarian is someone who does not eat meat, fish, or poultry or any product that contains these foods. They eat whole grains, legumes (pulses), nuts, seeds, vegetables and fruits with or without the use of dairy products and eggs. There are actually different types of vegetarians:

- **Semi-Vegetarian:** Does not eat red meats, but occasionally eats fish or poultry and dairy products. Semi-vegetarians are often people who are making a change to a vegetarian diet.
- **Lacto-Ovo Vegetarian:** Eats milk, dairy products, and eggs but not meat, fish, or poultry.
- **Lacto-Vegetarian:** Eats milk and other dairy products but not meat, fish, poultry, or eggs.
- **Pescetarian:** Eats a diet of fruits, vegetables, grains, legumes and includes fish. They may or may not eat eggs and dairy products.
- **Vegan:** Does not eat any animal products (meat, fish, poultry, eggs or dairy foods). A vegan eats only plant-based foods.

What are the health benefits of a vegetarian diet?

There are many reasons why people choose to follow a vegetarian diet, including financial reasons, ethical concerns, and religious beliefs. Some people choose to become vegetarian for health reasons, as well. A vegetarian diet may help reduce the risk of heart disease, high blood pressure, obesity, kidney disease, and cancer.

Can people with diabetes follow a vegetarian diet?

Yes. Vegetarian diet tends to be higher in carbohydrate and lower in protein than meat-based diets, so blood glucose levels may be affected. As a result, your healthcare provider may need to change the amount or type of your diabetes medication. Anyone interested in becoming a vegetarian, including people with diabetes, should work with a dietitian to make sure their nutritional needs are met.

Source: "Tips on Vegetarian Eating and Diabetes," Copyright 2011 by Joslin Diabetes Center. All rights reserved. Excerpted with permission from Joslin Diabetes Center's website (www.joslin.org). Please refer to the website for updates to this information.

Diabetes Snacking Habits

Your snacking habits with diabetes should depend on the type of diabetes medication you're taking and your diabetes meal plan. If you take oral diabetes medications, you may want to eat smaller meals and have more substantial snacks with protein, to keep you from getting hungry and overeating.

If you take insulin, Staum says it's better to eat the majority of your carbs at mealtimes, when you still have insulin coverage. Depending on your need for insulin, your snack should usually have 15 grams of carbs or less.

Snacks are beneficial for people with diabetes whose blood glucose tends to drop at a certain time of day even after adjusting their insulin regimen, Staum says. People with diabetes also benefit from carb-containing snacks pre- and post-exercise, when blood glucose can drop as well.

Key Ingredients In A Good Diabetes Snack

People with diabetes should choose snacks that are full of healthful nutrients such as protein, fiber, and vitamins and minerals. Snacks rich in protein and fiber make your snack more satisfying, Staum says. Snack ideas that contain protein can include choices such as:

- Natural peanut butter
- Low fat cheese or cottage cheese
- Unsalted nuts
- Egg
- Yogurt
- Milk

To get more fiber, and vitamins and minerals, try eating vegetables, fruits, or whole grain crackers or bread. Snacks for people with diabetes should also be heart-healthy, meaning low in sodium (140 mg per serving or less), low in saturated fat, and no trans fat.

Review your diabetes goals with your health care team to see how snacking can be incorporated into your diabetes meal plan.

Healthy Alternatives To Your Favorite Foods

Craving fast food? Have a sweet tooth? We talked to Elizabeth Staum, M.S., R.D., L.D.N., Nutrition Educator at Joslin Diabetes Center, to find healthy alternatives to your favorite foods. As always, it's important to keep in mind portion sizes of these healthier alternatives, and make sure that the calories per serving fit with the meal plan you're following.

Dining Out With Diabetes

In the real world, people with diabetes aren't going to be eating at home and preparing their own meals everyday. Dining out at restaurants is part of American culture. By planning ahead and ordering wisely, you can have an enjoyable dining experience with diabetes.

Planning Ahead

- Choose a restaurant with a large menu of healthy items. Many chains have nutritional information available online.
- Call restaurant ahead of time and ask if they can handle special requests.
- Ask your dinner companions to eat at the time you normally eat, but don't worry if you have to eat earlier or later.
- Have a small snack before going to a restaurant, so you aren't too hungry.

Tips On Ordering Meals With Diabetes

- If you are not sure how a food is prepared, ask your server.
- Watch your portion sizes. Order an appetizer for a main course, split an entrée, or eat half and take the rest home.
- Ask for substitutions. For example, get vegetables instead of french fries.
- Avoid breaded or fried foods, or foods in heavy sauces. Try fish or poultry that is grilled or boiled, without butter.
- Ask for salad dressing and sauces on the side.
- [Teens should not drink alcohol , and adults who do should] limit alcohol to one serving.
- Be careful of all-you-can-eat restaurants. If you do eat at a buffet, try to fill up on vegetable dishes.

"Choose foods that you really like," advises Nora Saul, M.S, R.D., L.D.N., C.D.E, Joslin Clinic. "Decide if it is really good and worth it, and if it is, make accommodations. If a place has very good bread, maybe have a roll, but skip the potato. If you like sweets, share a dessert with a few other people, and take a walk afterwards. Remember, dining out is also a social experience—concentrate on sharing time with family and friends."

When you want something sweet...

Instead of cake, cookies, or ice cream, try:

- Sugar-free Jell-O or hard candies (but always read the Nutrition Label on every food for serving size information)
- Sugar-free hot cocoa
- Fruit with cool whip
- Lower fat cookies like ginger snaps, vanilla wafers, graham crackers, animal crackers (again, observe serving size)
- No sugar added pudding or fudgsicles
- Eating very small portions of your favorite treat

When you want something salty and crunchy...

Instead of potato chips or tortilla chips, try:

- Low-sodium pretzels
- Air-popped popcorn
- Baked chips or baked tortilla chips
- Cut raw veggies with low fat dip, salsa, or low fat cream cheese
- Pickles

When you want something to drink...

Instead of soda or fruit punch, try:

- Diet soda
- Crystal light or other sugar-free beverages
- Seltzer with just an ounce or two of fruit juice
- Water with lemon juice

When you want fast food...

Instead of hamburgers or hotdogs, try:

- Grilled or broiled chicken sandwiches
- One slice of thin crust veggie pizza
- Low fat sub sandwiches

When you want "comfort food"...

Instead of high-fat, high-carb choices, try:

- Macaroni and cheese cooked with fat-free evaporated milk, low fat cheese, and egg substitute

- Mashed potatoes made with trans-fat free margarine and fat-free milk, or replace part of the potato with pureed cauliflower

- Meatloaf made with ground turkey and egg substitute

- Beef stew made with round cut beef, fewer potatoes, and more non-starchy vegetables like carrots, onions, green beans, and spinach

Chapter 24

Making Healthy Food Choices

Eating healthfully means getting the right balance of nutrients your body needs to perform every day. You can find out more about your nutritional needs by checking out the *Dietary Guidelines for Americans*. Published by the U.S. government, this publication explains how much of each type of food you should eat, along with great information on nutrition and physical activity. The guidelines suggest the number of calories you should eat daily based on your gender, age, and activity level. [Visit ChooseMyPlate.gov for the most recent recommendations and updated information about serving sizes and equivalents.]

According to the guidelines, a healthy eating plan includes the following components:

- Fruits and vegetables
- Fat-free or low-fat milk and milk products
- Lean meats, poultry, fish, beans, eggs, and nuts
- Whole grains

In addition, a healthy diet is low in saturated and trans fats, cholesterol, salt, and added sugars.

Fruits And Vegetables

Eat fruits and vegetables every day. When consumed as part of a well-balanced and nutritious eating plan, fruits and vegetables can help keep you healthy.

You may get your servings from fresh, frozen, dried, and canned fruits and vegetables. Teenagers who are consuming 2,000 calories per day should aim for two cups of fruit and two

About This Chapter: This chapter includes excerpts from "Take Charge of Your Health," Weight-Control Information Network (www.win.niddk.gov), August 2009.

and a half cups of vegetables every day. You may need fewer or more servings depending on your individual calorie needs, which your health care provider can help you determine.

Count Your Calcium

Calcium helps strengthen bones and teeth. This nutrient is very important, since getting enough calcium now can reduce the risk for broken bones later in life. Yet most teens get less than the recommended 1,200 mg of calcium per day. Aim for at least 3 one-cup equivalents of low-fat or fat-free calcium-rich foods and beverages each day.

Power Up With Protein

Protein builds and repairs body tissue like muscles and organs. Eating enough protein can help you grow strong and sustain your energy levels. Teens need 5½ one-ounce equivalents of protein-rich foods each day.

Go Whole Grain

Grain foods help give you energy. Whole-grain foods like whole-wheat bread, brown rice, and oatmeal usually have more nutrients than refined grain products. They give you a feeling of fullness and add bulk to your diet.

Try to get 6 one-ounce equivalents of grains every day, with at least 3 one-ounce equivalents coming from whole-grain sources.

Know Your Fats

Fat is also an important nutrient. It helps your body grow and develop, and it is a source of energy as well—it even keeps your skin and hair healthy. But be aware that some fats are better for you than others. Limit your fat intake to 25 to 35 percent of your total calories each day.

Unsaturated fat can be part of a healthy diet—as long as you do not eat too much since it is still high in calories. Good sources include the following choices:

- Olive, canola, safflower, sunflower, corn, and soybean oils
- Fish like salmon, trout, tuna, and whitefish
- Nuts like walnuts, almonds, peanuts, and cashews

Limit saturated fat, which can clog your arteries and raise your risk for heart disease. Saturated fat is found primarily in animal products and in a few plant oils like butter, full-fat cheese, whole milk, fatty meats, and coconut, palm, and palm kernel oils.

Limit trans fat, which is also bad for your heart. Trans fat is often found in baked goods like cookies, muffins, and doughnuts or snack foods like crackers and chips. It is also often found in vegetable shortening, stick margarine, and fried foods.

Look for words like "shortening," "partially hydrogenated vegetable oil," or "hydrogenated vegetable oil" in the list of ingredients. These ingredients tell you that the food contains trans fat. Packaged food products are required to list trans fat on their Nutrition Facts label.

Replenish Your Body With Iron

Teen boys need iron to support their rapid growth—most boys double their lean body mass between the ages of 10 and 17. Teen girls also need iron to support growth and replace blood lost during menstruation.

To get the iron you need, try eating these foods:

- Fish and shellfish
- Lean beef
- Iron-fortified cereals
- Enriched and whole-grain breads
- Cooked dried beans and peas like black beans, kidney beans, black-eyed peas, and chick-peas/garbanzo beans
- Spinach

Control Your Food Portions

The portion sizes that you get away from home at a restaurant, grocery store, or school event may contain more food than you need to eat in one sitting. Research shows that when people are served more food, they eat more food. So, how can you control your food portions? Try these tips:

- When eating out, share your meal, order a half-portion, or order an appetizer as a main meal. Be aware that some appetizers are larger than others and can have as many calories as an entree.
- Take at least half of your meal home.
- When eating at home, take one serving out of a package (read the Nutrition Facts to find out how big a serving is) and eat it off a plate instead of eating straight out of a box or bag.

Try These Healthy Eating Tips

- Take your time when you eat. It takes about 15 minutes for your stomach to tell your brain that you are full. So, wait 15 minutes before eating second helpings.
- Do not skip meals. Eat breakfast, lunch, and dinner, plus a snack. You will have a ready supply of energy and not get too hungry.
- For breakfast, try one or two slices of whole grain toast with a tablespoon of peanut butter, a hard-boiled egg, or a piece of low-fat cheese, along with a glass of low-fat or nonfat milk.
- Make a sandwich with turkey or lean beef for lunch. Use mustard or a little low-fat mayonnaise.
- Snack on a small bowl of whole-grain cereal with low-fat or nonfat milk and a piece of fruit.
- Don't "super-size" it! Order smaller, kid-sized meals and drink water or low-fat or nonfat milk. Share a larger meal with a friend.
- Fill up half of your plate with salad or vegetables. Use small amounts of low-fat salad dressing, mayonnaise, or margarine.

Source: Excerpted from "Tips for Teens: Lower Your Risk for Type 2 Diabetes," National Diabetes Education Program, November 1, 2007.

- Avoid eating in front of the TV or while you are busy with other activities. It is easy to lose track of how much you are eating if you eat while doing other things.

- Eat slowly so your brain can get the message that your stomach is full.

- Do not skip meals. Skipping meals may lead you to eat more high-calorie, high-fat foods at your next meal or snack. Eat breakfast every day.

Read Food Labels

When you read a food label, pay special attention to these items:

- **Serving Size:** Check the amount of food in a serving. Do you eat more or less? The "servings per container" line tells you the number of servings in the food package.

- **Calories And Other Nutrients:** Remember, the number of calories and other listed nutrients are for one serving only. Food packages often contain more than one serving.

- **Percent Daily Value:** Look at how much of the recommended daily amount of a nutrient (% DV) is in one serving of food—5% DV or less is low and 20% DV or more is high. For example, if your breakfast cereal has 25% DV for iron, it is high in iron.

Nutrition Facts

Serving Size 1 cup (228g)
Servings Per Container 2

Amount Per Serving

Calories 250	Calories from Fat 110

	% Daily Value*
Total Fat 12g	18%
Saturated Fat 3g	15%
Trans Fat 1.5g	
Cholesterol 30mg	10%
Sodium 470mg	20%
Total Carbohydrate 31g	10%
Dietary Fiber 0g	0%
Sugars 5g	
Protein 5g	

Vitamin A	4%
Vitamin C	2%
Calcium	20%
Iron	4%

* Percent Daily Values are based on a 2,000 calorie diet. Your Daily Values may be higher or lower depending on your calorie needs:

	Calories:	2,000	2,500
Total Fat	Less than	65g	80g
Sat Fat	Less than	20g	25g
Cholesterol	Less than	300mg	300mg
Sodium	Less than	2,400mg	2,400mg
Total Carbohydrate		300g	375g
Dietary Fiber		25g	30g

Figure 24.1. A Sample Food Label. Notice that this package contains two servings. Each serving has 250 calories. If you consume the entire package, that equals 500 calories. (Image from "How To Understand and Use the Nutrition Facts Label," U.S. Food and Drug Administration (www.fda.gov), June 2009.

Plan Meals And Snacks

You and your family have busy schedules, which can make eating healthfully a challenge. Planning ahead can help. Think about the meals and snacks you would like for the week—including bag lunches to take to school—and help your family make a shopping list. You may even want to go grocery shopping and cook together.

Jumpstart Your Day With Breakfast

Did you know that eating breakfast can help you do better in school? By eating breakfast you can increase your attention span and memory, have more energy, and feel less irritable and restless. A breakfast that is part of a healthy diet can also help you maintain an appropriate weight now and in the future.

Pack Your Lunch

Whether you eat lunch from school or pack your own, this meal should provide you with one-third of the day's nutritional needs. A lunch of chips, cookies, candy, or soda just gives you lots of calories, but not many nutrients. Instead of buying snacks from vending machines at school, bring food from home. Try packing your lunch with a lean turkey sandwich on whole-grain bread, healthy foods like fruits, vegetables, low-fat yogurt, and nuts.

Snack Smart

A healthy snack can contribute to a healthy eating plan and give you the energy boost you need to get through the day. Try these snack ideas, but keep in mind that most of these foods should be eaten in small amounts:

- Fruit—any kind—fresh, canned, dried, or frozen
- Peanut butter on rice cakes or whole-wheat crackers
- Baked potato chips or tortilla chips with salsa
- Veggies with low-fat dip
- String cheese, low-fat cottage cheese, or low-fat yogurt
- Frozen fruit bars, fruit sorbet, or low-fat frozen yogurt
- Vanilla wafers, graham crackers, animal crackers, or fig bars
- Popcorn (air popped or low-fat microwave)

Eat Dinner With Your Family

For many teens, dinner consists of eating on the run, snacking in front of the TV, or nonstop munching from after school to bedtime. Try to eat dinner as a family instead. Believe it or not, when you eat with your family you are more likely to get more fruits, vegetables, and other foods with the vitamins and minerals your body needs. Family meals also help you reconnect after a busy day. Talk to your family about fitting in at least a few meals together throughout the week.

Fast Food

Like many teens, you may eat at fast food restaurants often. If so, you are probably taking in a lot of extra calories from added sugar and fat. Just one value-sized fast food meal of a sandwich, fries, and sweetened soda can have more calories, fat, and added sugar than you need.

The best approach is to limit the amount of fast food you eat. If you do order fast food, try these tips:

- Skip "value-sized" or "super-sized" meals.

- Choose a grilled chicken sandwich or a plain, small burger.

- Use mustard instead of mayonnaise.

- Limit fried foods or remove breading from fried chicken, which can cut half the fat.

- Order garden or grilled chicken salads with light or reduced-calorie dressings.

- Choose water, fat-free, or low-fat milk instead of sweetened soda.

Rethink Your Drinks

Soda and other sugary drinks have replaced milk and water as the drinks of choice for teens and adults alike. Yet these drinks are actually more like desserts because they are high in added sugar and calories. In fact, soda and sugar-laden drinks may contribute to weight problems in kids and teens. Try sticking to water, low-fat milk, or fat-free milk.

Where can I learn about making a diabetes meal plan?

- Contact a registered dietitian to make a meal plan just for you.

- Visit the American Dietetic Association website to find a nutrition professional who can help you develop a healthy meal plan (www.eatright.org).

- Visit the American Association of Diabetes Educators to find a diabetes educator (www.diabeteseducator.org).

- Visit the American Diabetes Association website for more information on carbohydrate counting and the exchange method (www.diabetes.org).

Source: Excerpted from "Diabetes and Me: Eat Right," Centers for Disease Control and Prevention, June 4, 2010.

Chapter 25

Meal Plans And Diabetes

If you have diabetes, eating healthy meals helps you the same way it helps your best friend or the guy who sits next to you in math class. Good nutrition helps you grow properly, reach and maintain a weight that's right for your height, and stay healthy. But eating right also helps you keep your blood sugar levels on track—something that's important for people with diabetes. By eating well, you'll also help to prevent diabetes problems that can occur later in life, like heart disease.

People who have diabetes don't need to be on strict diets, but they do need to pay attention to when they eat and what's on their plates. Crack open the cookbooks and surf to your favorite recipe website because it's time to plan meals that you love!

Food Labels

Eating right means knowing what's in the foods you're eating. It's easy to guess what some foods contain, but others are more of a mystery. That's where food labels come in. Food labels list a food's ingredients, nutritional information, and calories per serving. This nutritional information includes carbohydrates (pronounced: kar-bo-hi-drates, and also known as carbs), sodium, and fats, all of which are important to people with diabetes.

Carbohydrates

The amount of carbohydrates you eat can help you control your diabetes. People with diabetes need to balance the amount of carbs they eat with their activity levels and insulin. A

About This Chapter: "Meal Plans and Diabetes," August 2010, reprinted with permission from www.kidshealth .org. Copyright © 2010 The Nemours Foundation. This information was provided by KidsHealth, one of the largest resources online for medically reviewed health information written for parents, kids, and teens. For more articles like this one, visit www.KidsHealth.org, or www.TeensHealth.org.

doctor or dietitian will show you how to do this and will tell you the amount of carbs you should have in your diet. Once you have this information, food labels will make it easy to track and meet your goals.

Food labels list carbohydrates in grams. You can figure out your carb intake in three steps:

1. Look on the food label for the serving size.

2. Look on the food label for the amount of carbohydrates per serving.

3. Calculate how many servings you ate.

For example, a food label might show that the serving size is ½ cup (120 milliliters) and the amount of carbohydrates per serving is 7 grams. If you ate 1 cup (240 milliliters) of that food, you ate 14 grams of carbs (7 grams per serving x 2 servings).

Sodium

Food labels also list how much sodium (salt) is in foods. Some people with diabetes have hypertension (high blood pressure), and eating too much salt can make it worse. If you have hypertension, you may need to check how much sodium is in the foods you eat so you can stick to the guidelines your doctor gives you. Even if you don't have hypertension, it's a good idea to go easy on sodium.

Fats

People with diabetes are also at greater risk of developing heart disease, especially if they have high levels of lipids (fats) in their blood. You can ask your doctor or dietitian if you need to limit your intake of saturated fats, cholesterol, and trans fats. Food labels list the amount and types of these fats that a food contains. All of these can contribute to the development of heart disease in people with or without diabetes.

Quick Tip

Aside from carbs, sodium, and fats, you might check food labels for the same reasons that everybody else does. Watching the calories you eat—and limiting the amount of high-calorie foods that you eat—can help you maintain a healthy weight. It's also important to make sure that you get enough vitamins, minerals, and fiber to stay healthy.

A quick-reference guide to food content can make choosing healthy foods a little easier if you're eating out or in situations where there's no food label. This guide contains details on the carbohydrate, fat, and sodium content of foods, along with other nutritional information. If you don't have one, you can get one from your doctor or dietitian.

Meal Planning

Just like everyone else, people with diabetes need to aim for each meal to be a good balance of nutrition and taste. Here are some estimates to shoot for over the course of a day:

- About 10% to 20% of the calories you eat should come from protein. Try to select lean meats like chicken or beef.

- Roughly 25% to 30% of calories should come from fat. Try to avoid foods with lots of trans and saturated fats (or eat them only in moderation).

- About 50% to 60% of the calories you eat should come from carbohydrates. Try to eat lots of green and orange vegetables in your daily diet—like carrots and broccoli. And choose vitamin-rich brown rice or sweet potatoes instead of white rice or regular potatoes.

Your diabetes health care team will teach you (and whoever prepares your meals, such as your mom or dad) meal planning guidelines. Your meal plan won't tell you specific foods to eat, but it may suggest mealtimes, food groups to select from, and the amounts to eat from these food groups.

There's no sense in having a boring diet you won't stick to, so your nutrition team will work to build the plan based on the foods that you usually eat. To find out what you like to eat, the team may ask you to keep a food diary or write down what you eat and drink for three days to get a good idea of your tastes.

Your meal plan will probably look different from someone else's because it depends on your needs and health goals. For example, if you need to lose weight, then the team will help you focus on controlling the number of calories and fat grams you eat.

Three Ways To Plan Meals

Some people with diabetes, especially people who've just developed it, use a program called the exchange meal plan as a guide for what they eat each day. The exchange meal plan is really useful for people with diabetes who are overweight or who need to pay close attention to the balance of calories and nutrients they eat each day.

For this meal plan, foods are divided into six groups: starch, fruit, milk, fat, vegetable, and meat. The plan sets a serving size (amount) for foods in each group. And each serving has a similar amount of calories, protein, carbohydrate, and fat. This allows a person some flexibility in planning meals because they can exchange, or substitute, choices from a food list. The number of servings from each food group recommended for each meal and snack is based on the total number of calories that the person needs each day.

The other two types of meal plans help make sure that the amount of carbohydrates that a person's eating matches up with the insulin or other diabetes medicines he or she is taking. Focusing on carbohydrate intake is important because carbs are mainly responsible for the rise in blood sugar that occurs after eating. With the constant carbohydrate meal plan, the person eats a certain amount of carbohydrates in each meal and snack. Then he or she takes insulin or other diabetes medicines at the same times and in the same amounts each day. This plan is easy to follow for people who usually eat and exercise about the same amount from day to day.

Another option is the carbohydrate counting meal plan. Many people with diabetes use carb counting to figure out the amount of carbohydrates in the foods they eat at each meal or snack. They then match their insulin dosage to that carb amount. This plan works best for people who take a dose of insulin (as a shot or with an insulin pump) with each meal. This meal plan works well for people who need more flexibility, because the person takes insulin when actually eating, rather than at a set time each day.

Helpful Tools

Keeping a written record of what you eat can help you and your diabetes health care team make changes to your diabetes management plan. One helpful tool is a blood glucose record. This record makes it easy to jot down your carbohydrate intake alongside your blood sugar readings and lets you see how well you're balancing your food and insulin. Then if you need to adjust your insulin dose, this written record can help you understand why and help you decide how much and what time you should have the new dosage.

It can also help to keep a few references handy, such as charts that show portion sizes and lists of how many carbohydrates various foods contain. Your diabetes health care team or a nutritionist can supply this information, and the American Diabetes Association offers it, too.

With your diabetes knowledge and the right tools, you'll be prepared to eat right for your health.

Chapter 26

Carbohydrate Counting

There are several different ways people with diabetes can manage their food intake to keep their blood glucose (sugar) as close to normal as possible, and one such method is *carbohydrate counting*. Carbohydrate counting is a method of calculating grams of carbohydrate consumed at meals and snacks. We count carbohydrates because they have the greatest effect on glucose. Before starting any new treatment or meal plan, you should always consult with your diabetes care professional.

What Are The Benefits Of Counting Carbs?

Counting carbohydrates is a good solution for many people with diabetes. Once you learn how to convert grams into their equivalent amount of carbohydrates, it is easier to incorporate a wider array of foods into your meal plan, including combination foods such as those in frozen dinners. For example, by consulting the Nutrition Facts on a frozen dinner, you can easily calculate the number of carbohydrates in the meal, rather than trying to calculate how that particular food fits into the more traditional exchange meal plan.

Another benefit of counting carbohydrates is that it can bring tighter control over your glucose readings. Being as precise as possible with your carb intake and medication will likely allow you to regulate blood glucose after a meal.

Lastly, counting carbohydrates may also allow you to adjust the amounts of carbohydrates you eat at each meal, rather than feeling like you have to eat a certain amount of carbohydrates, even if you do not want to.

Who Can Use Carbohydrate Counting?

Carbohydrate counting can be used by anyone with diabetes, not just people taking insulin.

This method is also useful for people who are using more aggressive methods of adjusting insulin to control diabetes. The amount of meal and snack carbohydrate is adjusted based on the pre-meal blood sugar reading. Depending on the reading, more or less carbohydrate may be eaten. Likewise, insulin may be adjusted based on what the person wants to eat. For example, if you want to eat a much larger meal than usual, carb counting can help you determine how much extra insulin to take. Depending on the situation, you must then adjust the amount of carbohydrates you eat at each subsequent meal to be certain it fits into your overall carbohydrate allowance, however, it does afford some flexibility with regard to how carbs are distributed throughout the day.

The following is an explanation of how to use carbohydrate meal planning. Copy these pages and discuss them with your nurse educator, dietitian, or physician at your next visit.

Tools Of The Trade

In order to count carbohydrates, you must begin by having a meal plan and also knowing the average carbohydrate values of various food groups. If you don't have some form of a meal plan developed by your health care team, you will be unable to figure out how many grams of carbohydrate you are supposed to eat at each meal and snack.

Good resources for exchange systems are "Joslin's Menu Planning—Simple!" (available online at http://www.joslin.harvard.edu/info/menu_planning_simple.html), *Joslin's Guide to Diabetes* (which also contains a chapter discussing meal planning, including carbohydrate counting; available at http://www.joslin.harvard.edu/jstore/the_joslin_guide_to_diabetes_revised_edition.html) or the *American Diabetes Association's Exchange Lists for Meal Planning*.

It is also helpful to have a carbohydrate counting reference book. We suggest: *Calorie King Calorie, Fat & Carbohydrate Counter* by Allan Borushek, *The Complete Book of Food Counts* by Corinne Netzer, *The Diabetes Carbohydrate and Fat Gram Guide* by Lea Holzmeister, *Calories and Carbohydrates* by Barbara Kraus, *Carbohydrate Guide to Brand Names and Basic Foods* by Barbara Kraus, *The Carbohydrate Addict's Gram Counter* by Richard Heller, and *The Restaurant Lovers' Fat Gram Counter* by Kalia Doner. Measuring equipment, such as a food scale, measuring cups and spoons, is essential. Probably the most frequently used tool will be food labels.

Step 1: Know your meal plan.

Indicate on the chart the number of servings from each food group planned as part of your meal plan. The last row will be completed in Step 2.

Food Groups	Breakfast	Snack	Lunch	Snack	Dinner	Snack
Starch						
Fruit						
Vegetable						
Milk						
Protein						
Fat						
Carbohydrates						

Chart 26.1. Your Meal Plan And Carbohydrates.

Step 2: Know your carbohydrates.

Most of the carbohydrates we eat come from three food groups: starch, fruit, and milk. Vegetables also contain some carbohydrates, but foods in the meat and fat groups contain very little carbohydrates. This list shows the average amount of carbohydrates in each food group per serving:

- Starch: 15 grams
- Fruit: 15 grams
- Milk: 12 grams
- Vegetable: 5 grams
- Meat: 0 grams
- Fat: 0 grams

To make things easy, many people begin carbohydrate counting by rounding the carbohydrate values of milk up to 15. In other words, one serving of starch, fruit, or milk all contain 15 grams of carbohydrates or one carbohydrate serving. Three servings of vegetable also contain 15 grams. One or two servings of vegetables do not need to be counted. Each meal and snack will contain a total number of grams of carbohydrates.

Complete the following list to test your understanding:

- 2 slices bread = _____grams of carbohydrates

- 1 whole banana (9" size) = _____grams of carbohydrates

- 1 cup oatmeal with 1 cup milk = _____grams of carbohydrates

Look back at your meal plan in Step 1. Total up the number of grams of carbohydrate for each meal and snack and write the totals in the last row. It is more important to know your carbohydrate allowance for each meal and snack than it is to know your total for the day. The amount of carbohydrates eaten at each meal should remain consistent (unless you learn to adjust your insulin for a change in the amount of carbohydrates eaten).

Step 3: Using carbohydrate counting in meal planning.

Here is an example to show how carbohydrate counting can make meal planning easier. Let's say your dinner meal plan contains five carbohydrate servings or 75 grams of carbohydrates. (This is based on a meal plan of three starch servings, four protein, one vegetable, one fruit, one milk, and three fat.) The label on a frozen dinner of beef enchiladas says it contains 62 grams of carbohydrate. Instead of calculating how many exchanges that converts to, just figure out how many more grams of carbohydrates you need to meet your 75 gram total. Add about 15 more grams of carbohydrates (one serving of fruit or milk, for example) and you have almost matched your total.

The Final Word On Carbohydrate Counting

Counting carbohydrates allows flexibility in your meal plan, but you can't abandon your meal plan and eat as many carbohydrates as you desire. Keep in mind your overall goals—to keep your carb intake at a certain amount each day, and keep your glucose as close to normal as possible—and you'll do well. Remember to consult your healthcare team before making any of the changes discussed here.

Chapter 27

Diabetes And Dietary Supplements

Introduction

Diabetes is a chronic condition affecting millions of Americans. Conventional medical treatments are available to control diabetes and its complications. However, some people also try complementary and alternative medicine—a group of diverse medical and health care systems, practices, and products that are not presently considered to be part of conventional medicine. Complementary medicine is used together with conventional medicine, and alternative medicine is used in place of conventional medicine. (CAM) therapies, including dietary supplements. This chapter sheet provides basic information on diabetes (with a focus on type 2), summarizes scientific research on the effectiveness and safety of selected supplements that people with diabetes sometimes use, and suggests sources for additional information.

About Diabetes

Diabetes encompasses a group of diseases. Type 2 diabetes accounts for 90 to 95 percent of all diagnosed cases and occurs more frequently in older people. Type 1 diabetes, which accounts for 5 to 10 percent of cases, usually strikes children and young adults. A third form, gestational diabetes, develops in some women during pregnancy.

In all forms of diabetes, the body's ability to convert food into energy is impaired. After a meal, the body breaks down most food into glucose (a kind of sugar), the main source of fuel for cells. In people with diabetes, the body does not make enough insulin—a hormone that helps glucose enter cells—or the cells do not respond to insulin properly. Often, both insulin

About This Chapter: From "Diabetes and CAM: A Focus on Dietary Supplements," National Center for Complementary and Alternative Medicine, October 2010.

production and insulin action are impaired. Without treatment, glucose builds up in the blood instead of moving into the cells, where it can be converted into energy. Over time, the high blood glucose levels caused by diabetes can damage many parts of the body, including the heart and blood vessels, eyes, kidneys, nerves, feet, and skin. Such complications can be prevented or delayed by controlling blood glucose, blood pressure, and cholesterol levels.

Type 2 diabetes most often is associated with older age (although it is increasingly being diagnosed in children), obesity (about 80 percent of people with type 2 diabetes are overweight), a family history of diabetes, and physical inactivity. Certain minority population groups are at greater risk, as are women who have had gestational diabetes. Type 2 diabetes usually begins as insulin resistance, a disorder in which cells do not use insulin properly. Symptoms develop gradually and may include fatigue, frequent urination, excessive thirst and hunger, weight loss, blurred vision, and slow-healing wounds or sores. However, it is possible to have type 2 diabetes without experiencing any symptoms.

People with diabetes should try to keep their blood glucose in a healthy range. The basic tools for managing type 2 diabetes are healthy eating, physical activity, and blood glucose monitoring. Many people also need to take prescription pills, insulin, or both.

Dietary Supplements And Type 2 Diabetes

Some people with diabetes use CAM therapies for their health condition. For example, they may try acupuncture or biofeedback (the use of electronic devices to help people learn to control body functions that are normally unconscious, such as breathing or heart rate) to help with painful symptoms. Some use dietary supplements in efforts to improve their blood glucose control, manage symptoms, and lessen the risk of developing serious complications such as heart problems.

Key Points

- In general, there is not enough scientific evidence to prove that dietary supplements have substantial benefits for type 2 diabetes or its complications.
- It is very important not to replace conventional medical therapy for diabetes with an unproven CAM therapy.
- Tell your health care providers about any complementary and alternative practices you use.
- The U.S. Food and Drug Administration has special labeling requirements for dietary supplements and treats them as foods, not drugs.

This chapter addresses what is known about a few of the many supplements used for diabetes, with a focus on some that have been studied in clinical trials, such as alpha-lipoic acid, chromium, omega-3 fatty acids (essential nutrients that the body cannot make on its own but can obtain from foods such as fish and flaxseed, or from dietary supplements), and polyphenols.

Alpha-Lipoic Acid

Alpha-lipoic acid (ALA, also known as lipoic acid or thioctic acid) is an antioxidant—a substance that protects against cell damage. ALA is found in certain foods, such as liver, spinach, broccoli, and potatoes. Some people with type 2 diabetes take ALA supplements in the hope of lowering blood glucose levels by improving the body's ability to use insulin; others use ALA to prevent or treat diabetic neuropathy (a nerve disorder). Supplements are marketed as tablets or capsules.

ALA has been researched for its effect on insulin sensitivity, glucose metabolism, and diabetic neuropathy. Some studies have found benefits, but more research is needed.

Because ALA might lower blood sugar too much, people with diabetes who take it must monitor their blood sugar levels very carefully.

Chromium

Chromium is an essential trace mineral—that is, the body requires small amounts of it to function properly. Some people with diabetes take chromium in an effort to improve their blood glucose control. Chromium is found in many foods, but usually only in small amounts; relatively good sources include meat, whole grain products, and some fruits, vegetables, and spices. In supplement form (capsules and tablets), it is sold as chromium picolinate, chromium chloride, and chromium nicotinate.

Chromium supplementation has been researched for its effect on glucose control in people with diabetes. Study results have been mixed. Some researchers have found benefits, but many of the studies have not been well designed. Additional, high-quality research is needed.

At low doses, short-term use of chromium appears to be safe for most adults. However, people with diabetes should be aware that chromium might cause blood sugar levels to go too low. High doses can cause serious side effects, including kidney problems—an issue of special concern to people with diabetes.

Omega-3 Fatty Acids

Omega-3 fatty acids are polyunsaturated fatty acids that come from foods such as fish, fish oil, vegetable oil (primarily canola and soybean), walnuts, and wheat germ. Omega-3 supplements are available as capsules or oils (such as fish oil). Omega-3s are important in a number of bodily functions, including the movement of calcium and other substances in and out of cells, the relaxation and contraction of muscles, blood clotting, digestion, fertility, cell division, and growth. In addition, omega-3s are thought to protect against heart disease, reduce inflammation, and lower triglyceride levels.

Omega-3 fatty acids have been researched for their effect on controlling glucose and reducing heart disease risk in people with type 2 diabetes. Studies show that omega-3 fatty acids lower triglycerides, but do not affect blood glucose control, total cholesterol, or HDL (good) cholesterol in people with diabetes. In some studies, omega-3 fatty acids also raised LDL (bad) cholesterol. Additional research, particularly long-term studies that look specifically at heart disease in people with diabetes, is needed.

Omega-3s appear to be safe for most adults at low-to-moderate doses. Safety questions have been raised about fish oil supplements, because some species of fish can be contaminated by substances such as mercury, pesticides, or PCBs. In high doses, fish oil can interact with certain medications, including blood thinners and drugs used for high blood pressure.

Polyphenols

Polyphenols—antioxidants found in tea and dark chocolate, among other dietary sources—are being studied for possible effects on vascular health (including blood pressure) and on the body's ability to use insulin.

Laboratory studies suggest that EGCG, a polyphenol found in green tea, may protect against cardiovascular disease and have a beneficial effect on insulin activity and glucose control. However, a few small clinical trials studying EGCG and green tea in people with diabetes have not shown such effects.

No adverse effects of EGCG or green tea were discussed in these studies. Green tea is safe for most adults when used in moderate amounts. However, green tea contains caffeine, which can cause, in some people, insomnia, anxiety, or irritability, among other effects. Green tea also has small amounts of vitamin K, which can make anticoagulant drugs, such as warfarin, less effective.

Other Supplements

Other supplements are also being studied for diabetes-related effects. For example:

- Preliminary research has explored the use of garlic for lowering blood glucose levels, but findings have not been consistent.

- Studies of the effects of magnesium supplementation on blood glucose control have had mixed results, although researchers have found that eating a diet high in magnesium may lower the risk of diabetes.

- There is not enough evidence to evaluate the effectiveness of coenzyme Q10 supplementation as a CAM therapy for diabetes; studies of its ability to affect glucose control have had conflicting findings.

- Researchers are studying whether the herb ginseng and the trace mineral vanadium might help control glucose levels.

- Some people with diabetes may also try botanicals such as prickly pear cactus, gurmar, *Coccinia indica*, aloe vera, fenugreek, and bitter melon to control their glucose levels. However, there is limited research on the effectiveness of these botanicals for diabetes.

If You Have Diabetes And Are Thinking About Using A Dietary Supplement

- Tell your health care providers about any complementary and alternative practices you use. Give them a full picture of what you do to manage your health. This will help ensure coordinated and safe care. For tips about talking with your health care providers about CAM, see the National Center for Complementary and Alternative Medicine "Time to Talk" campaign at nccam.nih.gov/timetotalk. Medicines for diabetes and other health conditions may need to be adjusted if a person is also using a dietary supplement.

- Women who are pregnant or nursing, or people who are thinking of using supplements to treat a child, should consult their health care provider before using any dietary supplement.

- Do not replace scientifically proven treatments for diabetes with CAM treatments that are unproven. The consequences of not following one's prescribed medical regimen for diabetes can be very serious.

- Be aware that the label on a dietary supplement bottle may not accurately reflect what is inside. For example, some tests of dietary supplements have found that the contents did not match the dose on the label, and some herbal supplements have been found to be contaminated.

Chapter 28

Physical Activity And Diabetes

What can a physically active lifestyle do for me?

Research has shown that physical activity can help accomplish these goals:

- Lower your blood glucose and your blood pressure
- Lower your bad cholesterol and raise your good cholesterol
- Improve your body's ability to use insulin
- Lower your risk for heart disease and stroke
- Keep your heart and bones strong
- Keep your joints flexible
- Lower your risk of falling
- Help you lose weight
- Reduce your body fat
- Give you more energy
- Reduce your stress levels

Physical activity also plays an important part in preventing type 2 diabetes. A major government study, the Diabetes Prevention Program (DPP), showed that modest weight loss of five to seven percent—for example, 10 to 15 pounds for a 200-pound person—can delay and possibly prevent type 2 diabetes. People in the study used diet and exercise to lose weight.

About This Chapter: Excerpted from "What I Need to Know about Physical Activity and Diabetes," National Diabetes Information Clearinghouse, March 2008.

What kinds of physical activity can help me?

Four kinds of activity can help. You can be extra active every day, do aerobic exercise, do strength training, and stretch.

Extra Active: Being extra active can increase the number of calories you burn. Try these ways to be extra active, or think of other things you can do.

- Walk around while you talk on the phone.

- Play with younger siblings.

- Take the dog for a walk.

- Get up to change the TV channel instead of using the remote control.

- Work in the garden or rake leaves.

- Clean your room (or the whole house).

- Wash the car.

What's so important about being physically active?

Being active keeps your body healthy and strong and gives you more energy. It can help you think and be more alert in school. It can also help you stay at a healthy weight or help you lose weight slowly. Being active is an important part of a healthy lifestyle.

Physical activity can make you feel better if you are in a bad mood or stressed out. It can relax you and help you sleep well. It helps your body use blood glucose, also called blood sugar, for energy. Physical activity can help keep your blood glucose in a normal range.

There are many ways you can be active. Pick things you like to do.

- Take a walk, hike, or ride a bike.
- Skateboard, roller blade, or ice skate.
- Play some music and dance with your friends. If you like video games, try a dance or other active video game.
- Play basketball, baseball, softball, golf, soccer, tennis, volleyball, or your favorite sport.
- Go bowling.

Think of other things you like to do and just move! It is an easy way to have fun.

Source: Excerpted from "Tips for Teens with Diabetes: Be Active," National Diabetes Education Program, November 1, 2007.

- Stretch out your chores. For example, make two trips to take the laundry downstairs instead of one.

- Park at the far end of the shopping center parking lot and walk to the store.

- At the grocery store, walk down every aisle.

- Take the stairs instead of the elevator.

Can you think of other things you can do?

Aerobic Exercise: Aerobic exercise is activity that requires the use of large muscles and makes your heart beat faster. You will also breathe harder during aerobic exercise. Doing aerobic exercise for 30 minutes a day at least five days a week provides many benefits. You can even split up those 30 minutes into several parts. For example, you can take three brisk 10-minute walks, one after each meal.

If you haven't exercised lately, see your doctor first to make sure it's OK for you to increase your level of physical activity. Talk with your doctor about how to warm up and stretch before you exercise and how to cool down after you exercise. Then start slowly with five to ten minutes a day. Add a little more time each week, aiming for at least 150 minutes per week. Try some of these activities:

- Walking briskly

- Hiking

- Climbing stairs

- Swimming or taking a water-aerobics class

- Dancing

- Riding a bicycle outdoors or a stationary bicycle indoors

- Taking an aerobics class

- Playing basketball, volleyball, or other sports

- In-line skating, ice skating, or skate boarding

- Playing tennis

- Cross-country skiing

If you need more ideas, check out the suggestions offered by the Centers for Disease Control and Prevention at their "BAM! Body and Mind" website: www.bam.gov.

Strength Training: Doing exercises with hand weights, elastic bands, or weight machines three times a week builds muscle. When you have more muscle and less fat, you'll burn more calories because muscle burns more calories than fat, even between exercise sessions. Strength training can help make daily chores easier, improving your balance and coordination, as well as your bones' health. You can do strength training at home, at a fitness center, or in a class. Your health care team can tell you more about strength training and what kind is best for you.

Stretch: Stretching increases your flexibility, lowers stress, and helps prevent muscle soreness after other types of exercise. Your health care team can tell you what kind of stretching is best for you.

Can I exercise any time I want?

Your health care team can help you decide the best time of day for you to exercise. Together, you and your team will consider your daily schedule, your meal plan, and your diabetes medicines.

If you have type 1 diabetes, avoid strenuous exercise when you have ketones in your blood or urine. Ketones are chemicals your body might make when your blood glucose level is too high and your insulin level is too low. Too many ketones can make you sick. If you exercise when you have ketones in your blood or urine, your blood glucose level may go even higher.

If you have type 2 diabetes and your blood glucose is high but you don't have ketones, light or moderate exercise will probably lower your blood glucose. Ask your health care team whether you should exercise when your blood glucose is high.

What are some good types of physical activity for people with diabetes?

Walking vigorously, hiking, climbing stairs, swimming, aerobics, dancing, bicycling, skating, skiing, tennis, basketball, volleyball, or other sports are just some examples of physical activity that will work your large muscles, increase your heart rate, and make you breathe harder—important goals for fitness.

In addition, strength training exercises with hand weights, elastic bands, or weight machines can help you build muscle. Stretching helps to make you flexible and prevent soreness after other types of exercise.

Do physical activities you really like. The more fun you have, the more likely you will do it each day. It can be helpful to exercise with a family member or friend.

Source: Excerpted from "Diabetes and Me: Be Active," Centers for Disease Control and Prevention, June 4, 2010.

Are there any types of physical activity I shouldn't do?

If you have diabetes complications, some kinds of exercise can make your problems worse. For example, activities that increase the pressure in the blood vessels of your eyes, such as lifting heavy weights, can make diabetic eye problems worse. If nerve damage from diabetes has made your feet numb, your doctor may suggest that you try swimming instead of walking for aerobic exercise.

When you have numb feet, you might not feel pain in your feet. Sores or blisters might get worse because you don't notice them. Without proper care, minor foot problems can turn into serious conditions, sometimes leading to amputation. Make sure you exercise in cotton socks and comfortable, well-fitting shoes designed for the activity you are doing. After you exercise, check your feet for cuts, sores, bumps, or redness. Call your doctor if any foot problems develop.

Can physical activity cause low blood glucose?

Physical activity can cause low blood glucose, also called hypoglycemia, in people who take insulin or certain types of diabetes medicines. Ask your health care team whether your diabetes medicines can cause low blood glucose.

Low blood glucose can happen while you exercise, right afterward, or even up to a day later. It can make you feel shaky, weak, confused, grumpy, hungry, or tired. You may sweat a lot or get a headache. If your blood glucose drops too low, you could pass out or have a seizure.

However, you should still be physically active. These steps can help you be prepared for low blood glucose:

Before Exercise

- Ask your health care team whether you should check your blood glucose level before exercising.

- If you take diabetes medicines that can cause low blood glucose, ask your health care team whether you should change the amount you take before you exercise or if you should have a snack if your blood glucose level is below 100.

During Exercise

- Wear your medical identification (ID) bracelet or necklace or carry your ID in your pocket.

- Always carry food or glucose tablets so you'll be ready to treat low blood glucose.

- If you'll be exercising for more than an hour, check your blood glucose at regular intervals. You may need snacks before you finish.

After Exercise

- Check to see how exercise affected your blood glucose level.

Treating Low Blood Glucose

If your blood glucose is below 70, have one of the following right away:

- 3 or 4 glucose tablets
- 1 serving of glucose gel—the amount equal to 15 grams of carbohydrate
- 1/2 cup (4 ounces) of any fruit juice
- 1/2 cup (4 ounces) of a regular—not diet—soft drink
- 1 cup (8 ounces) of milk
- 5 or 6 pieces of hard candy
- 1 tablespoon of sugar or honey

After 15 minutes, check your blood glucose again. If it's still too low, have another serving. Repeat until your blood glucose is 70 or higher. If it will be an hour or more before your next meal, have a snack as well.

Source: Excerpted from "What I Need to Know about Physical Activity and Diabetes," National Diabetes Information Clearinghouse, March 2008.

What should I do before I start a physical activity program?

Check with your doctor. Always talk with your doctor before you start a new physical activity program. Ask about your medicines—prescription and over-the-counter—and whether you should change the amount you take before you exercise. If you have heart disease, kidney disease, eye problems, or foot problems, ask which types of physical activity are safe for you.

Decide exactly what you'll do and set some goals. Choose the type of physical activity you want to do, the clothes and items you'll need to get ready, and the days and times you'll add activity. You'll also need to make decisions about the length of each session and your plan for warming up, stretching, and cooling down for each session. In addition, you'll want a backup plan, such as where you'll walk if the weather is bad, and some way to measure your of progress.

Find an exercise buddy. Many people find they are more likely to do something active if a friend joins them. If you and a friend plan to walk together, for example, you may be more likely to do it.

Keep track of your physical activity. Write down when you exercise and for how long in your blood glucose record book. You'll be able to track your progress and see how physical activity affects your blood glucose.

Decide how you'll reward yourself. Do something nice for yourself when you reach your activity goals. For example, treat yourself to a movie or buy a new plant for the garden.

What can I do to make sure I stay active?

One of the keys to staying on track is finding some activities you like to do. If you keep finding excuses not to exercise, think about why. Are your goals realistic? Do you need a change in activity? Would another time be more convenient? Keep trying until you find a routine that works for you. Once you make physical activity a habit, you'll wonder how you lived without it.

But I hate to exercise—what can I do?

You do not have to play a sport or go to a gym. There are a lot of things you can do to be more active:

- Do sit-ups or jump rope while watching TV.
- Lift light weights to strengthen your muscles.
- Jog around the block or walk fast around the mall a few times.
- Help your mom or dad carry groceries, clean the house, cut grass, do garden work, rake leaves, or shovel snow.
- Take the stairs instead of the elevator.
- Take your dog for a walk.
- Ride your bike instead of driving or getting a ride from your parents or a friend.

Make a list of things you like to do to be physically active. Hang it in your room as a reminder. Keep track of your progress.

Source: Excerpted from "Tips for Teens with Diabetes: Be Active," National Diabetes Education Program, November 1, 2007.

Chapter 29

Sports, Exercise, And Diabetes

People with diabetes can exercise and play sports at the same level as everyone else. But some don't. Take Olympic gold-medal swimmer Gary Hall Jr., for instance. He definitely doesn't swim like an average person. Pro golfers Kelli Kuehne and Michelle McGann don't putt like the folks at your local mini golf, either. And Major League Baseball player Jason Johnson pitches a bit differently than, say, your math teacher. All of these athletes deal with diabetes while wiping out the competition.

Get the idea? Whether you want to go for the gold or just go hiking in your hometown, diabetes shouldn't hold you back.

How Exercise Helps People With Diabetes

Exercise offers many benefits. It:

- strengthens bones and muscles

- reduces your risk of heart disease and some types of cancer

- improves coordination, balance, strength, and endurance

- can increase your energy level

- helps insulin work better in the body, which helps blood sugar levels stay in a healthy range

- burns calories, which helps you reach and stay at a healthy weight

- teaches you about teamwork, competition, and courage

- helps boost self-esteem and confidence

- relieves tension and stress, relaxes you, and boosts your mood, too

- can even help you clear your mind and focus your attention better

All exercise is great—whether it's walking the dog or playing team sports. Just be sure to do it every day. Changing exercise habits can be hard for everyone at first. But most people say that once they start feeling the benefits, they're hooked. After that, it's a lot easier to keep going. But there are some facts you need to know about exercise and diabetes.

What Happens During Exercise?

The muscles need more energy during exercise, so the body releases extra sugar, or glucose. For people with diabetes, this can have some side effects. For example, if the body doesn't have enough insulin to use the glucose that's released during exercise, then the glucose stays in the blood, which leads to high blood sugar levels. This is called hyperglycemia (pronounced: hy-per-gly-see-me-uh).

Not having enough insulin to use the sugar in the blood can also cause the body to burn fat for fuel. When the body starts to burn fat for fuel, substances called ketones (pronounced: kee-tones) are produced. People with diabetes shouldn't exercise if they have high levels of ketones in their blood because this can make them really sick. If you have type 1 diabetes, your doctor will tell you how to check for ketones (you may need to take a urine test before exercising) and treat yourself to get back on track.

The body's need for extra glucose during exercise can also cause low blood sugar levels (called hypoglycemia, pronounced: hy-po-gly-see-me-uh). Low blood sugar can occur when the body uses up all the sugar that it's stored so there's no more to be released as glucose when the muscles demand it. This is especially true if insulin levels in the blood are still high after taking an injection. You may need to check blood sugar levels and have an extra snack to prevent low blood sugar levels. If you're starting a rigorous exercise schedule, like training for a sport, your doctor may recommend that you adjust your insulin dosage to prevent low blood sugar levels.

Exercise Tips For People With Diabetes

These tips can help you avoid diabetes problems during exercise:

- **Test Yourself:** Your doctor will tell you when to test your glucose levels—often you'll need to check them before, during, and after exercise.

Getting Ready To Exercise

All teens—not just those with diabetes—need to get a physical before they play a sport. Your doctor will let you know about any changes you should make to your testing schedule or medication while exercising or playing sports.

The doctor is likely to give the green light to any activities you want to start—after all, exercise is an important part of diabetes management. However, doctors may recommend that you steer clear of certain adventure sports like rock climbing, hang gliding, or scuba diving. That's because a person could be seriously hurt if he or she has low blood sugar levels while doing these sports.

- **Take The Right Dose Of Insulin:** Your doctor might recommend adjusting your insulin dosage for exercise or sports. If you inject insulin, you might not want to inject a part of your body used for your sport before exercise (like injecting your leg before soccer). This could cause the insulin to be absorbed too quickly. If you wear an insulin pump, be sure that it won't be in the way for exercise and that it won't get disconnected. Talk to your doctor about what you should do when you want to go without the pump.

- **Eat Right:** Your diabetes health care team will also help you adjust your meal plan so you have enough energy for exercise. For example, you might need to eat extra snacks before, during, or after working out. Be sure to maintain the proper diet for your diabetes—don't try strategies like loading up on extra carbs before running or cutting back on food or water to get down to a certain weight for wrestling. These activities can be dangerous for people with diabetes.

- **Bring Snacks And Water:** Whether you're playing football at the school or swimming in your backyard, keep snacks and water nearby.

- **Pack It Up:** If you'll be exercising away from home, pack your testing supplies, medications, medical alert bracelet, emergency contact information, and a copy of your diabetes management plan. Keep these items in a special bag that you don't have to pack and re-pack every time you go out.

- **Tell Your Coaches:** Be sure that your coaches know about your diabetes. Tell them about the things you need to do to control diabetes that might happen before, during, or after a game.

- **Take Control:** Don't hesitate to stop playing or take a break in your exercise routine if you need to eat a snack, drink water, or go to the bathroom. You should also take a break if you feel any signs that something is wrong.

What To Watch For

Your doctor will help you learn what blood sugar levels make it a good or bad time to exercise. He or she will also explain how to take action and get back in the game. If you notice any of the signs listed below, stop exercising and follow your diabetes management plan.

You may have low blood sugar if you are:

- sweating
- lightheaded
- shaky
- weak
- anxious
- hungry
- having a headache
- having problems concentrating
- confused

You may have high blood sugar if you:

- feel very thirsty
- have to pee a lot
- feel very tired
- have blurry vision

Also, keep an eye on any cuts, scrapes, or blisters, and talk to your doctor if they're really red, swollen, or are oozing pus—these could be signs of infection.

By being prepared and knowing how to follow your diabetes management plan, you'll be able to prevent diabetes problems during exercise. After all, professional athletes follow a training and nutrition program to keep them playing their best—just think of your diabetes management plan as your own personal roadmap to exercise success.

Chapter 30

Stay At A Healthy Weight

Tips For Staying At A Healthy Weight

Why is it good to be at a healthy weight?

Staying at a healthy weight as a teen may help you control your weight for life. Being at a healthy weight helps you feel fit, stay well, and feel good about the way you look. It can also help prevent health problems like heart disease and high blood pressure. If you have diabetes and are overweight, weight loss may improve your blood glucose, also called blood sugar, and make your diabetes easier to manage.

How can I get to a healthy weight?

If your doctor says that you should not gain more weight or that you should lose weight, you need to get more physical activity every day and eat fewer calories. Ask a dietitian or diabetes educator to help you decide what kinds of activities might fit into your busy life as a teen and help you and your family create a well-balanced meal plan and make healthy food choices.

Here are some things to try:

Be active every day for at least 60 minutes. This will help you burn up extra calories and get fit. Invite some friends over to dance to your favorite music. Play a sport or go for a bike ride instead of playing computer games or going to the movies. Ask a friend or family member to join you on a walk instead of watching TV after school.

About This Chapter: This chapter begins with information from "Tips for Teens with Diabetes: Stay at a Healthy Weight," National Diabetes Education Program (NDEP), November 1, 2007. It continues with "Weight-Loss and Nutrition Myths," Weight-control Information Network (WIN), a service of the National Institute of Diabetes and Digestive and Kidney Diseases, March 2009.

Cut some calories. The number of calories shows how much energy a food supplies. Calories that are not used up are stored as body fat. Calories are listed on food labels. Get in the habit of reading food labels. If you cut 100 to 200 calories a day, it can make a big difference. Here are some suggestions for things you can do and how many calories you could cut:

- Drink water instead of regular soda or a sweetened fruit drink: cut 150 calories
- Eat a piece of fruit instead of a candy bar or a bag of chips: cut 200 calories
- Eat a small serving of french fries or share a big one: cut 250 calories
- Eat one half cup of sugar-free, nonfat pudding instead of regular ice cream: cut 150 calories

Eat smaller amounts of food for meals and snacks. Try raw vegetables or fruit for a snack. To avoid "grazing," measure out your snacks for the day into baggies that are easy to carry.

If you eat less and are more physically active, you should lose about one or two pounds a month—and feel great. It is best to lose weight a little at a time because you are still growing. If you lose weight slowly, you are more likely to keep it off.

What are some healthy eating tips I can try?

- Take your time when you eat. It takes about 15 minutes for your stomach to tell your brain that you are full. So, wait 15 minutes before eating second helpings.

- Ask if you can help plan, make, or shop for the family meals sometimes.

- Drink a glass of water before you eat.

- Fill up half of your plate with salad or vegetables. Use small amounts of low-fat salad dressing, mayonnaise, or margarine.

- If you like to eat sugary foods, sweets, desserts, or candy, eat only a small serving at the end of a meal and not every day, then take an extra walk. The less you eat them, the less you may crave them!

Very low-calorie diets are not healthy for teens. If you do not eat enough of the right kinds of food, you may not grow or develop properly. Never make a drastic change in what you eat without talking with your dietitian or doctor. They can help you determine the right amounts of food to keep you healthy and happy.

What about breakfast?

Breakfast is a great way to start your day. It will help you focus and pay attention in school throughout the day.

- Have one bowl of whole grain cereal with nonfat or low-fat milk or yogurt and a piece of fruit.

- When you do not have much time, try a couple of whole grain crackers or slices of bread with a tablespoon of natural peanut butter, a hard-boiled egg, or a piece of low-fat cheese, along with a glass of nonfat or low-fat milk.

What about school lunches?

If you buy your lunch at school, try to steer clear of fried foods. Choose items such as the following:

- Small deli sandwiches or subs made with lean turkey, chicken without the skin, or beef with mustard or a little low-fat mayonnaise
- Nonfat or low-fat milk instead of chocolate milk
- A piece of fresh fruit instead of cookies or cake

If there is a salad bar, choose a variety of fresh vegetables and fruits. Use a small amount of low-calorie dressing.

Pack lunch at home the night before to save time. Use leftovers from dinner. Make a tuna sandwich. Add raw carrots and a piece of fruit.

Can I still have a snack?

Most teens need a snack after school. The trick is not eating too much. Use a small plate or bowl for your snack to help you control the portion size. It is best not to snack while watching TV or at the computer—it is easy to lose track and eat too much.

Here are some healthy snack ideas:

- A piece of fresh fruit
- A cup of veggies served with some salsa or a little low-fat salad dressing
- A small bowl of whole grain cereal with nonfat or low-fat milk
- A small bowl of vegetable soup and a few crackers
- One small tortilla with one or two slices of low-fat cheese or turkey
- Three cups of low-fat microwave popcorn or a single serving bag
- One handful of pretzels or crackers
- Drink a couple of glasses of water with your snack

Can I eat at fast-food restaurants?

Sure, but not every day. When you do, try these ideas:

- Don't "super-size" it! Order smaller, kid-sized meals and drink water or nonfat or low-fat milk. Share a larger meal with a friend.

- Choose a grilled chicken sandwich or a simple hamburger rather than a burger covered with sauce, cheese, and bacon. Add a small baked potato with a little butter or sour cream or a small serving of fries.

- If you are eating pizza, order thin or medium crust instead of deep dish or stuffed crust. Eat only one or two slices of plain cheese or vegetable pizza. Add a salad with a little low-fat dressing.

- Try a small bag or a handful of baked chips or pretzels instead of regular chips.

> **Remember**
>
> Reaching and staying at a healthy weight while you are a teen helps you stay fit as you get older. Encourage family members and friends to get fit too by making healthy food choices and joining you in physical activity.
>
> Source: NDEP, November 1, 2007.

Weight-Loss And Nutrition Myths

Myth: Fad diets work for permanent weight loss.

Fact: Fad diets are not the best way to lose weight and keep it off. Fad diets often promise quick weight loss or tell you to cut certain foods out of your diet. You may lose weight at first on one of these diets. But diets that strictly limit calories or food choices are hard to follow. Most people quickly get tired of them and regain any lost weight.

Fad diets may be unhealthy because they may not provide all of the nutrients your body needs. Also, losing weight at a very rapid rate (more than three pounds a week after the first couple of weeks) may increase your risk for developing gallstones (clusters of solid material in the gallbladder that can be painful). Diets that provide less than 800 calories per day also could result in heart rhythm abnormalities, which can be fatal.

Research suggests that losing one-half to two pounds a week by making healthy food choices, eating moderate portions, and building physical activity into your daily life is the best way to lose weight and keep it off. By adopting healthy eating and physical activity habits, you may also lower your risk for developing type 2 diabetes, heart disease, and high blood pressure.

Myth: High-protein/low-carbohydrate diets are a healthy way to lose weight.

Fact: The long-term health effects of a high-protein/low-carbohydrate diet are unknown. But getting most of your daily calories from high-protein foods like meat, eggs, and cheese is not a balanced eating plan. You may be eating too much fat and cholesterol, which may raise heart disease risk. You may be eating too few fruits, vegetables, and whole grains, which may lead to constipation due to lack of dietary fiber. Following a high-protein/low-carbohydrate diet may also make you feel nauseous, tired, and weak.

Eating fewer than 130 grams of carbohydrate a day can lead to the buildup of ketones in your blood. Ketones are partially broken-down fats. A buildup of these in your blood (called ketosis) can cause your body to produce high levels of uric acid, which is a risk factor for gout (a painful swelling of the joints) and kidney stones. Ketosis may be especially risky for pregnant women and people with diabetes or kidney disease. Be sure to discuss any changes in your diet with a health care professional, especially if you have health conditions such as cardiovascular disease, kidney disease, or type 2 diabetes.

High-protein/low-carbohydrate diets are often low in calories because food choices are strictly limited, so they may cause short-term weight loss. But a reduced-calorie eating plan that includes recommended amounts of carbohydrate, protein, and fat will also allow you to lose weight. By following a balanced eating plan, you will not have to stop eating whole classes of foods, such as whole grains, fruits, and vegetables—and miss the key nutrients they contain. You may also find it easier to stick with a diet or eating plan that includes a greater variety of foods.

Check It Out

- "Lose 30 pounds in 30 days!"
- "Eat as much as you want and still lose weight."
- "Try the thigh buster and lose inches fast."

And so on, and so on. With so many products and weight-loss theories out there, it is easy to get confused.

If you do not know whether or not to believe a weight-loss or nutrition claim, check it out! The Federal Trade Commission has information on deceptive weight-loss advertising claims. You can find this online at http://www.ftc.com or call 877-FTC-HELP (877-382-4357). You can also find out more about nutrition and weight loss by talking with a registered dietitian. To find a registered dietitian in your area, visit the American Dietetic Association online (http://www.eatright.org) or call 800-877-1600.

Source: WIN, March 2009.

Myth: Starches are fattening and should be limited when trying to lose weight.

Fact: Many foods high in starch, like bread, rice, pasta, cereals, beans, fruits, and some vegetables (like potatoes and yams) are low in fat and calories. They become high in fat and calories when eaten in large portion sizes or when covered with high-fat toppings like butter, sour cream, or mayonnaise. Foods high in starch (also called complex carbohydrates) are an important source of energy for your body.

A healthy eating plan is one that emphasizes fruits, vegetables, whole grains, and fat-free or low-fat milk and milk products. It also includes lean meats, poultry, fish, beans, eggs, and nuts and is low in saturated fats, trans fat, cholesterol, salt (sodium), and added sugars.

Myth: Certain foods, like grapefruit, celery, or cabbage soup, can burn fat and make you lose weight.

Fact: No foods can burn fat. Some foods with caffeine may speed up your metabolism (the way your body uses energy, or calories) for a short time, but they do not cause weight loss.

The best way to lose weight is to cut back on the number of calories you eat and be more physically active.

Myth: Natural or herbal weight-loss products are safe and effective.

Fact: A weight-loss product that claims to be "natural" or "herbal" is not necessarily safe. These products are not usually scientifically tested to prove that they are safe or that they work. For example, herbal products containing ephedra (now banned by the U.S. government) have caused serious health problems and even death. Newer products that claim to be ephedra-free are not necessarily danger-free, because they may contain ingredients similar to ephedra.

Talk with your health care provider before using any weight-loss product. Some natural or herbal weight-loss products can be harmful.

Myth: I can "lose weight while eating whatever I want."

Fact: To lose weight, you need to use more calories than you eat. It is possible to eat any kind of food you want and lose weight. You need to limit the number of calories you eat every day and/or increase your daily physical activity. Portion control is the key. Try eating smaller amounts of food and choosing foods that are low in calories.

When trying to lose weight, you can still eat your favorite foods—as long as you pay attention to the total number of calories that you eat.

Dieting Is Not The Answer

The best way to lose weight is to eat healthfully and be physically active. It is a good idea to talk with your health care provider if you want to lose weight.

Many teens turn to unhealthy dieting methods to lose weight, including eating very little, cutting out whole groups of foods (like grain products), skipping meals, and fasting. These methods can leave out important foods you need to grow. Other weight-loss tactics such as smoking, self-induced vomiting, or using diet pills or laxatives can lead to health problems.

In fact, unhealthy dieting can actually cause you to gain more weight because it often leads to a cycle of eating very little, then overeating or binge eating. Also, unhealthy dieting can put you at greater risk for growth and emotional problems.

Source: Excerpted from "Take Charge of Your Health," Weight-control Information Network, August 9, 2011.

Myth: Low-fat or fat-free means no calories.

Fact: A low-fat or fat-free food is often lower in calories than the same size portion of the full-fat product. But many processed low-fat or fat-free foods have just as many calories as the full-fat versions of the same foods—or even more calories. They may contain added sugar, flour, or starch thickeners to improve flavor and texture after fat is removed. These ingredients add calories.

Read the Nutrition Facts on a food package to find out how many calories are in a serving. Check the serving size too—it may be less than you are used to eating. For more information about reading food labels, visit the U.S. Food and Drug Administration online at http://www .cfsan.fda.gov/~dms/foodlab.html.

Calories Always Count

Many food labels say "low-fat," "reduced fat," or "light." That does not always mean the food is low in calories. Sometimes fat-free or low-fat muffins or desserts have even more sugar than the full-fat versions. Remember, fat-free does not mean calorie-free, and calories do count!

Source: "Celebrate the Beauty of Youth," Weight-control Information Network, September 2008.

Myth: Fast foods are always an unhealthy choice and you should not eat them when dieting.

Fact: Fast foods can be part of a healthy weight-loss program with a little bit of know-how. Avoid supersized combo meals, or split one with a friend. Sip on water or fat-free milk instead of soda. Choose salads and grilled foods, like a grilled chicken breast sandwich or small hamburger. Try a "fresco" taco (with salsa instead of cheese or sauce) at taco stands. Fried foods, like french fries and fried chicken, are high in fat and calories, so order them only once in a while, order a small portion, or split an order with a friend. Also, use only small amounts of high-fat, high-calorie toppings, like regular mayonnaise, salad dressings, bacon, and cheese.

Myth: Skipping meals is a good way to lose weight.

Fact: Studies show that people who skip breakfast and eat fewer times during the day tend to be heavier than people who eat a healthy breakfast and eat four or five times a day. This may be because people who skip meals tend to feel hungrier later on, and eat more than they normally would. It may also be that eating many small meals throughout the day helps people control their appetites.

Eat small meals throughout the day that include a variety of healthy, low-fat, low-calorie foods.

Out 'N' About

You can hang out with your friends and still make healthy food choices. Try these tips when you are out 'n' about:

- Encourage your friends to make healthy choices with you. If you are all on the same page, it might be easier for you—and your friends—to avoid temptation.
- Order vegetable toppings on pizza instead of salty, high-fat meats like pepperoni or sausage.
- Share popcorn (and skip the added butter) at the movies instead of getting your own bag, or order the smallest size. You will save money too!
- Choose bottled water instead of soda and other artificially sweetened beverages like punch or natural fruit juices.
- Munch on pretzels or vegetables at parties instead of fried chips or fatty dips.

Source: "Celebrate the Beauty of Youth," Weight-control Information Network, September 2008.

Myth: Eating after 8 p.m. causes weight gain.

Fact: It does not matter what time of day you eat. It is what and how much you eat and how much physical activity you do during the whole day that determines whether you gain, lose, or maintain your weight. No matter when you eat, your body will store extra calories as fat.

If you want to have a snack before bedtime, think first about how many calories you have eaten that day. And try to avoid snacking in front of the TV at night—it may be easier to overeat when you are distracted by the television.

Myth: Nuts are fattening and you should not eat them if you want to lose weight.

Fact: In small amounts, nuts can be part of a healthy weight-loss program. Nuts are high in calories and fat. However, most nuts contain healthy fats that do not clog arteries. Nuts are also good sources of protein, dietary fiber, and minerals including magnesium and copper.

Enjoy small portions of nuts. One-half ounce of mixed nuts has about 84 calories.

Myth: Eating red meat is bad for your health and makes it harder to lose weight.

Fact: Eating lean meat in small amounts can be part of a healthy weight-loss plan. Red meat, pork, chicken, and fish contain some cholesterol and saturated fat (the least healthy kind of fat). They also contain healthy nutrients like protein, iron, and zinc.

Choose cuts of meat that are lower in fat and trim all visible fat. Lower fat meats include pork tenderloin and beef round steak, tenderloin, sirloin tip, flank steak, and extra lean ground beef. Also, pay attention to portion size. Three ounces of meat or poultry is the size of a deck of cards.

Myth: Dairy products are fattening and unhealthy.

Fact: Low-fat and fat-free milk, yogurt, and cheese are just as nutritious as whole-milk dairy products, but they are lower in fat and calories. Dairy products have many nutrients your body needs. They offer protein to build muscles and help organs work properly, and calcium to strengthen bones. Most milk and some yogurt are fortified with vitamin D to help your body use calcium. The *Dietary Guidelines for Americans* recommends consuming three cups per day of fat-free/low-fat milk or equivalent milk products.

If you cannot digest lactose (the sugar found in dairy products), choose low-lactose or lactose-free dairy products, or other foods and beverages that offer calcium and vitamin D (listed below).

- **Calcium:** Soy-based beverage or tofu made with calcium sulfate; canned salmon; dark leafy greens like collards or kale

- **Vitamin D:** Soy-based beverage or cereal (getting some sunlight on your skin also gives you a small amount of vitamin D)

Myth: "Going vegetarian" means you are sure to lose weight and be healthier.

Fact: Research shows that people who follow a vegetarian eating plan, on average, eat fewer calories and less fat than nonvegetarians. They also tend to have lower body weights relative to their heights than nonvegetarians. Choosing a vegetarian eating plan with a low fat content may be helpful for weight loss. But vegetarians—like nonvegetarians—can make food choices that contribute to weight gain, like eating large amounts of high-fat, high-calorie foods or foods with little or no nutritional value.

Vegetarian diets should be as carefully planned as nonvegetarian diets to make sure they are balanced. Nutrients that nonvegetarians normally get from animal products, but that are not always found in a vegetarian eating plan, are iron, calcium, vitamin D, vitamin B12, zinc, and protein.

Choose a vegetarian eating plan that is low in fat and that provides all of the nutrients your body needs. Food and beverage sources of nutrients that may be lacking in a vegetarian diet are listed below.

- **Iron:** Cashews, spinach, lentils, garbanzo beans, fortified bread or cereal

- **Calcium:** Dairy products, fortified soy-based beverages, tofu made with calcium sulfate, collard greens, kale, broccoli

- **Vitamin D:** Fortified foods and beverages including milk, soy-based beverages, or cereal

- **Vitamin B12:** Eggs, dairy products, fortified cereal or soy-based beverages, tempeh, miso (tempeh and miso are foods made from soybeans)

- **Zinc:** Whole grains (especially the germ and bran of the grain), nuts, tofu, leafy vegetables (spinach, cabbage, lettuce)

- **Protein:** Eggs, dairy products, beans, peas, nuts, seeds, tofu, tempeh, soy-based burgers

Myth: Lifting weights is not good to do if you want to lose weight, because it will make you "bulk up."

Fact: Lifting weights or doing strengthening activities like push-ups and crunches on a regular basis can actually help you maintain or lose weight. These activities can help you build muscle, and muscle burns more calories than body fat. So if you have more muscle, you burn more calories—even sitting still. Doing strengthening activities two or three days a week will not "bulk you up." Only intense strength training, combined with a certain genetic background, can build very large muscles.

In addition to doing moderate-intensity physical activity (like walking two miles in 30 minutes) on most days of the week, try to do strengthening activities two to three days a week. You can lift weights, use large rubber bands (resistance bands), do push-ups or sit-ups, or do household or garden tasks that make you lift or dig. Strength training helps keep your bones strong while building muscle, which can help burn calories.

Tips On Moving More

Physical activity can be fun! Do things you enjoy:

- Dancing
- In-line skating
- Fast walking
- Playing sports
- Bicycling
- Swimming
- Group fitness classes, such as dance or aerobics

If you can, be physically active with a friend or a group. That way, you can cheer each other on, have a good time while being active, and feel safer when you are outdoors. Find a local school track or park where you can walk or run with your friends, or join a recreation center so you can work out or take a fun fitness class together.

Source: "Celebrate the Beauty of Youth," Weight-control Information Network, September 2008.

Part Four
Mental Health And Lifestyle Issues

Chapter 31

Diabetes And Your Feelings

Are you asking yourself, "Why me?" Getting used to living with diabetes can be a challenge, and that's true whether you've just been diagnosed or you've lived with diabetes for a while.

If You've Just Been Diagnosed

When people are first diagnosed with diabetes, they might be nervous about getting shots or medical tests and scared about how diabetes will affect their future health.

In the beginning, almost everyone thinks that they will never be able to do the blood sugar testing or insulin injections they need to stay healthy. But after working with doctors and learning more about diabetes, these things start feeling like less of a big deal. Over time, shots and checks can become like brushing teeth or taking a shower—just another daily routine you do to stay healthy. Eventually, some people even start to feel pretty good about the fact that they can do all the things they need to do to manage their diabetes on their own.

It's perfectly normal for people with diabetes to feel sad, angry, confused, upset, alone, embarrassed, and even jealous. It's common to think things like:

- "I feel embarrassed giving myself shots in front of people. One day I had to give myself an insulin shot in the bathroom at the train station and this guy looked at me like I was doing drugs. That felt humiliating."
- "Why do I have to go through this when my friends don't have to follow a meal plan, test their blood sugar levels, or have shots all the time?"

"Diabetes: Dealing With Feelings," August 2010, reprinted with permission from www.kidshealth.org. Copyright © 2010 The Nemours Foundation. This information was provided by KidsHealth, one of the largest resources online for medically reviewed health information written for parents, kids, and teens. For more articles like this one, visit www.KidsHealth.org, or www.TeensHealth.org.

- "I worry that I'm a burden on my family. I feel guilty that my dad has drive me to doctor's appointments and pay for it all."

- "I get angry at my mom. I know she worries about me, but she's always nagging me about what I eat and stuff. My kid sister has it easy."

- "Sometimes I feel like I must have done something bad to deserve this."

Dealing With Your Feelings

Here are a few things you can do to cope with the emotional side of diabetes:

Open up to people you trust. If you feel sad, mad, embarrassed, or worried, talk about it with a close friend, parent, or doctor. It might be hard at first to open up, and you may have trouble finding the words to talk about it. Try to name your feelings and say what's got you feeling that way. Many times, just telling someone who will listen and understand your feelings can lighten a difficult emotion and help it to pass. Make it a regular habit to talk about what you're going through with someone close to you. As time goes on, be sure to notice and talk about the positive feelings, too. With time, you may notice that you're feeling more calm and confident, or that you're proud of what you're learning to do.

Get more support if you need it. If you're having a really tough time, or if you think you may be depressed, let an adult know. (Some signs that it might be depression are you're sleeping or eating all the time or not at all, or you feel sad or angry for long periods.) Sometimes people need the added support and care of a counselor or a mental health professional. Your doctor, parent, or another trusted adult can put you in touch with a counselor or other mental health professional who works with teens that have diabetes. Get all the support you need and deserve.

Learn how to take care of yourself. When you take good care of yourself and manage your diabetes, you will probably get sick less often, need fewer extra shots or tests, and be able to do the same activities as everyone else. When you can participate and feel well enough to get exercise (which is a great mood booster), you'll feel better, too.

If you're ready to take charge of tracking your blood sugar levels, adjusting and taking your insulin injections, and taking responsibility for preparing your meals and snacks, talk to your parents and doctor about how you can start making these changes. Again, taking charge of these practical tasks can give you more of a sense of control and power over diabetes. You might begin to feel proud—even amazed—that you're doing things you didn't think you'd be able to do.

Tell your teachers about your diabetes. Telling your teachers that you have diabetes can make things a little easier for you at school—for example, you might tell your teacher that you need to check your blood sugar level or have a snack at a certain time each day. That way you can just leave class without drawing extra attention to yourself. By knowing you have diabetes, your teacher also can be on the lookout for symptoms of diabetes problems and can call for medical help if you need it.

If you're not sure how to bring it up on your own or don't know what to say, ask your doctor to give you a note that covers the basics for your teacher. That can get the conversation started.

Get organized. There can be a lot to keep track of if you have diabetes. How much insulin did you take this morning? What did you eat at school? Did you pack your medicines? Getting organized can help you feel less worried about how diabetes will affect your health. Every night before going to school or work, check to make sure you have the snacks and medicines you'll need for the next day. You'll begin to feel prepared and in charge.

Focus on your strengths. It's easy to get lost in all the negative ways diabetes affects your world. If you feel like it's taking over your life, it can help to write down your strengths—and the stuff you love. Who are you? Are you a reader, a hockey player, a music lover, a math whiz, a spelling champ? Are you a son or daughter, a sister or brother, a grandchild, student, friend, babysitter? Are you a future astronomer, teacher, doctor, or poet? Diabetes is really only a small part of who you are. Keep track of your dreams and hopes, and find time for the people and things you enjoy.

Stick to the plan. Many people with diabetes get sick of dealing with it once in a while. And sometimes people who have learned to manage their illness feel so healthy and strong that they wonder whether they need to keep following their diabetes management plan. For example, you might wonder whether you can skip a meal when you're at the mall or check your blood sugar after the game instead of before. But skipping medicines, veering off the meal plan, or not checking your blood sugar can have disastrous results if you have diabetes. If you feel like throwing in the towel, talk to your doctor. Together you can find solutions that fit your life and help you stay healthy, too.

Take Your Time

Your feelings about diabetes will change over time—today you might feel worried about the future and different from your friends, but next year you might wonder why you were so upset. As you learn to manage diabetes on your own and take a more active role in your health, you may find it's a little easier dealing with the ups and downs.

Your Family's Feelings

Just as you can get emotional about your diabetes, so can parents and other family members. Seeing a parent get upset can be hard. It can help to remind yourself that the diabetes is not your fault, nor is it your parents' fault. Just as you feel upset from time to time, it's natural for your parents to feel that way, too.

When a parent or other family member is worried, it may show up in strange ways. For example, a parent may get angry at a doctor. Or your mom or dad may constantly ask how you feel, whether you're eating right, and whether you've taken your medication. Sure, you understand that they are doing this because they love you. But it can help to explain how this makes you feel. Find a good time to talk about it calmly and openly. Sometimes family counseling or joining a family support group can help families work through the emotional ups and downs of dealing with diabetes.

Other family members like grandparents, aunts, and uncles may also want to know if you're feeling OK—and all this attention can feel like prying or nosiness, especially when you just want to be treated like everyone else. If you're close to the person, you may be able to talk to him or her about how you feel. If not, you may just have to let it go and realize that your relative is trying to show concern; even if it's done clumsily, it's an expression of caring.

You may envy a brother or sister who doesn't have diabetes, but your sibling may feel envious of you because of the extra attention you're getting. Again, it can help to talk about this openly—and recognize that your sibling's feelings might show up in strange ways, such as anger at you.

Your Friends

It's up to you whether you tell friends or classmates about your diabetes. For some people, opening up can help them feel less embarrassed. They don't have to worry what friends think when they see them doing things to take care of the diabetes—like checking blood sugar levels or wearing an insulin pump.

If you choose to tell your friends, be prepared for them to ask questions about what having diabetes means and how it makes you feel. Some of their questions may seem silly or funny to you. But ultimately, friends who know about your health problem can be a source of support as you deal with your feelings about diabetes. Having friends who are willing to listen when you're depressed, angry, and frustrated—even if they don't have diabetes themselves—can definitely help you feel better.

It's wise to be aware of how friends and family feel, but your first priority is dealing with your own emotions. The teen years can be an emotionally tough time to start with—hormones can put anyone's emotions on a roller-coaster—without adding a health condition to the mix.

It's only human to let off some steam if you're going through a difficult adjustment—like dealing with diabetes—and the strong feelings that go with it. But if you find your emotions are getting the best of you, if you're feeling really down or really angry, or if you're having a tough time managing your health routines, let your doctor know. Together you can work out a plan for getting you situation under control.

It can take a long time to deal with having diabetes and there's no set adjustment period—some people accept it and adapt quickly whereas others need more time. One thing's for sure, though: Even people who have lived with the condition for a while can still experience strong emotions, such as fear or sadness, from time to time or when faced with new situations. It's normal to feel overwhelmed occasionally.

Positive emotions can be part of the adjustment process, too. Don't be surprised if, as you adapt to your diabetes, you find yourself feeling proud, confident, determined, hopeful, interested, relieved, relaxed, loved, supported, strong—and yes, even happy.

In time, you can become an expert at recognizing and dealing with your emotions, and doing your part to care for your health. In fact, having diabetes might even teach you ways to cope with and adjust to life's challenges in a way that many teens can't.

Chapter 32

Tips For Handling The Ups And Downs Of Diabetes

Feelings

Many teens like you deal with diabetes everyday. Most of the time, it's not a problem, you just deal with it. But sometimes, you may just want it to go away.

Do you ever ask "why me?" Do you ever think you're the only one who feels sad, mad, alone, afraid, or different? Do you get tired of others teasing you if you are overweight? Or do you ever blame yourself or your family for your diabetes?

All of these feelings are normal. Lots of teens who have diabetes feel the same way. It's okay to get angry, feel sad, or think you're different every now and then. But then you need to take charge and do something to feel better.

Everyone feels down sometimes. You are not alone.

Still Down?

Reach out for help. Talk to someone in your family or where you worship, a friend, a school counselor, teacher, or your doctor or diabetes educator. It might help to write down your feelings in a journal. If you still feel down or sad, ask your parents to help you find a counselor. It is okay to ask for help.

Speak Up

There are many people who care about you and want to help you stay healthy and happy. Your health care team (diabetes educator, dietitian, doctor, nurse, psychologist, and social worker)

About This chapter: From "Tips for Teens with Diabetes: Dealing with the Ups and Downs of Diabetes," National Diabetes Education Program, November 1, 2007.

can help you learn how to make healthy food choices, be more active, and feel good about yourself. Stay in touch with them. Let your health care team know how you feel and what you need.

Remember to also let your school know what's up. You or your parents need to give the school nurse, teacher, or other school staff a copy of your diabetes care plan. Let people at your school know you have diabetes and that you need to eat healthy foods, eat your meals, take your medicine on time, and be physically active.

Don't let diabetes stop you from joining in school activities. You can do all the things your friends do and then some!

Family Members

It's easier to manage diabetes when the whole family works at it with you. So, ask your family to choose the same healthy foods you eat—fruits and vegetables; whole grain breads; and low-fat meats, milk, and cheese. Ask them to keep healthy foods in the house and not tempt you with cookies, cake, candy, or regular soda.

Get everyone moving by being more physically active. Play hard. Shoot hoops, throw a ball, ride bikes, or go for a walk—together. Being active can also help you relax and lower stress. What's healthy for you is healthy for everyone in your family.

Other Teens

Want to meet other teens who feel like you do?

- Programs and support groups for teens with diabetes can be found in clinics, health centers, or hospitals. Ask your diabetes educator or doctor for help to find one that works for you.

True Or False?

Nobody wants to hear about your problems. When you are feeling down, you should keep it to yourself.

FALSE. You need to talk about your emotions with friends, family, or your healthcare provider. Sometimes just talking about a problem will help you solve it...and loved ones can help you gain perspective.

Source: From "Healthy Coping," © 2009. Reprinted with permission of the American Association of Diabetes Educators. All Rights Reserved. May not be reproduced or distributed without the written approval of AADE.

Did You Know?

Physical activity can influence your mood. If you are sad, anxious, stressed or upset, go for a walk, stand up and stretch, or take a bicycle ride. Exercise actually increases the chemicals in your brain that help make you feel good!

Source: From "Healthy Coping," © 2009. Reprinted with permission of the American Association of Diabetes Educators. All Rights Reserved. May not be reproduced or distributed without the written approval of AADE.

- Head to a diabetes or weight loss summer camp. You will do all the things that other campers do: swim, hike, dance, and more. But the best part is that everyone has diabetes or is there to lose weight, just like you. Some groups may have funds to help pay for teens to attend summer camps.

- Find a pen pal or e-mail buddy. Sometimes it is good to share how you feel about having diabetes with someone else.

Friends

Ever worry that your friends may have wrong ideas about diabetes? Tell them that you have diabetes. You don't have to keep it to yourself. The more people know about diabetes, the more they will understand. Explain that your body needs help to use the food you eat. Be sure everyone knows that no one can catch diabetes from you.

Good friends help each other out. They understand your needs and offer support. Hang on to friends who help you make healthy food choices when you are eating out.

Ever have kids make fun of you about your diabetes or weight? Teasing hurts. The best thing is to just walk away. Talk to someone, write down your feelings in a journal, write to a pen pal, e-mail a buddy, stay in touch with people who support you.

Take Action

It's time for YOU to do something about your diabetes care.

Set goals for what you will do. Start small and work your way up. For example: "I will cut down on regular soda and drink water instead." When that's going well, take the next step. Add another goal, such as "I will dance or bike ride a couple of times a week." Then add a new goal: "I will eat smaller servings of cookies, burgers, and fries." Try to make each new goal just a bit harder. After you shoot hoops twice a week, try adding another activity on three other days. Raise the goal until you reach a level that works for you.

Avoid goals that will be too hard to meet. For example, rather than saying you'll never eat a burger or a candy bar again, say you'll only eat one a week. Tell your family or friends about your goals. Maybe they'll be active with you or help out some other way.

Reward yourself when you reach each goal. Keep in mind that rewards can be anything—not just food. You do not have to reach all your goals at once. Start with one or two, then add more.

Write down your top three goals. Be sure to choose goals that you really can meet. Record in the date when you set the goal and when you met it.

Take it one step at a time. Make healthy food choices, be more active, and work towards a healthy weight. Soon you'll see progress and feel great.

Chapter 33

The Link Between Diabetes And Depression

A key report demonstrated that people with diabetes have at least twice the risk of developing depression compared to those without diabetes.[1] It is also thought that depression increases the risk of developing type 2 diabetes.[2] The most recent research on diabetes and depression indicates that having both these conditions increases the risk of developing diabetes complications, such as cardiovascular disease. Depression can also have a significant effect on blood glucose control, diabetes self-management, and overall quality of life. People with diabetes and depression are also more likely to die at an early age.

Furthermore, clinical depression may recur more frequently, episodes may last longer, and the long-term recovery rate may be much lower. A recent international report has clearly shown that the co-existence of diabetes and depression has the greatest negative impact on quality of life compared to diabetes or depression alone, or other chronic conditions.[3]

Depression may be linked to blood glucose control either through hormonal dysregulation, or—more likely—via its negative effects on diabetes self-care behavior, which include provoking low levels of physical activity, increased smoking and alcohol intake, and poor blood glucose monitoring. Recent evidence has also shown an association between depression and increased risk of weight gain and obesity.

These stark statistics, and the concerns for the mental well-being of people with diabetes, have led to national and international guidelines for detecting depression and recommendations for its care and treatment. For example, the International Diabetes Federation has published guidelines for the care of people with type 2 diabetes which include the assessment of psychological status and referral to mental healthcare professionals.[4]

About This Chapter: Text in this chapter is from "The effects of diabetes on depression and depression on diabetes," by Cathy Lloyd, in *DiabetesVoice*, March 2008, Volume 53, Issue 1. © 2008 International Diabetes Federation (www.diabetesvoice.org); reprinted with permission.

Defining Depression

Depression is usually defined by the number of symptoms found: in order to diagnose a person with major depression, a clinical interview is conducted and a number of symptoms have to be present. The *Diagnostic and Statistical Manual of Mental Disorders, 4th edition*[5] lists clear criteria for diagnosing depression (see Table 33.1).

In many clinical settings, and when researching the prevalence of depression in large-scale studies, a range of different self-reported instruments are used for detecting depression or depressive symptoms. Factors such as time and training often militate against the use of clinical diagnostic interviews. Depressive symptoms (Table 33.2) and clinical depression are not mutually exclusive in terms of criteria; most instruments that are used measure symptoms that approximate clinical levels of depression.[5]

Whether psychological distress increases the risk of developing diabetes and/or its complications, whether diabetes and/or diabetes complications increase the risk of depression, or whether these two are merely coincidental, they have serious consequences for both people with diabetes and the healthcare providers involved in their care. However, despite its higher prevalence, depression in people with diabetes seems poorly recognized. One recent estimate suggests that more than three-quarters of cases may go undetected.[6] It may be that there is both under-reporting and under-diagnosis of depressive symptoms in people with diabetes because psychological problems are often seen as secondary to diabetes by both the affected person and the healthcare provider.

Table 33.1. Criteria For Diagnosing Depression[5]

At least five symptoms present nearly every day for two weeks, including:

- Depressed mood
- Diminished interest in daily activities
- Significant weight loss/gain or decreased appetite
- Insomnia or hypersomnia
- Psychomotor agitation or retardation
- Fatigue or loss of energy
- Feelings of worthlessness/guilt
- Diminished ability to concentrate/make decisions
- Recurrent thoughts of death or suicide

Table 33.2. Depressive Symptoms—Often Measured Using Self-Report Instruments

- Feeling sad/depressed mood
- Inability to sleep
- Early waking
- Lack of interest/enjoyment
- Tiredness/lack of energy
- Loss of appetite
- Feelings of guilt/worthlessness
- Recurrent thoughts about death/suicide

Treatment

Some people with diabetes suffer from clinically recognized levels of depression; others may experience low levels of mood disturbance, or mild depressive symptoms. While literature on the treatment of depression in people with diabetes is still scarce, there is evidence that cognitive behavior therapy and anti-depressant medication are as effective in those with diabetes as in those without the condition, and have additional beneficial effects on blood glucose control. A recent study found that improved diabetes control during depression treatment was associated with improvements in mood and body mass index. In the longer term, improved self-care also had an important role to play.[9]

Summary

While depression is significantly more common in people with diabetes compared to those without diabetes, it can be treated effectively. Depression increases the risk of developing diabetes, impacts on blood glucose control, and increases the risk of developing diabetes complications. It is associated with increased body weight or obesity, and poorer diabetes self-management. It is important to recognize that although diabetes and depression are separate conditions they often co-exist and any treatment offered must reflect this in order to maximize the benefits to the person with diabetes. Recent studies have demonstrated the positive effects of treatment for depression on diabetes outcomes as well as quality of life.

Recently, there has been a surge of interest in psychological and psychosocial aspects of chronic disease management, and research in depression and diabetes has gained greater recognition. This has been in light of evidence of the serious impact of psychological problems on people with chronic conditions such as diabetes, their impact on day-to-day living, and the high costs to both the individual and society.

References

1. Anderson RJ, Freedland KE, Clouse RE, Lustman PJ. The prevalence of co-morbid depression in adults with diabetes. *Diabetes Care* 2001; 24: 1069-78.

2. Knol MJ, Twisk JWR, Beekman ATF, et al. Depression as a risk factor for the onset of type 2 diabetes mellitus. A meta-analysis. *Diabetologia* 2006; 49: 837-45.

3. Moussavi S, Chatterji S, Verdes E, et al. Depression, chronic disease, and decrements in health: results from the World Health Surveys. *Lancet* 2007; 370: 851-8.

4. International Diabetes Federation Clinical Guidelines Task Force. *Global guideline for type 2 diabetes*. IDF. Brussels, 2005.

5. American Psychiatric Association. *Diagnostic and Statistical Manual of Mental Disorders, 4th Edition*. American Psychiatric Association. Arlington, 2000.

6. Hermanns N, Kulzer B, Krichbaum M, et al. How to screen for depression and emotional problems in patients with diabetes: comparison of screening characteristics of depression questionnaires, measurement of diabetes-specific emotional problems and standard clinical assessment. *Diabetologia* 2006; 49: 469-77.

7. Pouwer F, Skinner TC, Pibernik-Okanovic M, et al. Serious diabetes-specific emotional problems and depression in a Croatian-Dutch-English Survey from the European Depression in Diabetes Research Consortium. *Diabetes Res Clin Pract* 2005; 70: 166-73.

8. Lloyd CE, Dyer PH, Barnett AH. Prevalence of symptoms of depression and anxiety in a diabetes clinic population. *Diabet Med* 2000; 17: 198-202.

Chapter 34

Diabetes And Eating Disorders

The daily management of diabetes and the focus on eating and nutrition has the potential to create a preoccupation with food. Sometimes this preoccupation becomes an obsession, building momentum until food is almost viewed as dangerous. Worrying about eating the wrong foods and using terms such as "cheating" are unhealthy perspectives that can contribute to the development of an eating disorder.

Disordered eating, or eating disorders, are serious illnesses that take their toll both emotionally and physically. For people with diabetes, the price of this condition is particularly high—resulting in uncontrolled blood glucose levels and increasing the risk for diabetes complications.

Diabetes may also contribute to the triggering factors that lead to an eating disorder—namely low self-esteem, depression, anxiety, and loneliness. In many of these cases, the person with diabetes may chose to obsessively control their food and/or weight in efforts to manage their emotions.

Teens, in particular, are vulnerable to eating disorders. A teenager with diabetes may learn that poor glucose control leads to weight loss and that well-controlled glucose levels may contribute to weight gain. The term "diabulimia" has cropped up over the last few years, referencing a frightening trend within the diabetes community. This term refers to the method of weight loss by which a person with diabetes intentionally skips insulin therapy in order to keep their blood sugar elevated to a dangerous level, thus causing them to lose weight. Unfortunately, the long-term effects of uncontrolled blood sugars are often viewed as unimportant in the mind of a person with diabetes who is battling an eating disorder.

About This Chapter: "Diabetes and Eating Disorders," reprinted with permission from www.dlife.com. © 2010 LifeMed Media, Inc. All rights reserved.

There are ways to minimize the catalysts for eating disorders, potentially preventing them entirely.

- Focus on food choices rather than food restrictions. Don't expect perfection in diet compliance.

- Avoid emotional or judgmental labels for foods or eating behaviors. Do not categorize foods as "good or bad," or say that a person is "good or bad" based on how or what they eat.

- Make exercise a part of your life, not just a method of calorie burning. Becoming involved in life-long recreational sports like hiking or tennis makes exercise more fun and can help remove the exercise obsession as it relates to diabetes management.

- Also, keep talking. Isolating and discussing the stressors in your life may help to alleviate them. Talking with family members, loved ones, or seeking professional counseling is an option. If you or your loved one exhibits the signs of an eating disorder, don't be afraid to talk about it.

Signs Of An Eating Disorder

What are the signs of an eating disorder, clinically known as disordered eating?

Diabulimia is characterized by a person with diabetes intentionally skipping insulin therapy to keep blood glucose levels elevated, which in turn causes dangerous weight loss. Signs and symptoms may include:

- Excessive exercise
- Intentionally skipped or drastically lowered insulin doses
- Decreased blood glucose monitoring
- Rapid weight loss
- Excessive urination
- Vomiting
- Extreme concern with body weight and shape

Anorexia nervosa is characterized by self-starvation and excessive weight loss.

Signs and symptoms may include:

- Refusal to maintain body weight at or above a minimally normal weight for height, body type, age, and activity level

- Intense fear of weight gain or being "fat"

- Feeling "fat" or overweight despite dramatic weight loss

- Loss of menstrual periods

- Extreme concern with body weight and shape

Bulimia is characterized by a secretive cycle of binge eating followed by purging. Bulimia includes eating large amounts of food—more than most people would eat in one meal—in short periods of time, then getting rid of the food and calories through vomiting, laxative abuse, or over-exercising. Signs and symptoms may include:

- Repeated episodes of binging and purging

- Feeling out of control during a binge and eating beyond the point of comfortable fullness

- Purging after a binge (typically by self-induced vomiting, abuse of laxatives, diet pills and/or diuretics, excessive exercise, or fasting)

- Frequent dieting

- Extreme concern with body weight and shape

Eating disorders are serious medical conditions. Combined with diabetes, they can cause illness, long-term complications, and even death. If you suspect that you or your loved one may have an eating disorder, talk to your doctor today about treatment options.

Chapter 35

Diabetes Support In Schools: Improvement Needed

In primary school, children with diabetes face a range of tasks and problems that are beyond their level of cognitive development, including regulating blood glucose levels with insulin, adjusting insulin doses in relation to food intake and physical exercise, and giving attention to symptoms. Many children of this age are unable to read, write, calculate, or think in abstract terms, so they clearly need to be able to rely on an adult with adequate knowledge of diabetes management. Even with the benefits of new types of therapy,[1,2] the need to calculate blood glucose and insulin doses presents a challenge for both children and parents which needs to be handled sensitively and in different ways for different age groups.[3]

As older children and adolescents have learned to manage much of their diabetes therapy by themselves, they are likely to need help only when acute complications like hypoglycemia arise, or in difficult therapeutic situations.[3] Teachers' attitudes or school policy constraints can present obstacles to therapeutic needs, such as not allowing blood glucose measurement, insulin injections, or pump therapy during school time. Indeed, it is essential that teachers and other school personnel know the danger signs of acute diabetes-related conditions and how to deal with them.[4]

How Big Is The Problem?

The DAWN Youth Web Talk survey was an innovative online survey that aimed to explore the views of young people with type 1 diabetes aged between 18 and 25 years (1905 from eight countries), parents or carers of children and adolescents with type 1 diabetes aged up to 18 years (4099), and pediatric healthcare professionals (785). The average age of diagnosis of the young people responding was 12 years, and for the children whose parents were responding, it was 6 years.

About This Chapter: Text in this chapter is from "The DAWN verdict on diabetes support in schools: could do better," by Karin Lange, in *DiabetesVoice*, October 2008, Volume 53, Special Issue. © 2008 International Diabetes Federation (www.diabetesvoice.org); reprinted with permission.

The survey was conducted between July and December 2007 in Spain, Brazil, Denmark, Germany, Italy, Japan, the Netherlands and the U.S. The 25- to 30-minute online structured questionnaire, which was endorsed by the International Diabetes Federation (IDF) and the International Society for Pediatric and Adolescent Diabetes (ISPAD), covered regimen adherence, psychological well-being, psychosocial adjustment, perceived support from different sources, healthcare (teams, relationships, access), the school environment, involvement in youth organizations or activities, and particular needs. The results featured in this article focus on the findings relating to diabetes in the school environment.

At the time of the survey, 25% of the young people with diabetes who participated in the survey were in full-time education and 85% of the parents had a child in full-time education—with significant differences between the countries due to the educational systems.

Low Rates Of Success In Managing Diabetes In School

- Only 35% of the healthcare professionals believed that the young people in their care were managing their diabetes well at school most of or almost all the time—in terms of practical difficulties, not emotional problems.

- For the young people with diabetes, the level of satisfaction with the support received from school (3.6) was lower than for support received from their friends (3.7), healthcare professionals (3.9) or family (4.0). Scores were on a scale of 1 (very dissatisfied) to 5 (very satisfied).

- For the parents of young children with diabetes, the level of satisfaction with the support their child received from school (3.2) was lower than for support received from the child's friends (3.7) or healthcare professionals (4.0).

- 19% of the young adults with diabetes said they were dissatisfied or very dissatisfied with the way they were being treated or had been treated at school.

Impact Of Diabetes On School Performance And Family Activities

- Around 75% of the parents surveyed had their work disrupted to some extent by their child's diabetes (62% somewhat or a lot; 18% a little). Many reported having to reduce their hours or give up work in order to care for a school-age child.

- An average of 40% of the young people with diabetes had missed educational activities some or half of the time because of their diabetes, with clear differences between countries.

- 39% of the parents reported a major-to-moderate impact of diabetes on the school performance of their children; 24% of the young people felt this level of impact on their own performance.

Who Do Young People Rely On?

- The young adults with diabetes felt most supported regarding their condition by parents or carers (3.3) and spouses or partners (3.3), and least supported by schools or colleges (1.8) and society in general (2.1)—with higher scores for the local community (2.4), classmates (2.5), siblings (2.6) and friends (2.9). Scores were on a scale of 1 (not at all supportive) to 4 (very supportive).

- School friends (69%) and teachers other than their class teacher (27%) were the two groups that young people were most likely to rely on if they required help managing their diabetes at school. Lower scores were given for class teachers, concierges, school nurses/health workers, head teachers, office personnel, or others. Teachers were clearly of low importance to the young people as a source of practical help in secondary schools.

- 76% of the young adults reported that all or most of their school friends knew about their diabetes.

- Class teachers (63%) and school friends (49%) were the two groups that parents thought their children were most likely to rely on if they required help managing their diabetes at school.

- Class teachers (85%), other teachers (38%) and school friends (64%) were the groups that healthcare professionals felt children and adolescents were most likely to rely on if they required help managing their diabetes at school.

How Do Schools Compare With Other Sources Of Support?

Of all the different categories of resources, services, and support available for children and adolescents with diabetes and their families, major or moderate improvements in support and understanding from schools was called for by a large proportion of healthcare professionals (86% in all countries).

Other factors that were ranked with high importance included improvements in the transition from pediatric to adult care (82% all countries) and psychosocial support from healthcare teams (81%). Improved opportunities for diabetes camps and networking opportunities (70%), age-appropriate self-management education (68%) and medical management (49%) also generated support, but at a lower level.

The young adults with diabetes and the parents of children with diabetes thought that having teachers who are better informed about diabetes was more important than seeing improvements in a wide range of other possible factors at school (Figure 35.1). This related to better teacher knowledge of how to deal with an emergency diabetes event, as well as better understanding about diabetes in general—in terms of practical management and support.

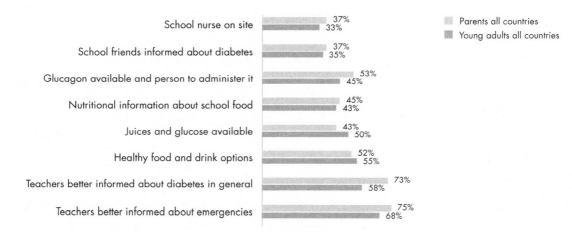

Proportions of young adults and parents supporting each factor

Figure 35.1. Areas For Urgent Improvement In School Diabetes Support

Discussion

The results of the DAWN Youth Web Talk survey have substantiated the suspicion that schools are a key area where improvements should be made to help young people with diabetes. Because of the chronic nature of diabetes, and the complex management needed—which only gradually can be assumed by the young people themselves—it is critical that every effort be made to provide a supportive environment in which they can develop a positive attitude and good skills to effectively manage their condition.

It is no surprise that the survey revealed 25% of young people with diabetes missing school activities and 25% (or 40% in young children, according to their parents) experiencing a significant impact on their educational performance due to their condition.

While the provision of nurses is understandably limited (less than 10% of parents said that they could rely on a school nurse or health worker to assist their child), there is much scope for improving the provision of diabetes education to school teachers. The urgent need for older children is in dealing with emergencies. However, improved overall knowledge of diabetes among school personnel would significantly help young people and particularly young children with day-to-day diabetes-related tasks and stresses.[4]

Inspiration in this direction might be taken from Sweden. Swedish schools do not rely on nurses; because the legal responsibility for overseeing self-care lies with the schools, the teacher of any class that includes a child with a medical condition is required to know how to support the child in the same way as his or her parents.

Teachers learn basic care management skills as part of their university training, and are supported by 24-hour telephone contact with children's hospitals. In the case of diabetes, teachers are able to help with the calculation of insulin doses, administering injections, and balancing insulin with food intake and physical exercise.[5] Putting such a system in place requires the proper legal basis, enhanced education for teachers, and adequate insurance protection.

References

1. Bangstad HJ, Danne T, Deeb LC, et al; International Society for Pediatric and Adolescent Diabetes (ISPAD). Insulin treatment. ISPAD clinical practice consensus guidelines 2006-2007. *Pediatr Diabetes* 2007; 8: 88-102.

2. Danne T, Lange K, Kordonouri O. New developments in the treatment of type 1 diabetes in children. *Arch Dis Child* 2007; 92: 1015-9.

3. Lange K, Sassmann H, von Schütz W, et al. Prerequisites for age-appropriate education in type 1 diabetes: a model programme for paediatric diabetes education in Germany. *Pediatr Diabetes* 2007; 8(Suppl 6): S63-S71.

4. American Diabetes Association. Diabetes care in the school and day care setting. *Diabetes Care* 2006; 29(Suppl 1): S49-S55.

5. Swedish National Agency for Education, Legal Secretariat. What is self-care and what is healthcare? 2007 Health and Welfare Board's Regulations and General Guidelines (Socialstyrelsens töreskrifter och allmänna råd). *SOSFS* 1997; 14: (M).

Chapter 36

Tips For Dealing With Diabetes At School

You probably spend about six hours or more at school each day—more than one third of your waking hours. If you have diabetes, chances are you'll need to check your blood sugar levels or give yourself an insulin injection during that time. So how do you deal with diabetes at school?

Talking To Teachers And School Staff About Diabetes

Maybe you just found out you have diabetes. Perhaps you've been living with it for a while but switched to a new school. Your first step is to let school staff know.

Set up a meeting with your school principal's office. Your mom or dad should be there, and you may want to suggest the school nurse join you.

Give your school nurse, teacher, and principal's office a copy of your diabetes management plan. This plan talks about what you will need to do during the school day, like test your blood sugar, give yourself injections, or eat lunch at a certain time each day. Your diabetes management plan also contains contact info for your doctors and diabetes health care team, so the school will know how to get in touch if you're sick.

Some schools might work with you to create a special plan for managing your diabetes at school. This may mean letting you eat lunch a little early or having a school nurse help with insulin injections if you need it.

About This Chapter: "School and Diabetes," 2010, reprinted with permission from www.kidshealth.org. Copyright © 2010 The Nemours Foundation. This information was provided by KidsHealth, one of the largest resources online for medically reviewed health information written for parents, kids, and teens. For more articles like this one, visit www.KidsHealth.org, or www.TeensHealth.org.

Tell your teachers. When your teachers know what needs to be done, they can schedule time for you to do stuff like test your blood glucose levels or get shots. Some teachers don't allow you to eat in class, which is why it's good to let your teacher know what's going on.

Ask to meet your teacher before or after class to talk about what you might need to do. If teachers know you have diabetes, they can watch for symptoms of diabetes problems and can call for medical help if you need it.

Teachers are busy. You might need to remind them once in a while about what you have to do to take care of your diabetes. If you have a substitute teacher, let him or her know that you have diabetes and may need to do things like go to the bathroom or get a snack.

If you feel uncomfortable talking to teachers or school staff about your diabetes, write a note or letter that goes over what you'll need to do to take care of your diabetes.

Taking Care Of Diabetes At School

Keep a stock of medications, testing equipment, and other supplies at school. You'll need the same supplies and equipment that you use at home. You'll probably need to keep these in the school nurse's office, but your school may want you to store them somewhere else. Ask the principal's office what your school's policy is.

Keep a copy of your diabetes management plan with you. Even if your school has your plan, it's good to keep one in your purse, backpack, locker, or car as well. If you run into any diabetes problems at school or start having symptoms of hypoglycemia or hyperglycemia, do what your plan tells you to do. That may mean having a snack, checking your blood glucose levels, or heading to the nurse's office—whatever your plan says.

Prepare to handle different situations. What if the school nurse isn't in? Is there someone else who can help? Who do you call if something unexpected happens—your doctor or your parent? Which kinds of problems can wait until after school and which ones should you handle right away?

Get To Know Your School Nurse

At many schools, students with diabetes need to get their diabetes medicines or test blood sugar levels in the nurse's office. Most schools won't let students carry needles or medications with them. Don't let that worry you, though. Even in an emergency, the extra time needed to get to the school nurse won't cause a problem.

Ask your doctor what you need to know about managing diabetes in school and how to handle special situations. Write down what you should do and who you should go to and keep this information with your management plan. Knowing what to do can help you feel more confident if you do have a problem at school.

Talking To Friends And Classmates About Diabetes

It's your call whether you tell friends and classmates about your diabetes. If they know, it can mean less worry for you about what they think when they see you doing things like leaving class to go to the nurse's office for a blood sugar level check.

But what about teasing? Some kids will tease anyone who seems the slightest bit different from anyone else. If this happens to you, you're definitely not alone: About one in three kids and teens with problems like diabetes have had to deal with bullying.

What can you do when people tease you? Get your friends' help to remind people that diabetes is no big deal. Ignoring a bully is a good strategy too. Bullies thrive on the reaction they get, and if you walk away, you're telling the bully that you just don't care. Sooner or later the bully will probably get bored with trying to bother you.

It may also help to talk to a guidance counselor, teacher, or friend—anyone who can give you the support you need. Talking can be a good outlet for the fears and frustrations that can build when you're being bullied.

Whatever happens, though, don't try to hide your condition by skipping treatments or eating foods that aren't on your meal plan—it'll just make you feel worse and risk getting sick at school.

Chapter 37

Driving When You Have Diabetes

For most people, driving represents freedom, control, and competence. Driving enables most people to get to the places they want or need to go. For many people, driving is important economically—some drive as part of their job or to get to and from work.

Driving is a complex skill. Our ability to drive safely can be affected by changes in our physical, emotional, and mental condition. This chapter is designed to give you the information you need to talk to your health care team about driving and diabetes.

How can having diabetes affect my driving?

In the short term, diabetes can make your blood glucose (sugar) levels too high or too low. As a result, diabetes can make you feel sleepy or dizzy, feel confused, have blurred vision, or even lose consciousness or have a seizure.

In the long run, diabetes can lead to problems that affect driving. Diabetes may cause nerve damage in your hands, legs and feet, or eyes. In some cases, diabetes can cause blindness or lead to amputation.

Can I still drive with diabetes?

Yes, people with diabetes are able to drive unless they are limited by certain complications of diabetes. These include severe low blood glucose levels or vision problems. If you are experiencing diabetes-related complications, you should work closely with your diabetes health care team to find out if diabetes affects your ability to drive. If it does, discuss if there are actions you can take to continue to drive safely.

About This Chapter: From "Driving When You Have Diabetes," National Highway Traffic Safety Administration, 2003. Updated by David A. Cooke, MD, FACP, August 2011.

While diabetes will not prevent you from regular driving, be aware that it may be an issue if you are applying for a commercial drivers' license (CDL). This is a special license required for professional drivers such as truck, bus, or limousine drivers. If you need this type of licensing, you should contact the U.S. Department of Transportation and your state licensing agency regarding whether you can qualify.

What can I do to ensure that I can drive safely with diabetes?

Insulin and some oral medications can cause blood glucose levels to become dangerously low (hypoglycemia). Do not drive if your blood glucose level is too low. If you do, you might not be able to make good choices, focus on your driving, or control your car. Your health care team can help you determine when you should check your blood glucose level before driving and how often you should check while driving.

Make sure you always carry your blood glucose meter and plenty of snacks (including a quick-acting source of glucose) with you. Pull over as soon as you feel any of the signs of a low blood glucose level. Check your blood glucose.

If your glucose level is low, eat a snack that contains a fast-acting sugar such as juice, soda with sugar (not diet), hard candy, or glucose tablets. Wait 15 minutes, and then check your blood glucose again. Treat again as needed. Once your glucose level has risen to your target range, eat a more substantial snack or meal containing protein. Do not continue driving until your blood glucose level has improved.

Most people with diabetes experience warning signs of a low blood glucose level. However, if you experience hypoglycemia without advance warning, you should not drive. Talk to your health care team about how glycemic awareness training might help you sense the beginning stages of hypoglycemia.

In extreme situations, high blood glucose levels (hyperglycemia) also may affect driving. Talk to your health care team if you have a history of very high glucose levels to determine at what point such levels might affect your ability to be a safe driver.

The key to preventing diabetes-related eye problems is good control of blood glucose levels, good blood pressure control, and good eye care. A yearly exam with an eye care professional is essential.

Improving your driving skills could help keep you and others around you safe. To find a specialist near you, call the Association of Driver Rehabilitation Specialists at 800-290-2344 or go to their website at www.aded.net. You also can call hospitals and rehabilitation facilities to find an occupational therapist who can help with the driving skills assessment.

Driving And Long-Term Diabetes Complications

Some people experience long-term complications of diabetes such as vision or sensation problems or they require an amputation. In people with these concerns, their diabetes health care team can refer them to a driving specialist. This specialist can give on and off-road tests to see if, and how, their diabetes is affecting their driving. The specialist also may offer training to improve driving skills.

What if I have to cut back or give up driving?

You can keep your independence even if you have to cut back or give up on your driving. It may take planning ahead on your part, but planning will help get you to the places you need to go and to the people you want to see.

- Consider rides with family and friends, taxi cabs, shuttle buses or vans, public buses, trains and subways; and walking.

- Contact your regional transit authority to find out which bus or train to take.

- Call Easter Seals Project ACTION (Accessible Community Transportation In Our Nation) at 800-659-6428 or go to their website http://projectaction.easterseals.com.

What else should I know about driving and safety?

Always wear your safety belt when you are driving or riding in a car. Make sure that every person who is riding with you also is buckled up. Wear your safety belt even if your car has air bags.

Chapter 38

Traveling When You Have Diabetes

Heading out of town? Leaving your troubles behind? Whenever you travel, your diabetes comes along with you. And while having diabetes shouldn't stop you from traveling in style, you will have to do some careful planning. Here are some helpful diabetes travel tips from the National Diabetes Education Program.

Plan Ahead

- Get all your immunizations. Find out what's required for where you're going, and make sure you get the right shots, on time.

- Control your ABCs: A1C, blood pressure, and cholesterol. See your health care provider for a check-up four to six weeks before your trip to make sure your ABCs are under control and in a healthy range before you leave.

- Ask your health care provider for a prescription and a letter explaining your diabetes medications, supplies, and any allergies. Carry this with you at all times on your trip. The prescription should be for insulin or diabetes medications and could help in case of an emergency.

- Wear identification that explains you have diabetes. The identification should be written in the languages of the places you are visiting.

- Plan for time zone changes. Make sure you'll always know when to take your diabetes medicine, no matter where you are. Remember: Eastward travel means a shorter day. If you inject insulin, less may be needed. Westward travel means a longer day, so more insulin may be needed.

About This Chapter: From "Have Diabetes. Will Travel." National Diabetes Education Program, March 2011.

- Find out how long the flight will be and whether meals will be served. However, you should always carry enough food to cover the entire flight time in case of delays or unexpected schedule changes.

Pack Properly

- Take twice the amount of diabetes medication and supplies that you'd normally need. Better safe than sorry.

- Keep your insulin cool by packing it in an insulated bag with refrigerated gel packs.

- Keep snacks, glucose gel, or tablets with you in case your blood glucose drops.

- If you use insulin, make sure you also pack a glucagon emergency kit.

- Make sure you keep your medical insurance card and emergency phone numbers handy.

- Don't forget to pack a first aid kit with all the essentials.

If You Are Flying

- Plan to carry all your diabetes supplies in your carry-on luggage. Don't risk a lost suitcase.

- Have all syringes and insulin delivery systems (including vials of insulin) clearly marked with the pharmaceutical preprinted label that identifies the medications. The FAA recommends that patients travel with their original pharmacy labeled packaging. Keep your diabetes medications and emergency snacks with you at your seat—don't store them in an overhead bin.

- If the airline offers a meal for your flight call ahead for a diabetic, low fat, or low cholesterol meal. Wait until your food is about to be served before you take your insulin. Otherwise, a delay in the meal could lead to low blood glucose.

- If no food is offered on your flight, bring a meal on board yourself.

- If you plan on using the restroom for insulin injections, ask for an aisle seat for easier access.

- Don't be shy about telling the flight attendant that you have diabetes—especially if you are traveling alone.

- When drawing up your dose of insulin, don't inject air into the bottle (the air on your plane will probably be pressurized).

If You Are Traveling Abroad

Because prescription laws may be very different in other countries, write for a list of International Diabetes Federation groups: IDF, 1 rue Defaeqz, B-1000, Belgium or visit http://www.idf.org. You may also want to get a list of English-speaking foreign doctors in case of an emergency. Contact the American Consulate, American Express, or local medical schools for a list of doctors.

Insulin in foreign countries comes in different strengths. If you purchase insulin in a foreign country, be sure to use the right syringe for the strength. An incorrect syringe may cause you to take too much or too little insulin.

On A Road Trip

- Don't leave your medications in the trunk, glove compartment, or near a window—they might overheat. If possible, carry a cooler in the car to keep medications cool.

- Bring extra food with you in the car in case you can't find a restaurant.

General Traveling Tips

- Stay comfortable and reduce your risk for blood clots by moving around every hour or two.

- Always tell at least one person traveling with you about your diabetes.

- Protect your feet. Never go barefoot in the shower or pool.

- Check your blood glucose often. Changes in diet, activity, and time zones can affect your blood glucose in unexpected ways.

You may not be able to leave your diabetes behind, but you can manage it and have a relaxing, safe trip. To learn more about managing your diabetes or to order free resources, visit the National Diabetes Education Program at www.YourDiabetesInfo.org or call 888-693-NDEP (888-693-6337); TTY: 866-569-1162.

Chapter 39

Handling Diabetes When You're Sick

Whether your head feels like it's stuffed with cotton because you have a cold or you're spending a lot of time on the toilet because of a stomach bug, being sick is no fun for anyone.

For people with diabetes, being sick can also affect blood sugar levels. The good news is that taking a few extra precautions can help you keep your blood sugar levels under control.

How Illness Affects Blood Sugar Levels

When you get sick—whether it's a minor illness like a sore throat or cold or a bigger problem like dehydration or surgery—the body perceives the illness as stress. To relieve the stress, the body fights the illness. This process requires more energy than the body normally uses.

On one hand, this is good because it helps supply the extra fuel the body needs. On the other hand, in a person with diabetes, this can lead to high blood sugar levels. Some illnesses cause the opposite problem, though. If you don't feel like eating or have nausea or vomiting, and you're taking the same amount of insulin you normally do, you can develop blood sugar levels that are too low.

Blood sugar levels can be very unpredictable when you're sick. Because you can't be sure how the illness will affect your blood sugar levels, it's important to check blood sugar levels often on sick days and adjust your insulin doses as needed.

About This Chapter: "Handling Diabetes When You're Sick," August 2010, reprinted with permission from www .kidshealth.org. Copyright © 2010 The Nemours Foundation. This information was provided by KidsHealth, one of the largest resources online for medically reviewed health information written for parents, kids, and teens. For more articles like this one, visit www.KidsHealth.org, or www.TeensHealth.org.

Planning For Sick Days

Your diabetes management plan will help you know what to do when you're sick. The plan might tell you:

- how to monitor your blood glucose levels and ketones when you're sick;

- which medicines are OK to take;

- what changes you might make to your food and drink and diabetes medications;

- when to call your doctor.

In addition, people with diabetes should get the pneumococcal vaccine, which protects against some serious infections. You should also get a flu shot every year. These vaccines may help you keep your diabetes under better control and cut down on the number of sick days you have.

What To Do When You're Sick

Your doctor will give you specific advice when you're sick. But here are some general guidelines:

- **Stay on track.** Unless your doctor tells you to make a change, keep taking the same diabetes medications. You need to keep taking insulin when you're sick, even if you're not eating as much as you usually do. That's because your liver makes and releases glucose into your blood—even when you're stuck channel surfing on the couch—so you always need insulin. Some people with diabetes need more insulin than usual on sick days. Even some people with type 2 diabetes who don't usually take insulin may need some on sick days.

- **Check blood sugar and ketone levels often.** Your doctor will tell you how often to check your blood sugar and ketone levels—usually you'll need to check more frequently while you're sick.

- **Pay special attention to nausea and vomiting.** People with diabetes sometimes catch a bug that causes nausea or vomiting. But nausea and vomiting are also symptoms of ketoacidosis. If you feel sick to your stomach or are throwing up, it's important to keep a close eye on your blood glucose and ketone levels and seek medical help according to the guidelines in your diabetes management plan. The best approach is to stick to your insulin schedule, check ketones regularly, and follow your doctor's advice about when to get help.

- **Prevent dehydration.** Be sure to drink plenty of fluids, even if you have nausea or vomiting. Your doctor can recommend the types and amounts of fluids to drink that can help you manage both your illness and your blood sugar levels.

- **Use over-the-counter (OTC) medications wisely.** People sometimes take OTC medications for illnesses like the cold or flu. But these have ingredients that can raise or lower blood sugar or cause symptoms that look similar to high or low blood sugar. Follow your doctor's advice about taking an OTC medication. Your doctor might even include common medications that are OK for you in your diabetes management plan and can also explain the things to check for on medication labels.

- **Take notes.** Your doctor might have a lot of questions about your illness and the symptoms you've had. You can answer these questions more easily if you write down your symptoms, medications and doses, what food and drink you had, and whether you kept the food down. Also, tell the doctor if you've lost weight or had a fever and have the record of your blood sugar and ketone level test results handy.

Get Some Rest

People need rest when they're sick. It helps your body focus its energy on fighting illness. If you think you need to, let a parent take over managing your diabetes for a day or two. Your mom or dad can keep track of your blood sugar levels and figure out the best insulin dosage—and you can get some sleep!

When To Call Your Doctor

Your diabetes management plan will explain when you may need medical help. It will tell you what to do and whom to call. Here are some general reasons for calling the doctor:

- All the same reasons you normally would call about diabetes management, as well as for any questions you have about being sick

- If you have no appetite or you can't eat or drink

- If your blood sugar level is low because you haven't been eating much—but remember to take steps at home to bring your blood sugar back up

- If you keep vomiting or having diarrhea

- If your blood sugar levels are high for several checks or don't decrease when you take extra insulin

- If you have moderate or large amounts of ketones in the urine

- If you think you might have ketoacidosis

- If you can't eat or drink because you're having a medical test like an X-ray, surgery, or a dental procedure

Any time you have questions or concerns, ask your doctor for advice.

Chapter 40

If Your Friend Or Family Member Has Diabetes

Friends With Diabetes

Let me give you the straight scoop on talking to a friend who has diabetes. Guess what— it's just like talking to anyone else! Someone with diabetes is just as likely to like the same books, movies, and activities you do—but they do have some special things they need to think about every day.

It can be hard to have a serious disease, and your friend may feel strange about bringing up all the new things he or she has to do—they may worry that you think it's gross when they stick their finger to test blood sugar or if they have to give themselves a shot. One of the best things you can do is give them a chance to talk to you about how they feel and what they worry about. Another thing that can help is learning more about their disease, and how you can help them manage it, including warning signs that their blood sugar may be too low. It may be a big relief for them to know that someone else is helping to look out for them.

And here's the inside scoop— two big things that every person with diabetes needs to think of every day.

First, food. While everyone should try and eat mostly healthy meals and snacks, it's REALLY important for someone with diabetes. Since some carbohydrates can affect blood sugar really quickly, people with diabetes need to make sure they eat mostly complex carbs like whole grain bread and pasta, fruits and vegetables, and low-fat dairy products. These are broken down more

About This Chapter: This chapter begins with "Friends With Diabetes," excerpted from "Diabetes, Xpert's Opinion," BAM! Body and Mind, Centers for Disease Control and Prevention, 2005. Reviewed by David A. Cooke, MD, FACP, August 2011. It continues with "Help a Loved One with Diabetes," National Diabetes Education Program, February 2011.

slowly by the body and help keep blood sugar stable. Carbs like white bread, juice, soda, or candy can send blood sugar soaring—just what people with diabetes need to avoid. Eating small meals every few hours also helps keep blood sugar levels from going up and down too much.

So, if a friend turns down cake at your birthday, don't take it personally or try to make him eat it anyway. And, it's even better if you can plan ahead to make sure that you have plenty of stuff they can eat there, too—there are even special cake recipes that use artificial sweetener that people with diabetes (and everyone else, too) can eat.

Is my grandma's diabetes the same as my friend's diabetes?

I've heard of different names for diabetes—my grandma calls it "sugar," and my friend has juvenile diabetes. Are these the same thing?

There are two types of diabetes. While both have similar effects—your body can't process glucose right—different things cause them.

Juvenile diabetes got its name because most people who got this type of the disease got it when they were children (even though adults can get it, too). Now, it is called type 1 diabetes. This kind of diabetes happens when the immune system attacks the cells that make insulin in a body organ called the pancreas. Without insulin, you develop diabetes.

The other kind of diabetes is called—you guessed it—type 2 diabetes. With this kind, your body makes insulin, but it either doesn't make enough, or something prevents your body from using it right.

Until recently, most cases of type 2 diabetes were in older people and adults who were overweight. In the last few years, though, more and more kids are being diagnosed with this kind of diabetes. Most likely, this is because kids today are more likely to be overweight and not get enough exercise than they were in the past. Children who are African-American, Hispanic, Asian, or Native American are more likely to develop type 2 diabetes than others.

Because diabetes causes people to have too much glucose, or sugar, in their blood, a lot of people call it sugar or sugar diabetes. No matter the name, though, it's all the same disease.

Scientists do not know exactly how many kids have diabetes, but they do know that doctors are seeing more and more cases of diabetes in kids. And most of these cases are now type 2 diabetes, which used to be very rare among kids.

Source: Excerpted from "Diabetes: Questions Answered," BAM! Body and Mind, Centers for Disease Control and Prevention, 2005. Reviewed by David A. Cooke, MD, FACP, August 2011.

Next, physical activity. Physical activity is important for everyone, and it's even MORE important that people with diabetes get plenty of activity, because it helps them to keep their blood sugar down.

And if you don't have diabetes, don't think you're off the hook. Being active can help prevent diabetes, because keeping your weight at the level that's right for you is one way to reduce the chance of getting type 2 diabetes. So, if you've got a friend with diabetes, it's great for both of you to get out and play some basketball, walk the dog, or check out other ideas to get moving.

Help A Loved One With Diabetes

There are many things you can do to help your loved one—a family member or friend—with diabetes. Use these tips to get started today.

Learn: There is a lot to learn about living well with diabetes. Use what you learn to help your loved one manage his or her diabetes.

Join a support group about living with diabetes. Check with your doctor, hospital, or area health clinic. Read about diabetes online. For help go to www.YourDiabetesInfo.org for more information. Or, ask your loved one's diabetes health care team how you can learn more.

Talk: Talk to your loved one about coping with diabetes. Ask questions like these:

- What things are hard for him or her to manage?
- What things are easy?
- Does your loved one set self-care goals?
- How does he or she stay on track to reach these goals?
- How can you help with diabetes care tasks?
- Does your loved one feel down sometimes?
- What can you do to help him or her feel better?
- Does your loved one talk to his or her doctor or other health care team members about feeling down?

Ask your loved one about what is needed:

- What do I do that helps you with your diabetes?
- What do I do that makes it harder for you to manage your diabetes?
- What can I do to help you more than I do now?

Find Ways To Help: Nagging will not help either you or your loved one. If it fits his or her lifestyle, you could offer to help your loved one with these issues:

- Figure out how to manage diabetes in his or her daily life.
- Keep track of visits to the health care team.
- Make a list of questions for the health care team.
- Go on a visit to his or her health care team.
- Find where to buy healthy, low-cost foods.
- Prepare tasty, healthy meals.
- Find a safe place to walk or to be more active.

When you have found one way to help, add another way. Diabetes is a hard disease to handle alone. You can have a big effect on how well your loved one copes with diabetes. Get started today.

Part Five
The Physical Complications
Of Diabetes

Chapter 41

Diabetes-Related Health Concerns

Questions About Diabetes And Health

Diabetes can affect any part of your body. The good news is that you can prevent most of these problems by keeping your blood glucose (blood sugar) under control, eating healthy, being physical active, working with your health care provider to keep your blood pressure and cholesterol under control, and getting necessary screening tests.

How can diabetes affect cardiovascular health?

Cardiovascular disease is the leading cause of early death among people with diabetes. Adults with diabetes are two to four times more likely than people without diabetes to have heart disease or experience a stroke. At least 65% of people with diabetes die from heart disease or stroke. About 70% of people with diabetes also have high blood pressure.

How are cholesterol, triglyceride, weight, and blood pressure problems related to diabetes?

People with type 2 diabetes have high rates of cholesterol and triglyceride abnormalities, obesity, and high blood pressure, all of which are major contributors to higher rates of cardiovascular disease. Many people with diabetes have several of these conditions at the same time. This combination of problems is often called metabolic syndrome (formerly known as syndrome X).

About This Chapter: This chapter begins with excerpts from "Diabetes and Me: Diabetes Health Concerns," Centers for Disease Control and Prevention, June 2010. It continues with "Complications of Diabetes in the United States," excerpted from "National Diabetes Fact Sheet, 2007," Centers for Disease Control and Prevention, 2008.

The metabolic syndrome is often defined as the presence of any three of the following conditions: 1) excess weight around the waist; 2) high levels of triglycerides; 3) low levels of HDL, or "good," cholesterol; 4) high blood pressure; and 5) high fasting blood glucose levels.

If you have one or more of these conditions, you are at an increased risk for having one or more of the others. The more conditions that you have, the greater the risk to your health.

How can I be "heart healthy" and avoid cardiovascular disease if I have diabetes?

To protect your heart and blood vessels, eat right, get physical activity, don't smoke, and maintain healthy blood glucose, blood pressure, and cholesterol levels. Choose a healthy diet, low in salt. Work with a dietitian to plan healthy meals. If you're overweight, talk about how to safely lose weight. Ask about a physical activity or exercise program. Quit smoking if you currently do. Get a hemoglobin A1C test at least twice a year to determine what your average blood glucose level was for the past two to three months. Get your blood pressure checked at every doctor's visit, and get your cholesterol checked at least once a year. Take medications if prescribed by your doctor.

How can diabetes affect the eyes?

In diabetic eye disease, high blood glucose and high blood pressure cause small blood vessels to swell and leak liquid into the retina of the eye, blurring the vision and sometimes leading to blindness. People with diabetes are also more likely to develop cataracts (a clouding of the eye's lens) and glaucoma (optic nerve damage). Laser surgery can help these conditions.

How can I keep my eyes healthy if I have diabetes?

There's a lot you can do to prevent eye problems. A recent study shows that keeping your blood glucose level closer to normal can prevent or delay the onset of diabetic eye disease. Keeping your blood pressure under control is also important. Finding and treating eye problems early can help save sight.

It is best to have an eye doctor give you a dilated eye exam at least once a year. The doctor will use eye drops to enlarge (dilate) your pupils to examine the backs of your eyes. Your eyes will be checked for signs of cataracts or glaucoma, problems that people with diabetes are more likely to get.

Because diabetic eye disease may develop without symptoms, regular eye exams are important for finding problems early. Some people may notice signs of vision changes. If you're having trouble reading, if your vision is blurred, or if you're seeing rings around lights, dark spots, or flashing lights, you may have eye problems. Be sure to tell your health care team or eye doctor about any eye problems you may have.

How can diabetes affect the kidneys?

In diabetic kidney disease (also called diabetic nephropathy), cells and blood vessels in the kidneys are damaged, affecting the organs' ability to filter out waste. Waste builds up in your blood instead of being excreted. In some cases this can lead to kidney failure. When the kidneys fail, a person has to have his or her blood filtered through a machine (a treatment called dialysis) several times a week or has to get a kidney transplant.

How can I keep my kidneys healthy if I have diabetes?

There's a lot you can do to prevent kidney problems. A recent study shows that controlling your blood glucose can prevent or delay the onset of kidney disease. Keeping your blood pressure under control is also important.

Diabetic kidney disease happens slowly and silently, so you might not feel that anything is wrong until severe problems have developed. Therefore, it is important to get your blood and urine checked for kidney problems each year.

Your doctor can learn how well your kidneys are working by testing every year for micro-albumin (a protein) in the urine. Microalbumin in the urine is an early sign of diabetic kidney disease. Your doctor can also do a yearly blood test to measure your kidney function.

Go to the doctor if you develop a bladder or kidney infection; symptoms include cloudy or bloody urine, pain or burning when you urinate, an urgent need to urinate often, back pain, chills, or fever.

How can diabetes affect nerve endings?

Having high blood glucose for many years can damage the blood vessels that bring oxygen to some nerves as well as the nerve coverings. Damaged nerves may stop sending messages, or send messages too slowly or at the wrong times. Numbness, pain, and weakness in the hands, arms, feet, and legs may develop. Problems may also occur in various organs, including the digestive tract, heart, and sex organs. Diabetic neuropathy is the medical term for damage to the nervous system from diabetes. The most common type is peripheral neuropathy, which affects the arms and legs.

An estimated 50% of those with diabetes have some form of neuropathy, but not all with neuropathy have symptoms. People with diabetes can develop nerve problems at any time, but the longer a person has diabetes, the greater the risk. The highest rates of neuropathy are among people who have had the disease for at least 25 years.

Diabetic neuropathy also appears to be more common in people who have had problems controlling their blood glucose levels, in those with high levels of blood fat and blood pressure, in overweight people, and in people over the age of 40.

How can I prevent nerve damage if I have diabetes?

You can help keep your nervous system healthy by keeping your blood glucose as close to normal as possible, getting regular physical activity, not smoking, taking good care of your feet each day, having your health care provider examine your feet at least four times a year, and getting your feet tested for nerve damage at least once a year.

Why is it especially important to take care of my feet if I have diabetes?

Nerve damage, circulation problems, and infections can cause serious foot problems for people with diabetes. Sometimes nerve damage can deform or misshape your feet, causing pressure points that can turn into blisters, sores, or ulcers. Poor circulation can make these injuries slow to heal. Sometimes this can lead to amputation of a toe, foot, or leg.

What should I do on a regular basis to take care of my feet?

Look for cuts, cracks, sores, red spots, swelling, infected toenails, splinters, blisters, and calluses on the feet each day. Call your doctor if such wounds do not heal after one day.

If you have corns and calluses, ask your doctor or podiatrist about the best way to care for them. Here are some additional tips for caring for your feet:

- Wash your feet in warm—not hot—water and dry them well.

- Cut your toenails once a week or when needed. Cut toenails when they are soft from washing. Cut them to the shape of the toe and not too short. File the edges with an emery board.

- Rub lotion on the tops and bottoms of feet—but not between the toes—to prevent cracking and drying.

- Wear shoes that fit well. Break in new shoes slowly, by wearing them one to two hours each day for the first one to two weeks.

- Wear stockings or socks to avoid blisters and sores.

- Wear clean, lightly padded socks that fit well; seamless socks are best.

- Always wear shoes or slippers, because when you are barefoot it is easy to step on something and hurt your feet.

- Protect your feet from extreme heat and cold.

- When sitting, keep the blood flowing to your lower limbs by propping your feet up and moving your toes and ankles for a few minutes at a time.

- Avoid smoking, which reduces blood flow to the feet.

And, remember, for your feet and your overall health, keep your blood sugar, blood pressure, and cholesterol under control by eating healthy foods, staying active, and taking your diabetes medicines.

How can diabetes affect the digestion?

Gastroparesis, otherwise known as delayed gastric emptying, is a disorder where, due to nerve damage, the stomach takes too long to empty itself. It frequently occurs in people with either type 1 or type 2 diabetes.

Symptoms of gastroparesis include heartburn, nausea, vomiting of undigested food, an early feeling of fullness when eating, weight loss, abdominal bloating, erratic blood glucose levels, lack of appetite, gastroesophageal reflux, and spasms of the stomach wall.

How can diabetes affect oral health?

Because of high blood glucose, people with diabetes are more likely to have problems with their teeth and gums. And like all infections, dental infections can make your blood glucose go up. Sore, swollen, and red gums that bleed when you brush your teeth are a sign of a dental problem called gingivitis. Another problem, called periodontitis, happens when your gums shrink or pull away from your teeth.

People with diabetes can have tooth and gum problems more often if their blood glucose stays high. Also, smoking makes it more likely for you to get a bad case of gum disease. People with diabetes are also prone to other mouth problems, like fungal infections, poor post-surgery healing, and dry mouth.

How can I keep my mouth, gums, and teeth healthy if I have diabetes?

You can help maintain your oral health by keeping your blood glucose as close to normal as possible, brushing your teeth at least twice a day, and flossing once a day. Keep any dentures clean. Get a dental cleaning and exam twice a year, and tell your dentist that you have diabetes. Call your dentist with any problems, such as gums that are red, sore, bleeding, or pulling away from the teeth; any possible tooth infection; or soreness from dentures.

How can diabetes affect sexual responses?

Many people with diabetic nerve damage have trouble having sex. For example, men can have trouble maintaining an erection and ejaculating. Women can have trouble with sexual response and vaginal lubrication. Both men and women with diabetes can get urinary tract infections and bladder problems more often than average.

How can diabetes affect mood?

Several studies suggest that diabetes doubles the risk of depression, although it's still unclear why. The psychological stress of having diabetes may contribute to depression, but diabetes' metabolic effect on brain function may also play a role. At the same time, people with depression may be more likely to develop diabetes.

The risk of depression increases as more diabetes complications develop. When you are depressed, you do not function as well, physically or mentally; this makes you less likely to eat properly, exercise, and take your medication regularly.

Psychotherapy, medication, or a combination of both can treat depression effectively. In addition, studies show that successful treatment for depression also helps improve blood glucose control.

How does diabetes affect how I respond to a cold or flu?

Being sick by itself can raise your blood glucose. Moreover, illness can prevent you from eating properly, which further affects blood glucose.

In addition, diabetes can make the immune system more vulnerable to severe cases of the flu. People with diabetes who come down with the flu may become very sick and may even have to go to a hospital. You can help keep yourself from getting the flu by getting a flu shot every year. Everyone with diabetes—even pregnant women—should get a yearly flu shot. The best time to get one is between October and mid-November, before the flu season begins.

What should I do when I am sick?

Be sure to continue taking your diabetes pills or insulin. Don't stop taking them even if you can't eat. Your health care provider may even advise you to take more insulin during sickness.

Test your blood glucose every four hours, and keep track of the results. Drink extra (calorie-free) liquids, and try to eat as you normally would. If you can't, try to have soft foods and liquids containing the equivalent amount of carbohydrates that you usually consume.

Weigh yourself every day. Losing weight without trying is a sign of high blood glucose.

Check your temperature every morning and evening. A fever may be a sign of infection.

Call your health care provider or go to an emergency room if any of the following happen to you:

- You feel too sick to eat normally and are unable to keep down food for more than six hours.
- You're having severe diarrhea.
- You lose five pounds or more.
- Your temperature is over 101 degrees F.
- Your blood glucose is lower than 60 mg/dL or remains over 300 mg/dL.
- You have moderate or large amounts of ketones in your urine.
- You're having trouble breathing.
- You feel sleepy or can't think clearly.

Complications Of Diabetes In The United States

Heart Disease And Stroke

- In 2004, heart disease was noted on 68% of diabetes-related death certificates among people aged 65 years or older.
- In 2004, stroke was noted on 16% of diabetes-related death certificates among people aged 65 years or older.
- Adults with diabetes have heart disease death rates about two to four times higher than adults without diabetes.
- The risk for stroke is two to four times higher among people with diabetes.

High Blood Pressure

- In 2003–2004, 75% of adults with self-reported diabetes had blood pressure greater than or equal to 130/80 millimeters of mercury (mm Hg), or used prescription medications for hypertension.

Blindness

- Diabetes is the leading cause of new cases of blindness among adults aged 20–74 years.
- Diabetic retinopathy causes 12,000 to 24,000 new cases of blindness each year.

Kidney Disease

- Diabetes is the leading cause of kidney failure, accounting for 44% of new cases in 2005.
- In 2005, 46,739 people with diabetes began treatment for end-stage kidney disease in the United States and Puerto Rico.
- In 2005, a total of 178,689 people in the United States and Puerto Rico with end-stage kidney disease due to diabetes were living on chronic dialysis or with a kidney transplant.

Nervous System Disease

- About 60% to 70% of people with diabetes have mild to severe forms of nervous system damage. The results of such damage include impaired sensation or pain in the feet or hands, slowed digestion of food in the stomach, carpal tunnel syndrome, erectile dysfunction, or other nerve problems.
- Almost 30% of people with diabetes aged 40 years or older have impaired sensation in the feet (that is, at least one area that lacks feeling).
- Severe forms of diabetic nerve disease are a major contributing cause of lower-extremity amputations.

Amputations

- More than 60% of nontraumatic lower-limb amputations occur in people with diabetes.
- In 2004, about 71,000 nontraumatic lower-limb amputations were performed in people with diabetes.

Dental Disease

- Periodontal (gum) disease is more common in people with diabetes. Among young adults, those with diabetes have about twice the risk of those without diabetes.
- Persons with poorly controlled diabetes (A1C greater than 9%) were nearly three times more likely to have severe periodontitis than those without diabetes.
- Almost one-third of people with diabetes have severe periodontal disease with loss of attachment of the gums to the teeth measuring 5 millimeters or more.

Complications Of Pregnancy

- Poorly controlled diabetes before conception and during the first trimester of pregnancy among women with type 1 diabetes can cause major birth defects in 5% to 10% of pregnancies and spontaneous abortions in 15% to 20% of pregnancies.

- Poorly controlled diabetes during the second and third trimesters of pregnancy can result in excessively large babies, posing a risk to both mother and child.

Other Complications

- Uncontrolled diabetes often leads to biochemical imbalances that can cause acute life-threatening events, such as diabetic ketoacidosis and hyperosmolar (nonketotic) coma.

- People with diabetes are more susceptible to many other illnesses. Once they acquire these illnesses, they often have worse prognoses. For example, they are more likely to die with pneumonia or influenza than people who do not have diabetes.

- Persons with diabetes aged 60 years or older are two to three times more likely to report an inability to walk one-quarter of a mile, climb stairs, do housework, or use a mobility aid compared with persons without diabetes in the same age group.

How To Reduce Your Risk Of Health Complications

Having diabetes puts you at a higher risk for developing other health problems. However, if you understand the risks, you can take steps now to lower your chance of diabetes-related complications.

Talk to your diabetes educator and healthcare provider about potential health issues such as kidney damage, nerve damage and vision loss. They can explain why complications happen and how they can be avoided.

But don't rely on your healthcare team to identify areas of concern—you need to play an active role in reducing your risk. Make an effort to learn about complications and consistently track your overall health. You can reduce your risks for several complications by taking these precautions:

- Don't smoke.
- Schedule regular medical checkups and medical tests.
- See an ophthalmologist (eye doctor) at least once a year.
- Keep your feet dry and clean. Look out for redness or sores, and report these to your healthcare team as soon as you find them. If you have trouble seeing the bottom of your feet, ask a family member or friend to help you.
- Be sensitive to your body—recognize when you aren't feeling well, and contact your care team if you need help identifying the problem.

Source: From "Reducing Risks," © 2009. Reprinted with permission of the American Association of Diabetes Educators. All Rights Reserved. May not be reproduced or distributed without the written approval of AADE.

Chapter 42

Cardiovascular Disease And Diabetes

Having diabetes or pre-diabetes puts you at increased risk for heart disease and stroke. You can lower your risk by keeping your blood glucose (also called blood sugar), blood pressure, and blood cholesterol close to the recommended target numbers—the levels suggested by diabetes experts for good health.

Reaching your targets also can help prevent narrowing or blockage of the blood vessels in your legs, a condition called peripheral arterial disease. You can reach your targets by choosing foods wisely, being physically active, and taking medications if needed.

What is the connection between diabetes, heart disease, and stroke?

If you have diabetes, you are at least twice as likely as someone who does not have diabetes to have heart disease or a stroke. People with diabetes also tend to develop heart disease or have strokes at an earlier age than other people. Some studies suggest that people who are middle-aged and have type 2 diabetes have a chance of having a heart attack that is as high as someone without diabetes who has already had one heart attack. Women who have not gone through menopause usually have less risk of heart disease than men of the same age. But women of all ages with diabetes have an increased risk of heart disease because diabetes cancels out the protective effects of being a woman in her child-bearing years.

People with diabetes who have already had one heart attack run an even greater risk of having a second one. In addition, heart attacks in people with diabetes are more serious and more

About This Chapter: From "Diabetes, Heart Disease, and Stroke," National Institute of Diabetes and Digestive and Kidney Diseases (www.niddk.nih.gov), December 2005. Updated by David A. Cooke, MD, FACP, August 2011.

likely to result in death. High blood glucose levels over time can lead to increased deposits of fatty materials on the insides of the blood vessel walls. These deposits may affect blood flow, increasing the chance of clogging and hardening of blood vessels (atherosclerosis).

What are the risk factors for heart disease and stroke in people with diabetes?

Diabetes itself is a risk factor for heart disease and stroke. Also, many people with diabetes have other conditions that increase their chance of developing heart disease and stroke. These conditions are called risk factors. One risk factor for heart disease and stroke is having a family history of heart disease. If one or more members of your family had a heart attack at an early age (before age 55 for men or 65 for women), you may be at increased risk.

You can't change whether heart disease runs in your family, but you can take steps to control the other risk factors for heart disease listed here:

- **Having Central Obesity:** Central obesity means carrying extra weight around the waist, as opposed to the hips. A waist measurement of more than 40 inches for men and more than 35 inches for women means you have central obesity. Your risk of heart disease is higher because abdominal fat can increase the production of LDL (bad) cholesterol, the type of blood fat that can be deposited on the inside of blood vessel walls.

- **Having Abnormal Blood Fat (Cholesterol) Levels:** LDL cholesterol can build up inside your blood vessels, leading to narrowing and hardening of your arteries—the blood vessels that carry blood from the heart to the rest of the body. Arteries can then become blocked. Therefore, high levels of LDL cholesterol raise your risk of getting heart disease. Triglycerides are another type of blood fat that can raise your risk of heart disease when the levels are high. HDL (good) cholesterol removes deposits from inside your blood vessels and takes them to the liver for removal. Low levels of HDL cholesterol increase your risk for heart disease.

- **Having High Blood Pressure:** If you have high blood pressure, also called hypertension, your heart must work harder to pump blood. High blood pressure can strain the heart, damage blood vessels, and increase your risk of heart attack, stroke, eye problems, and kidney problems.

- **Smoking:** Smoking doubles your risk of getting heart disease. Stopping smoking is especially important for people with diabetes because both smoking and diabetes narrow blood vessels. Smoking also increases the risk of other long-term complications, such as eye problems. In addition, smoking can damage the blood vessels in your legs and increase the risk of amputation.

Why are my heart and blood vessels at risk?

Your heart and blood vessels make up your circulatory system. Your heart is a muscle that pumps blood through your body. Your heart pumps blood carrying oxygen to large blood vessels, called arteries, and small blood vessels, called capillaries. Other blood vessels, called veins, carry blood back to the heart.

Several things, including having diabetes, can make your blood cholesterol level too high. Cholesterol is a substance that is made by the body and used for many important functions. Cholesterol is also found in some food derived from animals. When cholesterol is too high, the insides of large blood vessels become narrowed or clogged. This problem is called atherosclerosis.

Narrowed and clogged blood vessels make it harder for enough blood to get to all parts of your body. This condition can cause problems.

When blood vessels become narrowed and clogged, you can have serious health problems:

- **Chest Pain** (also called angina): When you have angina, you feel pain in your chest, arms, shoulders, or back. You may feel the pain more when your heart beats faster, such as when you exercise. The pain may go away when you rest. You also may sweat a lot and feel very weak. If you do not get treatment, chest pain may happen more often. If diabetes has damaged your heart nerves, you may not feel the chest pain. If you have chest pain with activity, contact your doctor.

- **Heart Attack:** A heart attack happens when a blood vessel in or near your heart becomes blocked. Then your heart muscle can't get enough blood. When an area of your heart muscle stops working, your heart becomes weaker. During a heart attack, you may have chest pain along with nausea, indigestion, extreme weakness, and sweating. Or you may have no symptoms at all. If you have chest pain that persists, call 911. Delay in getting treatment may make a heart attack worse.

- **Stroke:** A stroke can happen when the blood supply to your brain is blocked. Then your brain can be damaged.

Source: Excerpted from "Prevent Diabetes Problems: Keep Your Heart and Blood Vessels Healthy," National Institute of Diabetes and Digestive and Kidney Diseases, April 2009.

What is metabolic syndrome and how is it linked to heart disease?

Metabolic syndrome is a grouping of traits and medical conditions that puts people at risk for both heart disease and type 2 diabetes. It is defined by the National Cholesterol Education Program as having any three of the following five traits and medical conditions:

- Elevated waist circumference: Waist measurement of 40 inches or more in men; 35 inches or more in women

- Elevated levels of triglycerides: 150 mg/dL or higher or taking medication for elevated triglyceride levels

- Low levels of HDL (good) cholesterol: Below 40 mg/dL in men; below 50 mg/dL in women; or taking medication for low HDL cholesterol levels

- Elevated blood pressure levels: 130 mm Hg or higher for systolic blood pressure or 85 mm Hg or higher for diastolic blood pressure or taking medication for elevated blood pressure levels

- Elevated fasting blood glucose levels: 100 mg/dL or higher or taking medication for elevated blood glucose levels

The source for these criteria is: Grundy SM, et al. Diagnosis and Management of the Metabolic Syndrome: An American Heart Association/National Heart, Lung, and Blood Institute Scientific Statement. *Circulation*. 2005;112:2735–2752. Other definitions of similar conditions have been developed by the American Association of Clinical Endocrinologists, the International Diabetes Federation, and the World Health Organization.

What types of heart and blood vessel disease occur in people with diabetes?

Two major types of heart and blood vessel disease, also called cardiovascular disease, are common in people with diabetes: coronary artery disease (CAD) and cerebral vascular disease. People with diabetes are also at risk for heart failure. Narrowing or blockage of the blood vessels in the legs, a condition called peripheral arterial disease, can also occur in people with diabetes.

Coronary Artery Disease: Coronary artery disease, also called ischemic heart disease, is caused by a hardening or thickening of the walls of the blood vessels that go to your heart. Your blood supplies oxygen and other materials your heart needs for normal functioning. If the blood vessels to your heart become narrowed or blocked by fatty deposits, the blood supply is reduced or cut off, resulting in a heart attack.

Cerebral Vascular Disease: Cerebral vascular disease affects blood flow to the brain, leading to strokes and TIAs (transient ischemic attacks). It is caused by narrowing, blocking, or hardening of the blood vessels that go to the brain or by high blood pressure.

A stroke results when the blood supply to the brain is suddenly cut off, which can occur when a blood vessel in the brain or neck is blocked or bursts. Brain cells are then deprived of oxygen and die. A stroke can result in problems with speech or vision or can cause weakness or paralysis. Most strokes are caused by fatty deposits or blood clots—jelly-like clumps of blood cells—that narrow or block one of the blood vessels in the brain or neck. A blood clot may stay where it formed or can travel within the body. People with diabetes are at increased risk for strokes caused by blood clots.

A stroke may also be caused by a bleeding blood vessel in the brain. Called an aneurysm, a break in a blood vessel can occur as a result of high blood pressure or a weak spot in a blood vessel wall.

TIAs are caused by a temporary blockage of a blood vessel to the brain. This blockage leads to a brief, sudden change in brain function, such as temporary numbness or weakness on one side of the body. Sudden changes in brain function also can lead to loss of balance, confusion, blindness in one or both eyes, double vision, difficulty speaking, or a severe headache. However, most symptoms disappear quickly and permanent damage is unlikely. If symptoms do not resolve in a few minutes, rather than a TIA, the event could be a stroke. The occurrence of a TIA means that a person is at risk for a stroke sometime in the future.

Heart Failure: Heart failure is a chronic condition in which the heart cannot pump blood properly—it does not mean that the heart suddenly stops working. Heart failure develops over a period of years, and symptoms can get worse over time. People with diabetes have at least twice the risk of heart failure as other people. One type of heart failure is congestive heart failure, in which fluid builds up inside body tissues. If the buildup is in the lungs, breathing becomes difficult.

Blockage of the blood vessels and high blood glucose levels also can damage heart muscle and cause irregular heart beats. People with damage to heart muscle, a condition called cardiomyopathy, may have no symptoms in the early stages, but later they may experience weakness, shortness of breath, a severe cough, fatigue, and swelling of the legs and feet. Diabetes can also interfere with pain signals normally carried by the nerves, explaining why a person with diabetes may not experience the typical warning signs of a heart attack.

Peripheral Arterial Disease: Another condition related to heart disease and common in people with diabetes is peripheral arterial disease (PAD). With this condition, the blood vessels in the legs are narrowed or blocked by fatty deposits, decreasing blood flow to the legs and feet. PAD increases the chances of a heart attack or stroke occurring. Poor circulation in the legs and feet also raises the risk of amputation. Sometimes people with PAD develop pain in the calf or other parts of the leg when walking, which is relieved by resting for a few minutes.

How will I know whether I have heart disease?

One sign of heart disease is angina, the pain that occurs when a blood vessel to the heart is narrowed and the blood supply is reduced. You may feel pain or discomfort in your chest, shoulders, arms, jaw, or back, especially when you exercise. The pain may go away when you rest or take angina medicine. Angina does not cause permanent damage to the heart muscle, but if you have angina, your chance of having a heart attack increases.

A heart attack occurs when a blood vessel to the heart becomes blocked. With blockage, not enough blood can reach that part of the heart muscle and permanent damage results. During a heart attack, you may have symptoms such as the following:

- Chest pain or discomfort
- Pain or discomfort in your arms, back, jaw, neck, or stomach
- Shortness of breath
- Sweating
- Nausea
- Light-headedness

Symptoms may come and go. However, in some people, particularly those with diabetes, symptoms may be mild or absent due to a condition in which the heart rate stays at the same level during exercise, inactivity, stress, or sleep. Also, nerve damage caused by diabetes may result in lack of pain during a heart attack.

How do narrowed blood vessels cause high blood pressure?

Narrowed blood vessels leave a smaller opening for blood to flow through. Having narrowed blood vessels is like turning on a garden hose and holding your thumb over the opening. The smaller opening makes the water shoot out with more pressure. In the same way, narrowed blood vessels lead to high blood pressure. In addition, normal blood vessels are quite elastic, and will stretch under high pressure, which limits sudden jumps in pressure. Narrowed vessels are very stiff and inflexible, which leads to higher pressures when the heart pumps. Other factors, such as kidney problems and being overweight, also can lead to high blood pressure.

Many people with diabetes also have high blood pressure. If you have heart, eye, or kidney problems from diabetes, high blood pressure can make them worse.

You will see your blood pressure written with two numbers separated by a slash. For example, your reading might be 120/70, said as "120 over 70." For people with diabetes, the target is to keep the first number below 130 and the second number below 80.

Source: Excerpted from "Prevent Diabetes Problems: Keep Your Heart and Blood Vessels Healthy," National Institute of Diabetes and Digestive and Kidney Diseases, April 2009. Updated by David A. Cooke, MD, FACP, August 2011.

Women may not have chest pain but may be more likely to have shortness of breath, nausea, or back and jaw pain. If you have symptoms of a heart attack, call 911 right away. Treatment is most effective if given within an hour of a heart attack. Early treatment can prevent permanent damage to the heart.

Your doctor should check your risk for heart disease and stroke at least once a year by checking your cholesterol and blood pressure levels and asking whether you smoke or have a family history of premature heart disease. The doctor can also check your urine for protein, another risk factor for heart disease. If you are at high risk or have symptoms of heart disease, you may need to undergo further testing.

How will I know whether I have had a stroke?

The following signs may mean that you have had a stroke:

- Sudden weakness or numbness of your face, arm, or leg on one side of your body
- Sudden confusion, trouble talking, or trouble understanding
- Sudden dizziness, loss of balance, or trouble walking
- Sudden trouble seeing out of one or both eyes or sudden double vision
- Sudden severe headache

If you have any of these symptoms, call 911 right away. You can help prevent permanent damage by getting to a hospital within an hour of a stroke. If your doctor thinks you have had a stroke, you may have tests such as a neurological examination to check your nervous system, special scans, blood tests, ultrasound examinations, or x-rays. You also may be given medication that dissolves blood clots.

What research is being done about cardiovascular disease and diabetes?

The National Institute of Diabetes and Digestive and Kidney Diseases (NIDDK) is one of the National Institutes of Health (NIH) under the U.S. Department of Health and Human Services. The NIDDK conducts and supports research in diabetes, glucose metabolism, and related conditions. Several studies related to diabetes, heart disease, and stroke are under way.

The Look AHEAD (Action for Health in Diabetes) trial is studying whether strategies for weight loss in obese people with type 2 diabetes can improve health. This trial is also sponsored by other NIH Institutes and by the Centers for Disease Control and Prevention. For more information on the Look AHEAD trial, visit the website at www.niddk.nih.gov/patient/SHOW/lookahead.htm.

The EDIC (Epidemiology of Diabetes Interventions and Complications) study is examining the long-term effects of prior intensive versus conventional blood glucose control. It is a follow-up study of patients who took part more than a decade ago in the Diabetes Control and Complications Trial (DCCT), a major clinical study funded by the National Institutes of Health.

The BARI 2D (Bypass Angioplasty Revascularization Investigation 2 Diabetes) trial, sponsored by the National Heart, Lung, and Blood Institute, in partnership with NIDDK, is studying approaches to the medical care of people with type 2 diabetes who also have coronary artery disease. For more information on the BARI 2D trial, visit the website at www.bari2d.org or call the nearest research center (listed on the website).

The ACCORD (Action to Control Cardiovascular Risk in Diabetes) trial is studying three approaches to preventing major cardiovascular events in individuals with type 2 diabetes. For more information on the ACCORD trial, visit the website at www.accordtrial.org or call 888-342-2380.

The NIDDK and other components of the NIH will continue to fund research on the best ways to enhance health promotion, self-management, and risk reduction in people with diabetes. For more information on current studies, check www.ClinicalTrials.gov or call the National Diabetes Information Clearinghouse at 800-860-8747.

Points To Remember

- If you have diabetes, you are at least twice as likely as other people to have heart disease or a stroke.
- Controlling the ABCs of diabetes—A1C (blood glucose), blood pressure, and cholesterol—can cut your risk of heart disease and stroke.
- Choosing foods wisely, being physically active, losing weight, quitting smoking, and taking medications (if needed) can all help lower your risk of heart disease and stroke.
- If you have any warning signs of a heart attack or a stroke, get medical care immediately—don't delay. Early treatment of heart attack and stroke in a hospital emergency room can reduce damage to the heart and the brain.

Source: National Institute of Diabetes and Digestive and Kidney Diseases (www.niddk.nih.gov), December 2005. Reviewed by David A. Cooke, MD, FACP, August 2011.

Chapter 43

Diabetic Nerve Damage

What are diabetic neuropathies?

Diabetic neuropathies are a family of nerve disorders caused by diabetes. People with diabetes can, over time, develop nerve damage throughout the body. Some people with nerve damage have no symptoms. Others may have symptoms such as pain, tingling, or numbness—loss of feeling—in the hands, arms, feet, and legs. Nerve problems can occur in every organ system, including the digestive tract, heart, and sex organs.

About 60 to 70 percent of people with diabetes have some form of neuropathy. People with diabetes can develop nerve problems at any time, but risk rises with age and longer duration of diabetes. The highest rates of neuropathy are among people who have had diabetes for at least 25 years. Diabetic neuropathies also appear to be more common in people who have problems controlling their blood glucose, also called blood sugar, as well as those with high levels of blood fat and blood pressure and those who are overweight.

What causes diabetic neuropathies?

The causes are probably different for different types of diabetic neuropathy. Researchers are studying how prolonged exposure to high blood glucose causes nerve damage. Nerve damage is likely due to a combination of factors:

- Metabolic factors, such as high blood glucose, long duration of diabetes, abnormal blood fat levels, and possibly low levels of insulin

About This Chapter: From "Diabetic Neuropathies: The Nerve Damage of Diabetes," National Institute of Diabetes and Digestive and Kidney Diseases, February 2009.

What does my nervous system do?

Nerves carry messages back and forth between the brain and other parts of the body. All of your nerves together make up the nervous system.

Some nerves tell the brain what is happening in the body. For example, when you step on a tack, the nerve in your foot tells the brain about the pain. Other nerves tell the body what to do. For example, nerves from the brain tell your stomach when it is time to move food into your intestines.

Source: Excerpted from "Prevent Diabetes Problems: Keep Your Nervous System Healthy," National Institute of Diabetes and Digestive and Kidney Diseases, April 2009.

- Neurovascular factors, leading to damage to the blood vessels that carry oxygen and nutrients to nerves

- Autoimmune factors that cause inflammation in nerves

- Mechanical injury to nerves, such as carpal tunnel syndrome

- Inherited traits that increase susceptibility to nerve disease

- Lifestyle factors, such as smoking or alcohol use

What are the symptoms of diabetic neuropathies?

Symptoms depend on the type of neuropathy and which nerves are affected. Some people with nerve damage have no symptoms at all. For others, the first symptom is often numbness, tingling, or pain in the feet. Symptoms are often minor at first, and because most nerve damage occurs over several years, mild cases may go unnoticed for a long time. Symptoms can involve the sensory, motor, and autonomic—or involuntary—nervous systems. In some people, mainly those with focal neuropathy, the onset of pain may be sudden and severe. The symptoms of nerve damage may include the following:

- Numbness, tingling, or pain in the toes, feet, legs, hands, arms, and fingers

- Wasting of the muscles of the feet or hands

- Indigestion, nausea, or vomiting

- Diarrhea or constipation

- Dizziness or faintness due to a drop in blood pressure after standing or sitting up

- Problems with urination

- Erectile dysfunction in men or vaginal dryness in women

- Weakness

Symptoms that are not due to neuropathy, but often accompany it, include weight loss and depression.

What are the types of diabetic neuropathy?

Diabetic neuropathy can be classified as peripheral, autonomic, proximal, or focal. Each affects different parts of the body in various ways.

- Peripheral neuropathy, the most common type of diabetic neuropathy, causes pain or loss of feeling in the toes, feet, legs, hands, and arms.

- Autonomic neuropathy causes changes in digestion, bowel and bladder function, sexual response, and perspiration. It can also affect the nerves that serve the heart and control blood pressure, as well as nerves in the lungs and eyes. Autonomic neuropathy can also cause hypoglycemia unawareness, a condition in which people no longer experience the warning symptoms of low blood glucose levels.

- Proximal neuropathy causes pain in the thighs, hips, or buttocks and leads to weakness in the legs.

- Focal neuropathy results in the sudden weakness of one nerve or a group of nerves, causing muscle weakness or pain. Any nerve in the body can be affected.

Neuropathy Affects Nerves Throughout the Body

- Peripheral neuropathy affects toes, feet, legs, hands, and arms.
- Autonomic neuropathy affects heart and blood vessels, digestive system, urinary tract, sex organs, sweat glands, eyes, and lungs.
- Proximal neuropathy affects thighs, hips, buttocks, and legs.
- Focal neuropathy affects eyes, facial muscles, ears, pelvis and lower back, chest, abdomen, thighs, legs, and feet.

Source: NIDDK, February 2009.

What is peripheral neuropathy?

Peripheral neuropathy, also called distal symmetric neuropathy or sensorimotor neuropathy, is nerve damage in the arms and legs. Your feet and legs are likely to be affected before your hands and arms. Many people with diabetes have signs of neuropathy that a doctor could note but feel no symptoms themselves. Symptoms of peripheral neuropathy may include numbness or insensitivity to pain or temperature; a tingling, burning, or prickling sensation; sharp pains or cramps; extreme sensitivity to touch, even light touch; or loss of balance and coordination. These symptoms are often worse at night.

Peripheral neuropathy may also cause muscle weakness and loss of reflexes, especially at the ankle, leading to changes in the way a person walks. Foot deformities, such as hammertoes and the collapse of the midfoot, may occur. Blisters and sores may appear on numb areas of the foot because pressure or injury goes unnoticed. If foot injuries are not treated promptly, the infection may spread to the bone, and the foot may then have to be amputated. Some experts estimate that half of all such amputations are preventable if minor problems are caught and treated in time.

What is autonomic neuropathy?

Autonomic neuropathy affects the nerves that control the heart, regulate blood pressure, and control blood glucose levels. Autonomic neuropathy also affects other internal organs, causing problems with digestion, respiratory function, urination, sexual response, and vision. In addition, the system that restores blood glucose levels to normal after a hypoglycemic episode may be affected, resulting in loss of the warning symptoms of hypoglycemia.

Hypoglycemia Unawareness: Normally, symptoms such as shakiness, sweating, and palpitations occur when blood glucose levels drop below 70 mg/dL. In people with autonomic neuropathy, symptoms may not occur, making hypoglycemia difficult to recognize. Problems other than neuropathy can also cause hypoglycemia unawareness.

Heart And Blood Vessels: The heart and blood vessels are part of the cardiovascular system, which controls blood circulation. Damage to nerves in the cardiovascular system interferes with the body's ability to adjust blood pressure and heart rate. As a result, blood pressure may drop sharply after sitting or standing, causing a person to feel light-headed or even to faint. Damage to the nerves that control heart rate can mean that your heart rate stays high, instead of rising and falling in response to normal body functions and physical activity.

Digestive System: Nerve damage to the digestive system most commonly causes constipation. Damage can also cause the stomach to empty too slowly, a condition called gastroparesis. Severe gastroparesis can lead to persistent nausea and vomiting, bloating, and loss of appetite. Gastroparesis can also make blood glucose levels fluctuate widely, due to abnormal food digestion.

Nerve damage to the esophagus may make swallowing difficult, while nerve damage to the bowels can cause constipation alternating with frequent, uncontrolled diarrhea, especially at night. Problems with the digestive system can lead to weight loss.

Urinary Tract And Sex Organs: Autonomic neuropathy often affects the organs that control urination and sexual function. Nerve damage can prevent the bladder from emptying completely, allowing bacteria to grow in the bladder and kidneys and causing urinary tract infections. When the nerves of the bladder are damaged, urinary incontinence may result because a person may not be able to sense when the bladder is full or control the muscles that release urine.

Autonomic neuropathy can also gradually decrease sexual response in men and women, although the sex drive may be unchanged. A man may be unable to have erections or may reach sexual climax without ejaculating normally. A woman may have difficulty with arousal, lubrication, or orgasm.

Sweat Glands: Autonomic neuropathy can affect the nerves that control sweating. When nerve damage prevents the sweat glands from working properly, the body cannot regulate its temperature as it should. Nerve damage can also cause profuse sweating at night or while eating.

Eyes: Finally, autonomic neuropathy can affect the pupils of the eyes, making them less responsive to changes in light. As a result, a person may not be able to see well when a light is turned on in a dark room or may have trouble driving at night.

What's It Mean?

The nervous system has four main parts—cranial, central, peripheral, and autonomic.

- Cranial nerves go from your brain to your eyes, mouth, ears, and other parts of your head.
- Central nerves are in your brain and spinal cord.
- Peripheral nerves go from your spinal cord to your arms, hands, legs, and feet.
- Autonomic nerves go from your spinal cord to your lungs, heart, stomach, intestines, bladder, and sex organs.

Source: Excerpted from "Prevent Diabetes Problems: Keep Your Nervous System Healthy," National Institute of Diabetes and Digestive and Kidney Diseases, April 2009.

What is proximal neuropathy?

Proximal neuropathy, sometimes called lumbosacral plexus neuropathy, femoral neuropathy, or diabetic amyotrophy, starts with pain in the thighs, hips, buttocks, or legs, usually on one side of the body. This type of neuropathy is more common in those with type 2 diabetes and in older adults with diabetes. Proximal neuropathy causes weakness in the legs and the inability to go from a sitting to a standing position without help. Treatment for weakness or pain is usually needed. The length of the recovery period varies, depending on the type of nerve damage.

What is focal neuropathy?

Focal neuropathy appears suddenly and affects specific nerves, most often in the head, torso, or leg. Focal neuropathy may cause an inability to focus the eye, double vision, or an aching behind one eye. It can lead to paralysis on one side of the face (called Bell's palsy); severe pain in the lower back or pelvis; pain in the front of a thigh; pain in the chest, stomach, or side; pain on the outside of the shin or inside of the foot; or chest or abdominal pain that is sometimes mistaken for heart disease, a heart attack, or appendicitis.

Focal neuropathy is painful and unpredictable and occurs most often in older adults with diabetes. However, it tends to improve by itself over weeks or months and does not cause long-term damage.

People with diabetes also tend to develop nerve compressions, also called entrapment syndromes. One of the most common is carpal tunnel syndrome, which causes numbness and tingling of the hand and sometimes muscle weakness or pain. Other nerves susceptible to entrapment may cause pain on the outside of the shin or the inside of the foot.

How can I prevent diabetic neuropathies?

The best way to prevent neuropathy is to keep your blood glucose levels as close to the normal range as possible. Maintaining safe blood glucose levels protects nerves throughout your body.

How can diabetes hurt my nervous system?

Having high blood glucose for many years can damage the blood vessels that bring oxygen to some nerves. High blood glucose can also hurt the covering on the nerves. Damaged nerves may stop sending messages. Or they may send messages too slowly or at the wrong times.

Diabetic neuropathy is the medical term for damage to the nervous system from diabetes.

Source: Excerpted from "Prevent Diabetes Problems: Keep Your Nervous System Healthy," National Institute of Diabetes and Digestive and Kidney Diseases, April 2009.

How are diabetic neuropathies diagnosed?

Doctors diagnose neuropathy on the basis of symptoms and a physical exam. During the exam, your doctor may check blood pressure, heart rate, muscle strength, reflexes, and sensitivity to position changes, vibration, temperature, or light touch.

Foot Exams: Experts recommend that people with diabetes have a comprehensive foot exam each year to check for peripheral neuropathy. People diagnosed with peripheral neuropathy need more frequent foot exams. A comprehensive foot exam assesses the skin, muscles, bones, circulation, and sensation of the feet. Your doctor may assess protective sensation or feeling in your feet by touching your foot with a nylon monofilament—similar to a bristle on a hairbrush—attached to a wand or by pricking your foot with a pin. People who cannot sense pressure from a pinprick or monofilament have lost protective sensation and are at risk for developing foot sores that may not heal properly. The doctor may also check temperature perception or use a tuning fork, which is more sensitive than touch pressure, to assess vibration perception.

Other Tests: The doctor may perform other tests as part of your diagnosis.

- Nerve conduction studies or electromyography are sometimes used to help determine the type and extent of nerve damage. Nerve conduction studies check the transmission of electrical current through a nerve. Electromyography shows how well muscles respond to electrical signals transmitted by nearby nerves. These tests are rarely needed to diagnose neuropathy.

- A check of heart rate variability shows how the heart responds to deep breathing and to changes in blood pressure and posture.

- Ultrasound uses sound waves to produce an image of internal organs. An ultrasound of the bladder and other parts of the urinary tract, for example, can show how these organs preserve a normal structure and whether the bladder empties completely after urination.

How are diabetic neuropathies treated?

The first treatment step is to bring blood glucose levels within the normal range to help prevent further nerve damage. Blood glucose monitoring, meal planning, physical activity, and diabetes medicines or insulin will help control blood glucose levels. Symptoms may get worse when blood glucose is first brought under control, but over time, maintaining lower blood glucose levels helps lessen symptoms. Good blood glucose control may also help prevent or delay the onset of further problems. As scientists learn more about the underlying causes of neuropathy, new treatments may become available to help slow, prevent, or even reverse nerve damage.

Additional treatment depends on the type of nerve problem and symptom. If you have problems with your feet, your doctor may refer you to a foot care specialist.

Pain Relief: Doctors usually treat painful diabetic neuropathy with oral medications, although other types of treatments may help some people. People with severe nerve pain may benefit from a combination of medications or treatments. Talk with your health care provider about options for treating your neuropathy.

The following medications are sometimes used to help relieve diabetic nerve pain:

- Tricyclic antidepressants, such as amitriptyline, imipramine, and desipramine (Norpramin, Pertofrane)

- Other types of antidepressants, such as duloxetine (Cymbalta), venlafaxine, bupropion (Wellbutrin), paroxetine (Paxil), and citalopram (Celexa)

- Anticonvulsants, such as pregabalin (Lyrica), gabapentin (Gabarone, Neurontin), carbamazepine, and lamotrigine (Lamictal)

- Opioids and opioid-like drugs, such as controlled-release oxycodone, an opioid; and tramadol (Ultram), an opioid that also acts as an antidepressant

Duloxetine and pregabalin are approved by the U.S. Food and Drug Administration specifically for treating painful diabetic peripheral neuropathy.

You do not have to be depressed for an antidepressant to help relieve your nerve pain. All medications have side effects, and some are not recommended for use in older adults or those with heart disease. Because over-the-counter pain medicines such as acetaminophen and ibuprofen may not work well for treating most nerve pain and can have serious side effects, some experts recommend avoiding these medications.

Treatments that are applied to the skin—typically to the feet—include capsaicin cream and lidocaine patches (Lidoderm, Lidopain). Studies suggest that nitrate sprays or patches for the feet may relieve pain. Studies of alpha-lipoic acid, an antioxidant, and evening primrose oil have shown that they can help relieve symptoms and may improve nerve function.

A device called a bed cradle can keep sheets and blankets from touching sensitive feet and legs. Acupuncture, biofeedback, or physical therapy may help relieve pain in some people. Treatments that involve electrical nerve stimulation, magnetic therapy, and laser or light therapy may be helpful but need further study. Researchers are also studying several new therapies in clinical trials.

Gastrointestinal Problems: To relieve mild symptoms of gastroparesis—indigestion, belching, nausea, or vomiting—doctors suggest eating small, frequent meals; avoiding fats;

and eating less fiber. When symptoms are severe, doctors may prescribe erythromycin to speed digestion, metoclopramide to speed digestion and help relieve nausea, or other medications to help regulate digestion or reduce stomach acid secretion.

To relieve diarrhea or other bowel problems, doctors may prescribe an antibiotic such as tetracycline, or other medications as appropriate.

Dizziness And Weakness: Sitting or standing slowly may help prevent the light-headedness, dizziness, or fainting associated with blood pressure and circulation problems. Raising the head of the bed or wearing elastic stockings may also help. Some people benefit from increased salt in the diet and treatment with salt-retaining hormones. Others benefit from high blood pressure medications. Physical therapy can help when muscle weakness or loss of coordination is a problem.

Urinary And Sexual Problems: To clear up a urinary tract infection, the doctor will probably prescribe an antibiotic. Drinking plenty of fluids will help prevent another infection. People who have incontinence should try to urinate at regular intervals—every three hours, for example—since they may not be able to tell when the bladder is full.

Points To Remember

- Diabetic neuropathies are nerve disorders caused by many of the abnormalities common to diabetes, such as high blood glucose.
- Neuropathy can affect nerves throughout the body, causing numbness and sometimes pain in the hands, arms, feet, or legs, and problems with the digestive tract, heart, sex organs, and other body systems.
- Treatment first involves bringing blood glucose levels within the normal range. Good blood glucose control may help prevent or delay the onset of further problems.
- Foot care is an important part of treatment. People with neuropathy need to inspect their feet daily for any injuries. Untreated injuries increase the risk of infected foot sores and amputation.
- Treatment also includes pain relief and other medications as needed, depending on the type of nerve damage.
- Smoking significantly increases the risk of foot problems and amputation. If you smoke, ask your health care provider for help with quitting.

Source: NIDDK, February 2009.

To treat erectile dysfunction in men, the doctor will first do tests to rule out a hormonal cause. Several methods are available to treat erectile dysfunction caused by neuropathy. Medicines are available to help men have and maintain erections by increasing blood flow to the penis. Some are oral medications and others are injected into the penis or inserted into the urethra at the tip of the penis. Mechanical vacuum devices can also increase blood flow to the penis. Another option is to surgically implant an inflatable or semirigid device in the penis.

Vaginal lubricants may be useful for women when neuropathy causes vaginal dryness. To treat problems with arousal and orgasm, the doctor may refer women to a gynecologist.

Foot Care: People with neuropathy need to take special care of their feet. The nerves to the feet are the longest in the body and are the ones most often affected by neuropathy. Loss of sensation in the feet means that sores or injuries may not be noticed and may become ulcerated or infected. Circulation problems also increase the risk of foot ulcers.

More than half of all lower-limb amputations in the United States occur in people with diabetes—86,000 amputations per year. Doctors estimate that nearly half of the amputations caused by neuropathy and poor circulation could have been prevented by careful foot care.

Chapter 44

Diabetic Eye Disease

What is diabetic eye disease?

Diabetic eye disease refers to a group of eye problems that people with diabetes may face as a complication of diabetes. All can cause severe vision loss or even blindness. Diabetic eye disease may include the following conditions:

- **Diabetic Retinopathy:** Damage to the blood vessels in the retina.

- **Cataract:** Clouding of the eye's lens. Cataracts develop at an earlier age in people with diabetes.

- **Glaucoma:** Increase in fluid pressure inside the eye that leads to optic nerve damage and loss of vision. A person with diabetes is nearly twice as likely to get glaucoma as other adults.

What is diabetic retinopathy?

Diabetic retinopathy is the most common diabetic eye disease and a leading cause of blindness in American adults. It is caused by changes in the blood vessels of the retina.

In some people with diabetic retinopathy, blood vessels may swell and leak fluid. In other people, abnormal new blood vessels grow on the surface of the retina. The retina is the light-sensitive tissue at the back of the eye. A healthy retina is necessary for good vision.

If you have diabetic retinopathy, at first you may not notice changes to your vision. But over time, diabetic retinopathy can get worse and cause vision loss. Diabetic retinopathy usually affects both eyes.

About This Chapter: From "Facts about Diabetic Retinopathy," National Eye Institute, August 2010.

What are the stages of diabetic retinopathy?

Diabetic retinopathy has four stages:

Mild Nonproliferative Retinopathy: At this earliest stage, microaneurysms occur. They are small areas of balloon-like swelling in the retina's tiny blood vessels.

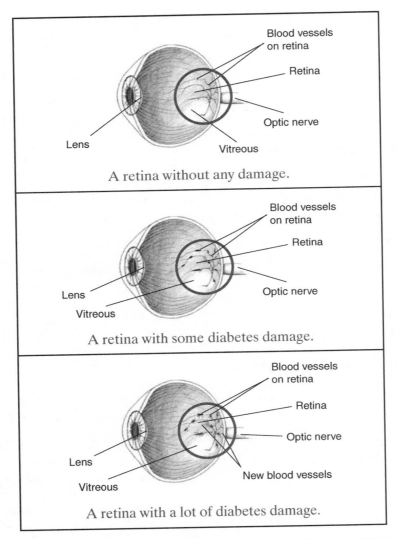

Figure 44.1. Diabetes can hurt the retinas of your eyes (Source: "Prevent Diabetes Problems: Keep Your Eyes Healthy," National Institute of Diabetes and Digestive and Kidney Diseases, November 2008.

Moderate Nonproliferative Retinopathy: As the disease progresses, some blood vessels that nourish the retina are blocked.

Severe Nonproliferative Retinopathy: Many more blood vessels are blocked, depriving several areas of the retina with their blood supply. These areas of the retina send signals to the body to grow new blood vessels for nourishment.

Proliferative Retinopathy: At this advanced stage, the signals sent by the retina for nourishment trigger the growth of new blood vessels. This condition is called proliferative retinopathy. These new blood vessels are abnormal and fragile. They grow along the retina and along the surface of the clear, vitreous gel that fills the inside of the eye. By themselves, these blood vessels do not cause symptoms or vision loss. However, they have thin, fragile walls. If they leak blood, severe vision loss and even blindness can result.

How does diabetic retinopathy cause vision loss?

Blood vessels damaged from diabetic retinopathy can cause vision loss in two ways:

Fragile, abnormal blood vessels can develop and leak blood into the center of the eye, blurring vision. This is proliferative retinopathy and is the fourth and most advanced stage of the disease.

Fluid can leak into the center of the macula, the part of the eye where sharp, straight-ahead vision occurs. The fluid makes the macula swell, blurring vision. This condition is called macular edema. It can occur at any stage of diabetic retinopathy, although it is more likely to occur as the disease progresses. About half of the people with proliferative retinopathy also have macular edema.

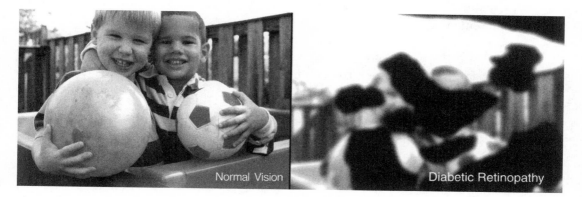

Normal Vision

Diabetic Retinopathy

Figure 44.2. Normal vision and the same scene viewed by a person with diabetic retinopathy (Source: "Facts about Diabetic Retinopathy," National Eye Institute, August 2010.)

Who is at risk for diabetic retinopathy?

All people with diabetes—both type 1 and type 2—are at risk. That's why everyone with diabetes should get a comprehensive dilated eye exam at least once a year. The longer someone has diabetes, the more likely he or she will get diabetic retinopathy. Between 40 to 45 percent of Americans diagnosed with diabetes have some stage of diabetic retinopathy. If you have diabetic retinopathy, your doctor can recommend treatment to help prevent its progression.

During pregnancy, diabetic retinopathy may be a problem for women with diabetes. To protect vision, every pregnant woman with diabetes should have a comprehensive dilated eye exam as soon as possible. Your doctor may recommend additional exams during your pregnancy.

What can I do to protect my vision?

If you have diabetes get a comprehensive dilated eye exam at least once a year and remember:

- Proliferative retinopathy can develop without symptoms. At this advanced stage, you are at high risk for vision loss.

- Macular edema can develop without symptoms at any of the four stages of diabetic retinopathy.

- You can develop both proliferative retinopathy and macular edema and still see fine. However, you are at high risk for vision loss.

- Your eye care professional can tell if you have macular edema or any stage of diabetic retinopathy. Whether or not you have symptoms, early detection and timely treatment can prevent vision loss.

If you have diabetic retinopathy, you may need an eye exam more often. People with proliferative retinopathy can reduce their risk of blindness by 95 percent with timely treatment and appropriate follow-up care.

The Diabetes Control and Complications Trial (DCCT) showed that better control of blood sugar levels slows the onset and progression of retinopathy. The people with diabetes who kept their blood sugar levels as close to normal as possible also had much less kidney and nerve disease. Better control also reduces the need for sight-saving laser surgery.

This level of blood sugar control may not be best for everyone, including some elderly patients, children under age 13, or people with heart disease. Be sure to ask your doctor if such a control program is right for you.

Other studies have shown that controlling elevated blood pressure and cholesterol can reduce the risk of vision loss. Controlling these will help your overall health as well as help protect your vision.

Does diabetic retinopathy have any symptoms?

Often there are no symptoms in the early stages of the disease, nor is there any pain. Don't wait for symptoms. Be sure to have a comprehensive dilated eye exam at least once a year.

Blurred vision may occur when the macula—the part of the retina that provides sharp central vision—swells from leaking fluid. This condition is called macular edema.

If new blood vessels grow on the surface of the retina, they can bleed into the eye and block vision.

What are the symptoms of proliferative retinopathy if bleeding occurs?

At first, you will see a few specks of blood, or spots, "floating" in your vision. If spots occur, see your eye care professional as soon as possible. You may need treatment before more serious bleeding occurs. Hemorrhages tend to happen more than once, often during sleep.

Sometimes, without treatment, the spots clear, and you will see better. However, bleeding can reoccur and cause severely blurred vision. You need to be examined by your eye care professional at the first sign of blurred vision, before more bleeding occurs.

If left untreated, proliferative retinopathy can cause severe vision loss and even blindness. Also, the earlier you receive treatment, the more likely treatment will be effective.

What's It Mean?

Retina: The retina is the lining at the back of the eye. The retina's job is to sense light coming into the eye.

Vitreous: The vitreous is a jelly-like fluid that fills the back of the eye.

Lens: The lens is at the front of the eye. The lens focuses light on the retina.

Optic nerve: The optic nerve is the eye's main nerve to the brain.

"Prevent Diabetes Problems: Keep Your Eyes Healthy," National Institute of Diabetes and Digestive and Kidney Diseases, November 2008.

How are diabetic retinopathy and macular edema detected?

Diabetic retinopathy and macular edema are detected during a comprehensive eye exam that includes:

- **Visual Acuity Test:** This eye chart test measures how well you see at various distances.

- **Dilated Eye Exam:** Drops are placed in your eyes to widen, or dilate, the pupils. This allows the eye care professional to see more of the inside of your eyes to check for signs of the disease. Your eye care professional uses a special magnifying lens to examine your retina and optic nerve for signs of damage and other eye problems. After the exam, your close-up vision may remain blurred for several hours.

- **Tonometry:** An instrument measures the pressure inside the eye. Numbing drops may be applied to your eye for this test.

Your eye care professional checks your retina for early signs of the disease, including leaking blood vessels; retinal swelling (macular edema); pale, fatty deposits on the retina—signs of leaking blood vessels; damaged nerve tissue; and any changes to the blood vessels.

If your eye care professional believes you need treatment for macular edema, he or she may suggest a fluorescein angiogram. In this test, a special dye is injected into your arm. Pictures are taken as the dye passes through the blood vessels in your retina. The test allows your eye care professional to identify any leaking blood vessels and recommend treatment.

How is diabetic retinopathy treated?

During the first three stages of diabetic retinopathy, no treatment is needed, unless you have macular edema. To prevent progression of diabetic retinopathy, people with diabetes should control their levels of blood sugar, blood pressure, and blood cholesterol.

Proliferative retinopathy is treated with laser surgery. This procedure is called scatter laser treatment. Scatter laser treatment helps to shrink the abnormal blood vessels. Your doctor places 1,000 to 2,000 laser burns in the areas of the retina away from the macula, causing the abnormal blood vessels to shrink. Because a high number of laser burns are necessary, two or more sessions usually are required to complete treatment. Although you may notice some loss of your side vision, scatter laser treatment can save the rest of your sight. Scatter laser treatment may slightly reduce your color vision and night vision.

Scatter laser treatment works better before the fragile, new blood vessels have started to bleed. That is why it is important to have regular, comprehensive dilated eye exams. Even if bleeding has started, scatter laser treatment may still be possible, depending on the amount of bleeding.

If the bleeding is severe, you may need a surgical procedure called a vitrectomy. During a vitrectomy, blood is removed from the center of your eye.

How is a macular edema treated?

Macular edema is treated with laser surgery. This procedure is called focal laser treatment. Your doctor places up to several hundred small laser burns in the areas of retinal leakage surrounding the macula. These burns slow the leakage of fluid and reduce the amount of fluid in the retina. The surgery is usually completed in one session. Further treatment may be needed.

A patient may need focal laser surgery more than once to control the leaking fluid. If you have macular edema in both eyes and require laser surgery, generally only one eye will be treated at a time, usually several weeks apart.

Focal laser treatment stabilizes vision. In fact, focal laser treatment reduces the risk of vision loss by 50 percent. In a small number of cases, if vision is lost, it can be improved. Contact your eye care professional if you have vision loss.

What happens during laser treatment?

Both focal and scatter laser treatment are performed in your doctor's office or eye clinic. Before the surgery, your doctor will dilate your pupil and apply drops to numb the eye. The area behind your eye also may be numbed to prevent discomfort.

The lights in the office will be dim. As you sit facing the laser machine, your doctor will hold a special lens to your eye. During the procedure, you may see flashes of light. These flashes eventually may create a stinging sensation that can be uncomfortable. You will need someone to drive you home after surgery. Because your pupil will remain dilated for a few hours, you should bring a pair of sunglasses.

For the rest of the day, your vision will probably be a little blurry. If your eye hurts, your doctor can suggest treatment.

Laser surgery and appropriate follow-up care can reduce the risk of blindness by 90 percent. However, laser surgery often cannot restore vision that has already been lost. That is why finding diabetic retinopathy early is the best way to prevent vision loss.

What is a vitrectomy?

If you have a lot of blood in the center of the eye (vitreous gel), you may need a vitrectomy to restore your sight. If you need vitrectomies in both eyes, they are usually done several weeks apart.

A vitrectomy is performed under either local or general anesthesia. Your doctor makes a tiny incision in your eye. Next, a small instrument is used to remove the vitreous gel that is clouded with blood. The vitreous gel is replaced with a salt solution. Because the vitreous gel is mostly water, you will notice no change between the salt solution and the original vitreous gel.

You will probably be able to return home after the vitrectomy. Some people stay in the hospital overnight. Your eye will be red and sensitive. You will need to wear an eye patch for a few days or weeks to protect your eye. You also will need to use medicated eyedrops to protect against infection.

Are scatter laser treatment and vitrectomy effective in treating proliferative retinopathy?

Yes. Both treatments are very effective in reducing vision loss. People with proliferative retinopathy have less than a five percent chance of becoming blind within five years when they get timely and appropriate treatment. Although both treatments have high success rates, they do not cure diabetic retinopathy.

Once you have proliferative retinopathy, you always will be at risk for new bleeding. You may need treatment more than once to protect your sight.

Treating Other Eye Problems

People with diabetes get cataracts and glaucoma more often and at a younger age than people without diabetes.

A cataract is a cloud over the lens of your eye, which is usually clear. The lens focuses light onto the retina. A cataract makes everything you look at seem cloudy. You need surgery to remove the cataract. During surgery your lens is taken out and a plastic lens, like a contact lens, is put in. The plastic lens stays in your eye all the time. Cataract surgery helps you see clearly again.

Glaucoma starts from pressure building up in the eye. Over time, this pressure damages your eye's main nerve—the optic nerve. The damage first causes you to lose sight from the sides of your eyes. Treating glaucoma is usually simple. Your eye care professional will give you special drops to use every day to lower the pressure in your eyes. Or your eye care professional may want you to have laser surgery.

Source: "Prevent Diabetes Problems: Keep Your Eyes Healthy," National Institute of Diabetes and Digestive and Kidney Diseases, November 2008.

What can I do if I already have lost some vision from diabetic retinopathy?

If you have lost some sight from diabetic retinopathy, ask your eye care professional about low vision services and devices that may help you make the most of your remaining vision. Ask for a referral to a specialist in low vision. Many community organizations and agencies offer information about low vision counseling, training, and other special services for people with visual impairments. A nearby school of medicine or optometry may provide low vision services.

What research is being done?

The National Eye Institute (NEI) is conducting and supporting research that seeks better ways to detect, treat, and prevent vision loss in people with diabetes. This research is conducted through studies in the laboratory and with patients.

For example, researchers are studying drugs that may stop the retina from sending signals to the body to grow new blood vessels. Someday, these drugs may help people control their diabetic retinopathy and reduce the need for laser surgery.

Chapter 45

Kidney Disease Of Diabetes

The Burden Of Kidney Failure

Each year in the United States, more than 100,000 people are diagnosed with kidney failure, a serious condition in which the kidneys fail to rid the body of wastes. Kidney failure is the final stage of chronic kidney disease (CKD).

Diabetes is the most common cause of kidney failure, accounting for nearly 44 percent of new cases. Even when diabetes is controlled, the disease can lead to CKD and kidney failure. Most people with diabetes do not develop CKD that is severe enough to progress to kidney failure. Nearly 24 million people in the United States have diabetes, and nearly 180,000 people are living with kidney failure as a result of diabetes.

People with kidney failure undergo either dialysis, an artificial blood-cleaning process, or transplantation to receive a healthy kidney from a donor. Most U.S. citizens who develop kidney failure are eligible for federally funded care.

African Americans, American Indians, and Hispanics/Latinos develop diabetes, CKD, and kidney failure at rates higher than Caucasians. Scientists have not been able to explain these higher rates. Nor can they explain fully the interplay of factors leading to kidney disease of diabetes—factors including heredity, diet, and other medical conditions, such as high blood pressure. They have found that high blood pressure and high levels of blood glucose increase the risk that a person with diabetes will progress to kidney failure.

About This Chapter: Text in this chapter is from "Kidney Disease of Diabetes," National Institute of Diabetes and Digestive and Kidney Diseases, September 2008.

The Course Of Kidney Disease

Diabetic kidney disease takes many years to develop. In some people, the filtering function of the kidneys is actually higher than normal in the first few years of their diabetes.

Over several years, people who are developing kidney disease will have small amounts of the blood protein albumin begin to leak into their urine. This first stage of CKD is called microalbuminuria. The kidney's filtration function usually remains normal during this period.

As the disease progresses, more albumin leaks into the urine. This stage may be called macroalbuminuria or proteinuria. As the amount of albumin in the urine increases, the kidneys' filtering function usually begins to drop. The body retains various wastes as filtration falls. As kidney damage develops, blood pressure often rises as well.

Overall, kidney damage rarely occurs in the first ten years of diabetes, and usually 15 to 25 years will pass before kidney failure occurs. For people who live with diabetes for more than 25 years without any signs of kidney failure, the risk of ever developing it decreases.

Diagnosis Of CKD

People with diabetes should be screened regularly for kidney disease. The two key markers for kidney disease are eGFR and urine albumin.

eGFR

eGFR stands for estimated glomerular filtration rate. Each kidney contains about one million tiny filters made up of blood vessels. These filters are called glomeruli. Kidney function can be checked by estimating how much blood the glomeruli filter in a minute. The calculation of eGFR is based on the amount of creatinine, a waste product, found in a blood sample. As the level of creatinine goes up, the eGFR goes down.

Kidney disease is present when eGFR is less than 60 milliliters per minute.

The American Diabetes Association (ADA) and the National Institutes of Health (NIH) recommend that eGFR be calculated from serum creatinine at least once a year in all people with diabetes.

Urine Albumin

Urine albumin is measured by comparing the amount of albumin to the amount of creatinine in a single urine sample. When the kidneys are healthy, the urine will contain large amounts of creatinine but almost no albumin. Even a small increase in the ratio of albumin to creatinine is a sign of kidney damage.

What do my kidneys do?

The kidneys act as filters to clean the blood. They get rid of wastes and send along filtered fluid. The tiny filters in the kidneys are called glomeruli.

When kidneys are healthy, the artery brings blood and wastes from the bloodstream into the kidneys. The glomeruli clean the blood. Then wastes and extra fluid go out into the urine through the ureter. Clean blood leaves the kidneys and goes back into the bloodstream through the vein.

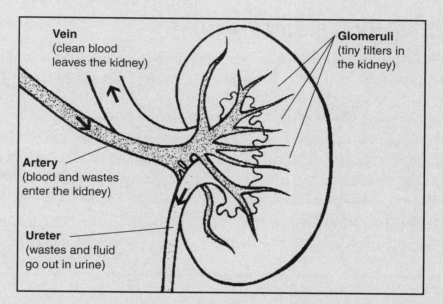

Figure 45.1. You have two kidneys. Your kidneys clean your blood and make urine. This drawing shows a cross section of a kidney.

Once you have kidney damage, you can slow it down or stop it from getting worse by controlling your blood glucose and blood pressure. Taking an ACE inhibitor or an ARB is important for both controlling your blood pressure and reducing kidney damage. (Pregnant women, however, should not take an ACE inhibitor or ARB.)

If you have diabetes, you should have your urine and blood tested regularly to see how well your kidneys are working. The test results should be given to you as your urine albumin and GFR results.

Source: Excerpted from "Prevent Diabetes Problems: Keep Your Kidneys Healthy," National Institute of Diabetes and Digestive and Kidney Diseases, February 2010.

Kidney disease is present when urine contains more than 30 milligrams of albumin per gram of creatinine, with or without decreased eGFR.

The ADA and the NIH recommend annual assessment of urine albumin excretion to assess kidney damage in all people with type 2 diabetes and people who have had type 1 diabetes for five years or more.

If kidney disease is detected, it should be addressed as part of a comprehensive approach to the treatment of diabetes.

Effects Of High Blood Pressure

High blood pressure, or hypertension, is a major factor in the development of kidney problems in people with diabetes. Both a family history of hypertension and the presence of hypertension appear to increase chances of developing kidney disease. Hypertension also accelerates the progress of kidney disease when it already exists.

Blood pressure is recorded using two numbers. The first number is called the systolic pressure, and it represents the pressure in the arteries as the heart beats. The second number is called the diastolic pressure, and it represents the pressure between heartbeats. In the past, hypertension was defined as blood pressure higher than 140/90, said as "140 over 90."

The ADA and the National Heart, Lung, and Blood Institute recommend that people with diabetes keep their blood pressure below 130/80.

How will I know if my kidneys fail?

At first, you cannot tell. Kidney damage from diabetes happens so slowly that you may not feel sick at all for many years. You will not feel sick even when your kidneys do only half the job of normal kidneys. You may not feel any signs of kidney failure until your kidneys have almost stopped working. However, getting your urine and blood checked every year can tell you how well your kidneys are working.

Once your kidneys fail, you may feel sick to your stomach and tired all the time. Your hands and feet may swell from extra fluid in your body.

Source: Excerpted from "Prevent Diabetes Problems: Keep Your Kidneys Healthy," National Institute of Diabetes and Digestive and Kidney Diseases, February 2010.

Hypertension can be seen not only as a cause of kidney disease but also as a result of damage created by the disease. As kidney disease progresses, physical changes in the kidneys lead to increased blood pressure. Therefore, a dangerous spiral, involving rising blood pressure and factors that raise blood pressure, occurs. Early detection and treatment of even mild hypertension are essential for people with diabetes.

Preventing And Slowing Kidney Disease

Blood Pressure Medicines

Scientists have made great progress in developing methods that slow the onset and progression of kidney disease in people with diabetes. Drugs used to lower blood pressure can slow the progression of kidney disease significantly. Two types of drugs, angiotensin-converting enzyme (ACE) inhibitors and angiotensin receptor blockers (ARBs), have proven effective in slowing the progression of kidney disease. Many people require two or more drugs to control their blood pressure. In addition to an ACE inhibitor or an ARB, a diuretic can also be useful. Beta blockers, calcium channel blockers, and other blood pressure drugs may also be needed.

An example of an effective ACE inhibitor is lisinopril (Prinivil, Zestril), which doctors commonly prescribe for treating kidney disease of diabetes. The benefits of lisinopril extend beyond its ability to lower blood pressure: it may directly protect the kidneys' glomeruli. ACE inhibitors have lowered proteinuria and slowed deterioration even in people with diabetes who did not have high blood pressure.

An example of an effective ARB is losartan (Cozaar), which has also been shown to protect kidney function and lower the risk of cardiovascular events.

Any medicine that helps patients achieve a blood pressure target of 130/80 or lower provides benefits. Patients with even mild hypertension or persistent microalbuminuria should consult a health care provider about the use of antihypertensive medicines.

Moderate-Protein Diets

In people with diabetes, excessive consumption of protein may be harmful. Experts recommend that people with kidney disease of diabetes consume the recommended dietary allowance for protein, but avoid high-protein diets. For people with greatly reduced kidney function, a diet containing reduced amounts of protein may help delay the onset of kidney failure. Anyone following a reduced-protein diet should work with a dietitian to ensure adequate nutrition.

Intensive Management Of Blood Glucose

Antihypertensive drugs and low-protein diets can slow CKD. A third treatment, known as intensive management of blood glucose or glycemic control, has shown great promise for people with diabetes, especially for those in the early stages of CKD.

The human body normally converts food to glucose, the simple sugar that is the main source of energy for the body's cells. To enter cells, glucose needs the help of insulin, a hormone produced by the pancreas. When a person does not make enough insulin, or the body does not respond to the insulin that is present, the body cannot process glucose, and it builds up in the bloodstream. High levels of glucose in the blood lead to a diagnosis of diabetes.

Intensive management of blood glucose is a treatment regimen that aims to keep blood glucose levels close to normal. The regimen includes testing blood glucose frequently, administering insulin throughout the day on the basis of food intake and physical activity, following a diet and activity plan, and consulting a health care team regularly. Some people use an insulin pump to supply insulin throughout the day.

A number of studies have pointed to the beneficial effects of intensive management of blood glucose. In the Diabetes Control and Complications Trial supported by the National Institute of Diabetes and Digestive and Kidney Diseases (NIDDK), researchers found a 50 percent decrease in both development and progression of early diabetic kidney disease in participants who followed an intensive regimen for controlling blood glucose levels. The intensively managed patients had average blood glucose levels of 150 milligrams per deciliter—about 80 milligrams per deciliter lower than the levels observed in the conventionally managed patients. The United Kingdom Prospective Diabetes Study, conducted from 1976 to 1997, showed conclusively that, in people with improved blood glucose control, the risk of early kidney disease was reduced by a third. Additional studies conducted over the past decades have clearly established that any program resulting in sustained lowering of blood glucose levels will be beneficial to patients in the early stages of CKD.

Dialysis And Transplantation

When people with diabetes experience kidney failure, they must undergo either dialysis or a kidney transplant. As recently as the 1970s, medical experts commonly excluded people with diabetes from dialysis and transplantation, in part because the experts felt damage caused by diabetes would offset benefits of the treatments. Today, because of better control of diabetes and improved rates of survival following treatment, doctors do not hesitate to offer dialysis and kidney transplantation to people with diabetes.

Currently, the survival of kidneys transplanted into people with diabetes is about the same as the survival of transplants in people without diabetes. Dialysis for people with diabetes also works well in the short run. Even so, people with diabetes who receive transplants or dialysis experience higher morbidity and mortality because of coexisting complications of diabetes—such as damage to the heart, eyes, and nerves.

Points To Remember

- Diabetes is the leading cause of chronic kidney disease (CKD) and kidney failure in the United States.

- People with diabetes should be screened regularly for kidney disease. The two key markers for kidney disease are estimated glomerular filtration rate (eGFR) and urine albumin.

- Drugs used to lower blood pressure can slow the progression of kidney disease significantly. Two types of drugs, angiotensin-converting enzyme (ACE) inhibitors and angiotensin receptor blockers (ARBs), have proven effective in slowing the progression of kidney disease.

- In people with diabetes, excessive consumption of protein may be harmful.

- Intensive management of blood glucose has shown great promise for people with diabetes, especially for those in the early stages of CKD.

What's It Mean?

Dialysis: Dialysis is a treatment that does some of the work your kidneys used to do. Two types of dialysis are available:

- **Hemodialysis:** In hemodialysis, your blood flows through a tube from your arm to a machine that filters out the waste products and extra fluid. The clean blood flows back to your arm.
- **Peritoneal Dialysis:** In peritoneal dialysis, your belly is filled with a special fluid. The fluid collects waste products and extra water from your blood. Then the fluid is drained from your belly and thrown away.

Source: Excerpted from "Prevent Diabetes Problems: Keep Your Kidneys Healthy," National Institute of Diabetes and Digestive and Kidney Diseases, February 2010.

Chapter 46

Gastroparesis

What is gastroparesis?

Gastroparesis, also called delayed gastric emptying, is a disorder in which the stomach takes too long to empty its contents. Normally, the stomach contracts to move food down into the small intestine for digestion. The vagus nerve controls the movement of food from the stomach through the digestive tract. Gastroparesis occurs when the vagus nerve is damaged and the muscles of the stomach and intestines do not work normally. Food then moves slowly or stops moving through the digestive tract.

What causes gastroparesis?

The most common cause of gastroparesis is diabetes. People with diabetes have high blood glucose, also called blood sugar, which in turn causes chemical changes in nerves and damages the blood vessels that carry oxygen and nutrients to the nerves. Over time, high blood glucose can damage the vagus nerve.

Some other causes of gastroparesis include surgery on the stomach or vagus nerve, viral infections, anorexia nervosa or bulimia, and medications (anticholinergics and narcotics) that slow contractions in the intestine. Diseases other than diabetes that can cause gastroparesis include gastroesophageal reflux disease, smooth muscle disorders (such as amyloidosis and scleroderma), nervous system diseases (including abdominal migraine and Parkinson's disease), and metabolic disorders (including hypothyroidism). Many people have what is

About This Chapter: Information in this chapter is from "Gastroparesis," National Institute of Diabetes and Digestive and Kidney Diseases, July 2007.

called idiopathic gastroparesis, meaning the cause is unknown and cannot be found even after medical tests.

What are the symptoms of gastroparesis?

The symptoms of gastroparesis may be mild or severe, depending on the person. Symptoms can happen frequently in some people and less often in others. Many people with gastroparesis experience a wide range of symptoms, and sometimes the disorder is difficult for the physician to diagnose. Symptoms include the following:

- Heartburn
- Pain in the upper abdomen
- Nausea
- Vomiting of undigested food—sometimes several hours after a meal
- Early feeling of fullness after only a few bites of food
- Weight loss due to poor absorption of nutrients or low calorie intake
- Abdominal bloating
- High and low blood glucose levels
- Lack of appetite
- Gastroesophageal reflux
- Spasms in the stomach area

Eating solid foods, high-fiber foods such as raw fruits and vegetables, fatty foods, or drinks high in fat or carbonation may contribute to these symptoms.

What are the complications of gastroparesis?

If food lingers too long in the stomach, it can cause bacterial overgrowth from the fermentation of food. Also, the food can harden into solid masses called bezoars that may cause nausea, vomiting, and obstruction in the stomach. Bezoars can be dangerous if they block the passage of food into the small intestine.

Gastroparesis can make diabetes worse by making blood glucose control more difficult. When food that has been delayed in the stomach finally enters the small intestine and is absorbed, blood glucose levels rise. Since gastroparesis makes stomach emptying unpredictable, a person's blood glucose levels can be erratic and difficult to control.

How is gastroparesis diagnosed?

After performing a full physical exam and taking your medical history, your doctor may order several blood tests to check blood counts and chemical and electrolyte levels. To rule out an obstruction or other conditions, the doctor may perform the following tests:

- **Upper Endoscopy:** After giving you a sedative to help you become drowsy, the doctor passes a long, thin tube called an endoscope through your mouth and gently guides it down the throat, also called the esophagus, into the stomach. Through the endoscope, the doctor can look at the lining of the stomach to check for any abnormalities.

- **Ultrasound:** To rule out gallbladder disease and pancreatitis as sources of the problem, you may have an ultrasound test, which uses harmless sound waves to outline and define the shape of the gallbladder and pancreas.

- **Barium X-Ray:** After fasting for 12 hours, you will drink a thick liquid called barium, which coats the stomach, making it show up on the x-ray. If you have diabetes, your doctor may have special instructions about fasting. Normally, the stomach will be empty of all food after 12 hours of fasting. Gastroparesis is likely if the x-ray shows food in the stomach. Because a person with gastroparesis can sometimes have normal emptying, the doctor may repeat the test another day if gastroparesis is suspected.

Once other causes have been ruled out, the doctor will perform one of the following gastric emptying tests to confirm a diagnosis of gastroparesis.

- **Gastric Emptying Scintigraphy:** This test involves eating a bland meal, such as eggs or egg substitute, that contains a small amount of a radioactive substance, called radioisotope, that shows up on scans. The dose of radiation from the radioisotope is not dangerous. The scan measures the rate of gastric emptying at one, two, three, and four hours. When more than 10 percent of the meal is still in the stomach at four hours, the diagnosis of gastroparesis is confirmed.

- **Breath Test:** After ingestion of a meal containing a small amount of isotope, breath samples are taken to measure the presence of the isotope in carbon dioxide, which is expelled when a person exhales. The results reveal how fast the stomach is emptying.

- **SmartPill:** Approved by the U.S. Food and Drug Administration (FDA) in 2006, the SmartPill is a small device in capsule form that can be swallowed. The device then moves through the digestive tract and collects information about its progress that is sent to a cell phone-sized receiver worn around your waist or neck. When the capsule is passed from the body with the stool in a couple of days, you take the receiver back to the doctor, who enters the information into a computer.

What medications are used to treat gastroparesis?

Several medications are used to treat gastroparesis. Your doctor may try different medications or combinations to find the most effective treatment. Discussing the risk of side effects of any medication with your doctor is important.

- **Metoclopramide (Reglan):** This drug stimulates stomach muscle contractions to help emptying. Metoclopramide also helps reduce nausea and vomiting. Metoclopramide is taken 20 to 30 minutes before meals and at bedtime. Side effects of this drug include fatigue, sleepiness, depression, anxiety, and problems with physical movement.

- **Erythromycin:** This antibiotic also improves stomach emptying. It works by increasing the contractions that move food through the stomach. Side effects include nausea, vomiting, and abdominal cramps.

- **Domperidone:** This drug works like metoclopramide to improve stomach emptying and decrease nausea and vomiting. The FDA is reviewing domperidone, which has been used elsewhere in the world to treat gastroparesis. Use of the drug is restricted in the United States.

- **Other Medications:** Other medications may be used to treat symptoms and problems related to gastroparesis. For example, an antiemetic can help with nausea and vomiting. Antibiotics will clear up a bacterial infection. If you have a bezoar in the stomach, the doctor may use an endoscope to inject medication into it to dissolve it.

How else is gastroparesis treated?

Dietary Changes: Changing your eating habits can help control gastroparesis. Your doctor or dietitian may prescribe six small meals a day instead of three large ones. If less food enters the stomach each time you eat, it may not become overly full. In more severe cases, a liquid or pureed diet may be prescribed.

Treating Gastroparesis

Treatment of gastroparesis depends on the severity of the symptoms. In most cases, treatment does not cure gastroparesis—it is usually a chronic condition. Treatment helps you manage the condition so you can be as healthy and comfortable as possible.

The doctor may recommend that you avoid high-fat and high-fiber foods. Fat naturally slows digestion—a problem you do not need if you have gastroparesis—and fiber is difficult to digest. Some high-fiber foods like oranges and broccoli contain material that cannot be digested. Avoid these foods because the indigestible part will remain in the stomach too long and possibly form bezoars.

Feeding Tube: If a liquid or pureed diet does not work, you may need surgery to insert a feeding tube. The tube, called a jejunostomy, is inserted through the skin on your abdomen into the small intestine. The feeding tube bypasses the stomach and places nutrients and medication directly into the small intestine. These products are then digested and delivered to your bloodstream quickly. You will receive special liquid food to use with the tube. The jejunostomy is used only when gastroparesis is severe or the tube is necessary to stabilize blood glucose levels in people with diabetes.

Parenteral Nutrition: Parenteral nutrition refers to delivering nutrients directly into the bloodstream, bypassing the digestive system. The doctor places a thin tube called a catheter in a chest vein, leaving an opening to it outside the skin. For feeding, you attach a bag containing liquid nutrients or medication to the catheter. The fluid enters your bloodstream through the vein. Your doctor will tell you what type of liquid nutrition to use.

This approach is an alternative to the jejunostomy tube and is usually a temporary method to get you through a difficult period with gastroparesis. Parenteral nutrition is used only when gastroparesis is severe and is not helped by other methods.

Gastric Electrical Stimulation: A gastric neurostimulator is a surgically implanted battery-operated device that releases mild electrical pulses to help control nausea and vomiting associated with gastroparesis. This option is available to people whose nausea and vomiting do not improve with medications. Further studies will help determine who will benefit most from this procedure, which is available in a few centers across the United States.

Botulinum Toxin: The use of botulinum toxin has been associated with improvement in symptoms of gastroparesis in some patients; however, further research on this form of therapy is needed.

What if I have diabetes and gastroparesis?

The primary treatment goals for gastroparesis related to diabetes are to improve stomach emptying and regain control of blood glucose levels. Treatment includes dietary changes, insulin, oral medications, and, in severe cases, a feeding tube and parenteral nutrition.

Dietary Changes: The doctor will suggest dietary changes such as six smaller meals to help restore your blood glucose to more normal levels before testing you for gastroparesis. In some cases, the doctor or dietitian may suggest you try eating several liquid or pureed meals a day until your blood glucose levels are stable and the symptoms improve. Liquid meals provide all the nutrients found in solid foods, but can pass through the stomach more easily and quickly.

Insulin For Blood Glucose Control: If you have gastroparesis, food is being absorbed more slowly and at unpredictable times. To control blood glucose, you may need to take insulin more often or change the type of insulin you take. You may also need to take your insulin after you eat instead of before and check your blood glucose levels frequently after you eat and administer insulin whenever necessary.

Your doctor will give you specific instructions for taking insulin based on your particular needs.

What research is underway?

The National Institute of Diabetes and Digestive and Kidney Diseases' Division of Digestive Diseases and Nutrition supports basic and clinical research into gastrointestinal motility disorders, including gastroparesis. Among other areas, researchers are studying whether experimental medications can relieve or reduce symptoms of gastroparesis, such as bloating, abdominal pain, nausea, and vomiting, or shorten the time the stomach needs to empty its contents following a meal.

Points To Remember

- Gastroparesis is the result of damage to the vagus nerve, which controls the movement of food through the digestive system. Instead of moving through the digestive tract normally, the food is retained in the stomach.

- Gastroparesis may occur in people with type 1 diabetes or type 2 diabetes. The vagus nerve becomes damaged after years of high blood glucose, resulting in gastroparesis. In turn, gastroparesis contributes to poor blood glucose control.

- Symptoms of gastroparesis include early fullness, abdominal pain, stomach spasms, heartburn, nausea, vomiting, bloating, gastroesophageal reflux, lack of appetite, and weight loss.

- Gastroparesis is diagnosed with tests such as x-rays, manometry, and gastric emptying scans.

- Treatment includes dietary changes, oral medications, adjustments in insulin injections for people with diabetes, a jejunostomy tube, parenteral nutrition, gastric neurostimulators, or botulinum toxin.

Chapter 47

Tooth And Gum Problems Caused By Diabetes

How can diabetes hurt my teeth and gums?

Tooth and gum problems can happen to anyone. A sticky film full of germs, called plaque, builds up on your teeth. High blood glucose helps germs, also called bacteria, grow. Then you can get red, sore, and swollen gums that bleed when you brush your teeth.

People with diabetes can have tooth and gum problems more often if their blood glucose stays high. High blood glucose can make tooth and gum problems worse. You can even lose your teeth.

Smoking makes it more likely for you to get a bad case of gum disease, especially for people who have diabetes and are age 45 or older.

Red, sore, and bleeding gums are the first sign of gum disease. These problems can lead to periodontitis. Periodontitis is an infection in the gums and the bone that holds the teeth in place. If the infection gets worse, your gums may pull away from your teeth, making your teeth look long.

Call your dentist if you think you have problems with your teeth or gums.

How do I know if I have damage to my teeth and gums?

If you have one or more of these problems, you may have tooth and gum damage from diabetes:

• Red, sore, swollen gums

• Bleeding gums

About This Chapter: Text in this chapter is from "Prevent Diabetes Problems: Keep Your Teeth and Gums Healthy," National Institute of Diabetes and Digestive and Kidney Diseases, April 2008.

- Gums pulling away from your teeth so your teeth look long

- Loose or sensitive teeth

- Bad breath

- A bite that feels different

- Dentures—false teeth—that do not fit well

How can I keep my teeth and gums healthy?

- Keep your blood glucose as close to normal as possible.

- Use dental floss at least once a day. Flossing helps prevent the buildup of plaque on your teeth. Plaque can harden and grow under your gums and cause problems. Using a sawing motion, gently bring the floss between the teeth, scraping from bottom to top several times.

- Brush your teeth after each meal and snack. Use a soft toothbrush. Turn the bristles against the gum line and brush gently. Use small, circular motions. Brush the front, back, and top of each tooth.

- If you wear false teeth, keep them clean.

- Call your dentist right away if you have problems with your teeth and gums.

- Call your dentist if you have red, sore, or bleeding gums; gums that are pulling away from your teeth; a sore tooth that could be infected; or soreness from your dentures.

Diabetes And Your Gums And Teeth

Diabetes can lead to infections in your gums and the bones that hold your teeth in place. Like all infections, gum infections can cause blood glucose to rise. Without treatment, teeth may become loose and fall out. Help prevent damage to your gums and teeth by taking these steps:

- Seeing your dentist twice a year.
- Brush and floss your teeth at least twice a day
- If you smoke, quit.
- Keep your blood glucose as close to normal as possible.
- Having regular checkups with your dentist. Be sure to tell your dentist that you have diabetes.

Source: Excerpted from "Your Guide to Diabetes: Type 1 and Type 2," National Institute of Diabetes and Digestive and Kidney Diseases, October 2008.

- Get your teeth cleaned and your gums checked by your dentist twice a year.

- If your dentist tells you about a problem, take care of it right away.

- Be sure your dentist knows that you have diabetes.

- If you smoke, talk with your doctor about ways to quit smoking.

How can my dentist take care of my teeth and gums?

Your dentist can help you take care of your teeth and gums by cleaning and checking your teeth twice a year. Your dentist can also help you learn the best way to brush and floss your teeth and telling you if you have problems with your teeth or gums and what to do about them. If you wear dentures, your dentist can make sure your false teeth fit well.

How can dental appointments affect diabetes management?

You may be taking a diabetes medicine that can cause low blood glucose, also called hypo-glycemia. Talk with your doctor and dentist before the visit about the best way to take care of your blood glucose during the dental work. You may need to bring some diabetes medicine and food with you to the dentist's office.

If your mouth is sore after the dental work, you might not be able to eat or chew for several hours or days. For guidance on how to adjust your normal routine while your mouth is healing, ask your doctor what foods and drinks you should have, how you should change your diabetes medicines, and how often you should check your blood glucose.

Chapter 48

Foot And Skin Problems Caused By Diabetes

How can diabetes hurt my feet?

High blood glucose from diabetes causes two problems that can hurt your feet:

- **Nerve Damage:** One problem is damage to nerves in your legs and feet. With damaged nerves, you might not feel pain, heat, or cold in your legs and feet. A sore or cut on your foot may get worse because you do not know it is there. This lack of feeling is caused by nerve damage, also called diabetic neuropathy. Nerve damage can lead to a sore or an infection.

- **Poor Blood Flow:** The second problem happens when not enough blood flows to your legs and feet. Poor blood flow makes it hard for a sore or infection to heal. This problem is called peripheral vascular disease, also called PVD. Smoking when you have diabetes makes blood flow problems much worse.

These two problems can work together to cause a foot problem. For example, you get a blister from shoes that do not fit. You do not feel the pain from the blister because you have nerve damage in your foot. Next, the blister gets infected. If blood glucose is high, the extra glucose feeds the germs. Germs grow and the infection gets worse. Poor blood flow to your legs and feet can slow down healing. Once in a while a bad infection never heals. The infection might cause gangrene. If a person has gangrene, the skin and tissue around the sore die. The area becomes black and smelly.

To keep gangrene from spreading, a doctor may have to do surgery to cut off a toe, foot, or part of a leg. Cutting off a body part is called an amputation.

About This Chapter: Text in this chapter is excerpted from "Prevent Diabetes Problems: Keep Your Feet and Skin Healthy," National Institute of Diabetes and Digestive and Kidney Diseases, May 2008.

What can I do to take care of my feet?

Look at your feet every day to check for problems.

- Wash your feet in warm water every day. Make sure the water is not too hot by testing the temperature with your elbow. Do not soak your feet. Dry your feet well, especially between your toes.

- Look at your feet every day to check for cuts, sores, blisters, redness, calluses, or other problems. Checking every day is even more important if you have nerve damage or poor blood flow. If you cannot bend over or pull your feet up to check them, use a mirror. If you cannot see well, ask someone else to check your feet.

- If your skin is dry, rub lotion on your feet after you wash and dry them. Do not put lotion between your toes.

- File corns and calluses gently with an emery board or pumice stone. Do this after your bath or shower.

- Cut your toenails once a week or when needed. Cut toenails when they are soft from washing. Cut them to the shape of the toe and not too short. File the edges with an emery board.

- Always wear slippers or shoes to protect your feet from injuries.

- Always wear socks or stockings to avoid blisters. Do not wear socks or knee-high stockings that are too tight below your knee.

- Wear shoes that fit well. Shop for shoes at the end of the day when your feet are bigger. Break in shoes slowly. Wear them one to two hours each day for the first few weeks.

- Before putting your shoes on, feel the insides to make sure they have no sharp edges or objects that might injure your feet.

How can my doctor help me take care of my feet?

- Tell your doctor right away about any foot problems.

- Your doctor should do a complete foot exam every year.

- Ask your doctor to look at your feet at each diabetes checkup. To make sure your doctor checks your feet, take off your shoes and socks before your doctor comes into the room.

- Ask your doctor to check how well the nerves in your feet sense feeling.

- Ask your doctor to check how well blood is flowing to your legs and feet.

Protect Your Feet

Protect your feet from hot and cold:

- Wear shoes at the beach or on hot pavement. Always protect your feet when walking on any hot surfaces.
- Put sunscreen on the top of your feet to prevent sunburn.
- Keep your feet away from radiators and open fires.
- Do not put hot water bottles or heating pads on your feet.
- Wear socks at night if your feet get cold. Lined boots are good in winter to keep your feet warm.
- Check your feet often in cold weather to avoid frostbite.

Keep the blood flowing to your feet:

- Put your feet up when you are sitting.
- Wiggle your toes for five minutes, two or three times a day. Move your ankles up and down and in and out to improve blood flow in your feet and legs.
- Don't cross your legs for long periods of time.
- Don't wear tight socks, elastic or rubber bands, or garters around your legs.
- Don't smoke. Smoking reduces blood flow to your feet. Ask for help to stop smoking.
- Work with your health care team to control your A1C (blood glucose), blood pressure, and cholesterol.

Source: Excerpted from "Take Care of Your Feet for a Lifetime," National Diabetes Education Program, July 2003. Despite the older date of this document, the foot care tips provided are still applicable.

- Ask your doctor to show you the best way to trim your toenails. Ask what lotion or cream to use on your legs and feet.

- If you cannot cut your toenails or you have a foot problem, ask your doctor to send you to a foot doctor. A doctor who cares for feet is called a podiatrist.

What are common diabetes foot problems?

Anyone can have corns, blisters, and other foot problems. If you have diabetes and your blood glucose stays high, these foot problems can lead to infections.

Corns and calluses are thick layers of skin caused by too much rubbing or pressure on the same spot. Corns and calluses can become infected.

Blisters can form if shoes always rub the same spot. Wearing shoes that do not fit or wearing shoes without socks can cause blisters. Blisters can become infected.

Ingrown toenails happen when an edge of the nail grows into the skin. The skin can get red and infected. Ingrown toenails can happen if you cut into the corners of your toenails when you trim them. You can also get an ingrown toenail if your shoes are too tight. If toenail edges are sharp, smooth them with an emery board.

A bunion forms when your big toe slants toward the small toes and the place between the bones near the base of your big toe grows big. This spot can get red, sore, and infected. Bunions can form on one or both feet. Pointed shoes may cause bunions. Bunions often run in the family. Surgery can remove bunions.

Plantar warts are caused by a virus. The warts usually form on the bottoms of the feet.

Hammertoes form when a foot muscle gets weak. Diabetic nerve damage may cause the weakness. The weakened muscle makes the tendons in the foot shorter and makes the toes curl under the feet. You may get sores on the bottoms of your feet and on the tops of your toes. The feet can change their shape. Hammertoes can cause problems with walking and finding shoes that fit well. Hammertoes can run in the family. Wearing shoes that are too short can also cause hammertoes.

Dry and cracked skin can happen because the nerves in your legs and feet do not get the message to keep your skin soft and moist. Dry skin can become cracked. Cracks allow germs to enter and cause infection. If your blood glucose is high, it feeds the germs and makes the infection worse.

Tips For Proper Footwear

- Proper footwear is very important for preventing serious foot problems. Athletic or walking shoes are good for daily wear. They support your feet and allow them to "breathe."
- Never wear vinyl or plastic shoes, because they don't stretch or "breathe."
- When buying shoes, make sure they are comfortable from the start and have enough room for your toes.
- Don't buy shoes with pointed toes or high heels. They put too much pressure on your toes.

Source: Excerpted from "Take Care of Your Feet for a Lifetime," National Diabetes Education Program, July 2003. Despite the older date of this document, the foot care tips provided are still applicable.

Athlete's foot is a fungus that causes itchiness, redness, and cracking of the skin. The cracks between the toes allow germs to get under the skin and cause infection. If your blood glucose is high, it feeds the germs and makes the infection worse. The infection can spread to the toenails and make them thick, yellow, and hard to cut.

Tell your doctor about any foot problem as soon as you see it.

How can special shoes help my feet?

Special shoes can be made to fit softly around your sore feet or feet that have changed shape. These special shoes help protect your feet. Medicare and other health insurance programs may pay for special shoes. Talk with your doctor about how and where to get them.

How can diabetes hurt my skin?

Diabetes can hurt your skin in two ways:

- If your blood glucose is high, your body loses fluid. With less fluid in your body, your skin can get dry. Dry skin can be itchy, causing you to scratch and make it sore. Also, dry skin can crack. Cracks allow germs to enter and cause infection. If your blood glucose is high, it feeds germs and makes infections worse. You may get dry skin on your legs, feet, elbows, and other places on your body.

- Nerve damage can decrease the amount you sweat. Sweating helps keep your skin soft and moist. Decreased sweating in your feet and legs can cause dry skin.

What can I do to take care of my skin?

- After you wash with a mild soap, make sure you rinse and dry yourself well. Check places where water can hide, such as under the arms, under the breasts, between the legs, and between the toes.

- Keep your skin moist by using a lotion or cream after you wash. Ask your doctor to suggest one.

- Drink lots of fluids, such as water, to keep your skin moist and healthy.

- Wear all-cotton underwear. Cotton allows air to move around your body better.

- Check your skin after you wash. Make sure you have no dry, red, or sore spots that might lead to an infection.

- Tell your doctor about any skin problems.

Chapter 49

Acanthosis Nigricans

Ruby is 17. At age 9, she started compulsively scrubbing and scrubbing at her neck and arms, almost until they were raw, because she thought she had dirt or a stain on her skin. What she actually had was acanthosis nigricans—a condition in which the skin thickens and darkens in places.

For Ruby, trying to maintain a healthy weight made the condition less noticeable, and getting the facts helped her avoid freaking out. "Learning what it was and what I could do about it was huge," she says.

What Is Acanthosis Nigricans?

OK, so the name is hard to pronounce (ay-can-tho-sis nyg-ruh-cans), but if you have it, you're probably more concerned about how it looks. You'll notice that your skin is thicker and darker, especially around joints and areas with lots of creases and folds, like your knuckles, armpits, elbows, knees, and neck.

Some people see thicker, darker skin on the palms of their hands, inner thighs, groin, lips, or other areas. The skin usually stays soft, which is why the word "velvety" is often used to describe the symptoms of acanthosis nigricans (AN).

AN is most common in people of African, Caribbean, and Hispanic descent but anyone can have it. Many people who develop AN have no other symptoms and are otherwise healthy. But because AN can be a sign of certain other medical conditions, it's a good idea for it to be checked out by a doctor.

About This Chapter: "Acanthosis Nigricans," March 2010, reprinted with permission from www.kidshealth.org. Copyright © 2010 The Nemours Foundation. This information was provided by KidsHealth, one of the largest resources online for medically reviewed health information written for parents, kids, and teens. For more articles like this one, visit www.KidsHealth.org, or www.TeensHealth.org.

What Causes AN?

People who are overweight or obese are more likely to develop AN, which often lessens or goes away with weight loss. Some people with the condition inherit it. Certain medicines—for example, birth control pills or hormone treatments—also can cause AN.

Sometimes, it's seen in people who have type 2 diabetes or who are at greater risk for getting this type of diabetes. In these cases, acanthosis nigricans itself isn't dangerous. But it can be a sign to doctors to check someone for diabetes or other health problems. Sometimes, finding and treating the health problem might make the person's skin condition improve or clear up.

Almost 75% of kids with type 2 diabetes develop AN, according to the American Diabetes Association. For many, getting their diabetes and weight (if they are overweight) under control goes a long way toward lessening the visibility of AN.

What To Do

First of all, don't panic. Acanthosis nigricans itself is not harmful or contagious but you should see a doctor to make sure it's not caused by something that does need attention. In some cases, AN can be a signal that you're at risk for diabetes. Whenever you notice a change in the color, thickness, or texture of your skin, it's wise to see a health professional.

What To Expect

If you're diagnosed with AN, your doctor might want you to have a blood test or other tests to try to determine what's causing it or to look for other conditions (like type 2 diabetes) that occur more often in people with AN.

Treatment For AN

If your doctor determines that your AN is not connected to a more serious medical condition, you don't need to treat it. But you might want to if your doctor thinks there is a way to help improve the appearance of your skin. Sometimes, AN fades on its own.

Your doctor may prescribe lotions, creams, or a medicine called isotretinoin, which is used to treat very severe acne. Ask as many questions as you need to in order to understand when and how to follow the treatment plan.

It's easy to fall into believing the hype about bleaches, skin scrubs, and over-the-counter exfoliating treatments. But these aren't likely to work and can irritate your skin, not to mention waste money and sometimes just boost your stress about AN!

Maintaining a healthy weight by staying physically active and eating well can help prevent or treat acanthosis nigricans in some cases.

You also should make plans to take care of yourself in other ways. Because this condition is visible, some teens with acanthosis nigricans feel self-conscious or embarrassed about the way their skin looks.

It can help to talk to a counselor, doctor, friend, or even peer support group to help you feel more confident. Your doctor or nurse probably can help you find local or online support groups. And don't be afraid to talk to your friends. Good friends are the best support!

Chapter 50

Sexual And Urologic Problems Of Diabetes

Troublesome bladder symptoms and changes in sexual function are common health problems as people age. Having diabetes can mean early onset and increased severity of these problems. Sexual and urologic complications of diabetes occur because of the damage diabetes can cause to blood vessels and nerves. Men may have difficulty with erections or ejaculation. Women may have problems with sexual response and vaginal lubrication. Urinary tract infections and bladder problems occur more often in people with diabetes. People who keep their diabetes under control can lower their risk of the early onset of these sexual and urologic problems.

Diabetes And Sexual Problems

Men and women with diabetes can develop sexual problems because of damage to nerves and small blood vessels. When a person wants to lift an arm or take a step, the brain sends nerve signals to the appropriate muscles. Nerve signals also control internal organs like the heart and bladder, but people do not have the same kind of conscious control over them as they do over their arms and legs. The nerves that control internal organs are called autonomic nerves, which signal the body to digest food and circulate blood without a person having to think about it. The body's response to sexual stimuli is also involuntary, governed by autonomic nerve signals that increase blood flow to the genitals and cause smooth muscle tissue to relax. Damage to these autonomic nerves can hinder normal function. Reduced blood flow resulting from damage to blood vessels can also contribute to sexual dysfunction.

About This Chapter: From "Sexual and Urologic Problems of Diabetes," National Institute of Diabetes and Digestive and Kidney Diseases," December 2008.

Erectile Dysfunction

Erectile dysfunction is a consistent inability to have an erection firm enough for sexual intercourse. The condition includes the total inability to have an erection and the inability to sustain an erection.

Estimates of the prevalence of erectile dysfunction in men with diabetes vary widely, ranging from 20 to 75 percent. Men who have diabetes are two to three times more likely to have erectile dysfunction than men who do not have diabetes. Among men with erectile dysfunction, those with diabetes may experience the problem as much as 10 to 15 years earlier than men without diabetes. Research suggests that erectile dysfunction may be an early marker of diabetes, particularly in men ages 45 and younger.

In addition to diabetes, other major causes of erectile dysfunction include high blood pressure, kidney disease, alcohol abuse, and blood vessel disease. Erectile dysfunction may also occur because of the side effects of medications, psychological factors, smoking, and hormonal deficiencies.

Men who experience erectile dysfunction should consider talking with a health care provider. The health care provider may ask about the patient's medical history, the type and frequency of sexual problems, medications, smoking and drinking habits, and other health conditions. A physical exam and laboratory tests may help pinpoint causes of sexual problems. The health care provider will check blood glucose control and hormone levels and may ask the patient to do a test at home that checks for erections that occur during sleep. The health care provider may also ask whether the patient is depressed or has recently experienced upsetting changes in his life.

Treatments for erectile dysfunction caused by nerve damage, also called neuropathy, vary widely and range from oral pills, a vacuum pump, pellets placed in the urethra, and shots directly into the penis, to surgery. All of these methods have advantages and disadvantages. Psychological counseling to reduce anxiety or address other issues may be necessary. Surgery to implant a device to aid in erection or to repair arteries is usually used as a treatment after all others fail.

Retrograde Ejaculation

Retrograde ejaculation is a condition in which part or all of a man's semen goes into the bladder instead of out the tip of the penis during ejaculation. Retrograde ejaculation occurs when internal muscles, called sphincters, do not function normally. A sphincter automatically opens or closes a passage in the body. With retrograde ejaculation, semen enters the bladder, mixes with urine, and leaves the body during urination without harming the bladder. A man experiencing retrograde ejaculation may notice that little semen is discharged during ejaculation or may become aware of the condition if fertility problems arise. Analysis of a urine sample after ejaculation will reveal the presence of semen.

Poor blood glucose control and the resulting nerve damage can cause retrograde ejaculation. Other causes include prostate surgery and some medications.

Retrograde ejaculation caused by diabetes or surgery may be helped with a medication that strengthens the muscle tone of the sphincter in the bladder. A urologist experienced in infertility treatments may assist with techniques to promote fertility, such as collecting sperm from the urine and then using the sperm for artificial insemination.

Women's Sexual Problems

Many women with diabetes experience sexual problems. Although research about sexual problems in women with diabetes is limited, one study found 27 percent of women with type 1 diabetes experienced sexual dysfunction. Another study found 18 percent of women with type 1 diabetes and 42 percent of women with type 2 diabetes experienced sexual dysfunction.

Sexual problems may include decreased vaginal lubrication, resulting in vaginal dryness, uncomfortable or painful sexual intercourse, decreased or no desire for sexual activity, and decreased or absent sexual response. Decreased or absent sexual response can include the inability to become or remain aroused, reduced or no sensation in the genital area, and the constant or occasional inability to reach orgasm.

Causes of sexual problems in women with diabetes include nerve damage, reduced blood flow to genital and vaginal tissues, and hormonal changes. Other possible causes include some medications, alcohol abuse, smoking, psychological problems such as anxiety or depression, gynecologic infections, other diseases, and conditions relating to pregnancy or menopause.

Women who experience sexual problems or notice a change in sexual response should consider talking with a health care provider. The health care provider will ask about the patient's medical history, any gynecologic conditions or infections, the type and frequency of sexual problems, medications, smoking and drinking habits, and other health conditions. The health care provider may ask whether the patient might be pregnant or has reached menopause and whether she is depressed or has recently experienced upsetting changes in her life. A physical exam and laboratory tests may also help pinpoint causes of sexual problems. The health care provider will also talk with the patient about blood glucose control.

Prescription or over-the-counter vaginal lubricants may be useful for women experiencing vaginal dryness. Techniques to treat decreased sexual response include changes in position and stimulation during sexual relations. Psychological counseling may be helpful. Kegel exercises that help strengthen the pelvic muscles may improve sexual response. Studies of drug treatments are under way.

Diabetes And Urologic Problems

Urologic problems that affect men and women with diabetes include bladder problems and urinary tract infections.

Bladder Problems

Many events or conditions can damage nerves that control bladder function, including diabetes and other diseases, injuries, and infections. More than half of men and women with diabetes have bladder dysfunction because of damage to nerves that control bladder function. Bladder dysfunction can have a profound effect on a person's quality of life. Common bladder problems in men and women with diabetes include the following:

- **Overactive Bladder:** Damaged nerves may send signals to the bladder at the wrong time, causing its muscles to squeeze without warning. The symptoms of overactive bladder include urinary frequency (urination eight or more times a day or two or more times a night), urinary urgency (the sudden, strong need to urinate immediately), and urge incontinence (leakage of urine that follows a sudden, strong urge to urinate).

Hope Through Research

The National Institute of Diabetes and Digestive and Kidney Diseases (NIDDK) conducts and supports research on diabetes, glucose metabolism, and related conditions. NIDDK-supported research on the sexual and urologic complications of diabetes includes research conducted as part of the Epidemiology of Diabetes Interventions and Complications (EDIC) study. The EDIC is an observational follow-up study of people who originally participated in the Diabetes Control and Complications Trial (DCCT). The DCCT showed that intensive blood glucose control can reduce the risk of complications of type 1 diabetes. EDIC study results suggest that tight glucose control can delay the onset of erectile dysfunction in men with type 1 diabetes.

A recent study focused on urinary incontinence in women at high risk for developing type 2 diabetes who participated in the NIDDK-sponsored Diabetes Prevention Program (DPP). The women had pre-diabetes, a condition in which blood glucose levels are higher than normal but not high enough for a diagnosis of diabetes. Women who were in the DPP group that used a lifestyle change approach to diabetes prevention and lost five to seven percent of their weight through dietary changes and increased physical activity were compared with those in other DPP groups who received standard education and maintained a stable weight. The women in the lifestyle intervention group had fewer problems with urinary incontinence than women in the other groups. This finding adds to other results of the DPP study that indicate the value of lifestyle changes for preventing or delaying the development of type 2 diabetes.

- **Poor Control Of Sphincter Muscles:** Sphincter muscles surround the urethra—the tube that carries urine from the bladder to the outside of the body—and keep it closed to hold urine in the bladder. If the nerves to the sphincter muscles are damaged, the muscles may become loose and allow leakage or stay tight when a person is trying to release urine.

- **Urine Retention:** For some people, nerve damage keeps their bladder muscles from getting the message that it is time to urinate or makes the muscles too weak to completely empty the bladder. If the bladder becomes too full, urine may back up and the increasing pressure may damage the kidneys. If urine remains in the body too long, an infection can develop in the kidneys or bladder. Urine retention may also lead to overflow incontinence—leakage of urine when the bladder is full and does not empty properly.

Diagnosis of bladder problems may involve checking both bladder function and the appearance of the bladder's interior. Tests may include x-rays, urodynamic testing to evaluate bladder function, and cystoscopy, a test that uses a device called a cystoscope to view the inside of the bladder.

Treatment of bladder problems due to nerve damage depends on the specific problem. If the main problem is urine retention, treatment may involve medication to promote better bladder emptying and a practice called timed voiding—urinating on a schedule—to promote more efficient urination. Sometimes people need to periodically insert a thin tube called a catheter through the urethra into the bladder to drain the urine. Learning how to tell when the bladder is full and how to massage the lower abdomen to fully empty the bladder can help as well. If urinary leakage is the main problem, medications, strengthening muscles with Kegel exercises, or surgery can help. Treatment for the urinary urgency and frequency of overactive bladder may involve medications, timed voiding, Kegel exercises, and surgery in some cases.

Urinary Tract Infections

Infections can occur when bacteria, usually from the digestive system, reach the urinary tract. If bacteria are growing in the urethra, the infection is called urethritis. The bacteria may travel up the urinary tract and cause a bladder infection, called cystitis. An untreated infection may go farther into the body and cause pyelonephritis, a kidney infection. Some people have chronic or recurrent urinary tract infections. Symptoms of urinary tract infections can include a frequent urge to urinate, pain or burning in the bladder or urethra during urination, or cloudy or reddish urine. In women, symptoms can include pressure above the pubic bone. In men, symptoms can include a feeling of fullness in the rectum.

If the infection is in the kidneys, a person may have nausea, feel pain in the back or side, and have a fever. Frequent urination can be a sign of high blood glucose, so results from recent blood glucose monitoring should be evaluated.

The health care provider will ask for a urine sample, which will be analyzed for bacteria and pus. Additional tests may be done if the patient has frequent urinary tract infections. An ultrasound exam provides images from the echo patterns of sound waves bounced back from internal organs. An intravenous pyelogram uses a special dye to enhance x-ray images of the urinary tract. Cystoscopy might be performed.

Early diagnosis and treatment are important to prevent more serious infections. To clear up a urinary tract infection, the health care provider will probably prescribe antibiotic treatment based on the type of bacteria in the urine. Kidney infections are more serious and may require several weeks of antibiotic treatment. Drinking plenty of fluids will help prevent another infection.

Risks Factors For Developing Sexual And Urologic Problems Of Diabetes

Risk factors are conditions that increase the chances of getting a particular disease. The more risk factors people have, the greater their chances of developing that disease or condition. Diabetic neuropathy and related sexual and urologic problems appear to be more common in people who have poor blood glucose control, have high levels of blood cholesterol, have high blood pressure, are overweight, are older than 40, smoke, and are physically inactive.

Points To Remember

The nerve damage of diabetes may cause sexual or urologic problems.

- Sexual problems in men with diabetes include erectile dysfunction and retrograde ejaculation.
- Sexual problems in women with diabetes include decreased vaginal lubrication and uncomfortable or painful intercourse, decreased or no sexual desire, and decreased or absent sexual response.
- Urologic problems in men and women with diabetes include bladder problems related to nerve damage, such as overactive bladder, poor control of sphincter muscles, and urine retention and urinary tract infections.
- Controlling diabetes through diet, physical activity, and medications as needed can help prevent sexual and urologic problems.
- Treatment is available for sexual and urologic problems.

People with diabetes can lower their risk of sexual and urologic problems by keeping their blood glucose, blood pressure, and cholesterol levels close to the target numbers their health care provider recommends. Being physically active and maintaining a healthy weight can also help prevent the long-term complications of diabetes. For those who smoke, quitting will lower the risk of developing sexual and urologic problems due to nerve damage and also lower the risk for other health problems related to diabetes, including heart attack, stroke, and kidney disease.

Chapter 51

The Diabetes Control And Complications Trial And Follow-Up Study

What is the DCCT?

The Diabetes Control and Complications Trial (DCCT) was a major clinical study conducted from 1983 to 1993 and funded by the National Institute of Diabetes and Digestive and Kidney Diseases. The study showed that keeping blood glucose levels as close to normal as possible slows the onset and progression of the eye, kidney, and nerve damage caused by diabetes. In fact, it demonstrated that any sustained lowering of blood glucose, also called blood sugar, helps, even if the person has a history of poor control.

The DCCT involved 1,441 volunteers, ages 13 to 39, with type 1 diabetes and 29 medical centers in the United States and Canada. Volunteers had to have had diabetes for at least one year but no longer than 15 years. They also were required to have no, or only early signs of, diabetic eye disease.

The study compared the effects of standard control of blood glucose versus intensive control on the complications of diabetes. Intensive control meant keeping hemoglobin A1C levels as close as possible to the normal value of six percent or less. The A1C blood test reflects a person's average blood glucose over the last two to three months. Volunteers were randomly assigned to each treatment group.

What is the EDIC?

When the DCCT ended in 1993, researchers continued to study more than 90 percent of participants. The follow-up study, called Epidemiology of Diabetes Interventions and

About This Chapter: Text in this chapter is from "DCCT and EDIC: The Diabetes Control and Complications Trial and Follow-up Study," National Institute of Diabetes and Digestive and Kidney Disease, March 2008.

Complications (EDIC), is assessing the incidence and predictors of cardiovascular disease events such as heart attack, stroke, or needed heart surgery, as well as diabetic complications related to the eye, kidney, and nerves. The EDIC study is also examining the impact of intensive control versus standard control on quality of life. Another objective is to look at the cost-effectiveness of intensive control.

How did intensive treatment affect diabetic eye disease?

All DCCT participants were monitored for diabetic retinopathy, an eye disease that affects the retina. Study results showed that intensive therapy reduced the risk for developing retinopathy by 76 percent. In participants who had some eye damage at the beginning of the study, intensive management slowed the progression of the disease by 54 percent.

The retina is the light-sensing tissue at the back of the eye. According to the National Eye Institute, one of the National Institutes of Health, as many as 24,000 people with diabetes lose their sight each year. In the United States, diabetic retinopathy is the leading cause of blindness in adults less than 65 years of age.

How did intensive treatment affect diabetic kidney disease?

Participants in the DCCT were tested to assess the development of diabetic kidney disease, or nephropathy. Findings showed that intensive treatment prevented the development and slowed the progression of diabetic kidney disease by 50 percent.

DCCT And EDIC Study Findings

DCCT Study Findings

Intensive blood glucose control reduces these risks:

- Eye disease: 76% reduced risk
- Kidney disease: 50% reduced risk
- Nerve disease: 60% reduced risk

EDIC Study Findings

Intensive blood glucose control reduces these risks:

- Any cardiovascular disease event: 42% reduced risk
- Nonfatal heart attack, stroke, or death from cardiovascular causes: 57% reduced risk

---

> ## Elements of Intensive Management in the DCCT
>
> - Testing blood glucose levels four or more times a day
> - Injecting insulin at least three times daily or using an insulin pump
> - Adjusting insulin doses according to food intake and exercise
> - Following a diet and exercise plan
> - Making monthly visits to a health care team composed of a physician, nurse educator, dietitian, and behavioral therapist

Diabetic kidney disease is the most common cause of kidney failure in the United States. After having diabetes for 15 years, one-third of people with type 1 diabetes develop kidney disease. Diabetes damages the small blood vessels in the kidneys, impairing their ability to filter impurities from blood for excretion in the urine. People with kidney failure must have a kidney transplant or rely on dialysis to cleanse their blood.

How did intensive treatment affect diabetic nerve disease?

Participants in the DCCT were examined to detect the development of nerve damage, or diabetic neuropathy. Study results showed the risk of nerve damage was reduced by 60 percent in people on intensive treatment.

Diabetic nerve disease can cause pain and loss of feeling in the feet, legs, and fingertips. It can also affect the parts of the nervous system that control blood pressure, heart rate, digestion, and sexual function. Neuropathy is a major contributing factor in foot and leg amputations among people with diabetes.

How did intensive treatment affect diabetes-related cardio-vascular disease?

People with type 1 diabetes have a tenfold greater risk of heart disease compared with nondiabetic patients because high blood glucose can damage the heart and blood vessels. That damage can lead to heart attacks and strokes, the leading causes of death for people with diabetes.

Another condition related to heart disease and common in people with diabetes is peripheral arterial disease (PAD), also called peripheral vascular disease (PVD). With this condition, the blood vessels in the legs are narrowed or blocked by fatty deposits, decreasing blood flow to the legs and feet. PAD is a sign of widespread atherosclerosis, and people with PAD are at increased risk of heart attack or stroke. Poor circulation in the legs and feet also raises the risk of amputation.

When the initial findings of the DCCT were announced in 1993, it was too early to detect the effects of the therapies on cardiovascular disease because patients were young. In 2005, however, EDIC researchers reported that the risk of any heart disease was reduced by 42 percent in people who had been in the intensive treatment group. Volunteers in the intensive treatment group also cut their risk of nonfatal heart attack, stroke, or death from cardiovascular causes by 57 percent.

Patients received the intensive therapy for an average of 6.5 years in the DCCT. More than 10 years after the DCCT ended, when both groups began receiving similar care, the benefits to the heart of the earlier treatment emerged. Moreover, the EDIC study found the benefits of tight glucose control on eye, kidney, and nerve problems persisted long after the DCCT ended. Researchers call the long-lasting benefit of tight control "metabolic memory." Following the DCCT, blood glucose levels in the intensive treatment group rose, and those of the conventional treatment group declined, so that blood glucose levels are now nearly the same between treatment groups.

What are the risks of intensive treatment?

In the DCCT, the most significant side effect of intensive treatment was an increase in the risk for hypoglycemia, also called low blood glucose, including episodes severe enough to require assistance from another person.

When blood glucose falls too low, a person can become confused, behave irrationally, have seizures, lose consciousness, or even die. The good news is that such episodes, while dangerous at the time, do not lead to a long-term loss of cognitive function—the ability to perceive, reason, and remember—as scientists originally feared. Researchers recently reported this finding after examining 1,144 of the original DCCT participants a mean of 18 years after enrollment in the DCCT.

The DCCT did not study intensive therapy in young children or in patients with severe complications, frequent hypoglycemia, or those with a limited life expectancy. While most patients benefit from keeping their blood glucose levels as close to normal as possible, less stringent goals may be appropriate for some patients.

DCCT researchers estimate that intensive management doubles the cost of managing diabetes because of increased visits to a health care professional and the need for more frequent blood testing at home. However, this cost is offset by the reduction in medical expenses related to long-term complications and by the improved quality of life of people with diabetes.

What are the most important factors in preventing diabetes complications?

Research studies have shown that control of blood glucose, blood pressure, and blood lipid levels helps prevent complications in people with type 1 or type 2 diabetes.

Where can I get more information about DCCT and EDIC?

Results of the DCCT are reported in the *New England Journal of Medicine*, 329(14), September 30, 1993.

Results of the EDIC are reported in the *New England Journal of Medicine*, 353(25), December 22, 2005.

Reprints of articles related to the DCCT or the EDIC can be ordered from the National Diabetes Information Clearinghouse at this address:

National Diabetes Information Clearinghouse
1 Information Way
Bethesda, MD 20892-3560
Phone: 800-860-8747
Fax: 703-738-4929
Internet: www.diabetes.niddk.nih.gov/statistics/reprints.htm
E-mail: http://www.diabetes.niddk.nih.gov/about/contact.htm

Part Six
If You Need More Information

Chapter 52

Resources For Diabetes Information

National Institute Of Diabetes And Digestive And Kidney Diseases (NIDDK)

Website: http://www2.niddk.nih.gov

The National Institute of Diabetes and Digestive and Kidney Diseases (NIDDK) is the government's lead agency for diabetes research. The NIDDK operates three Information Clearinghouses of potential interest to people seeking diabetes information and funds six Diabetes Research and Training Centers and eight Diabetes Endocrinology Research Centers.

National Diabetes Information Clearinghouse (NDIC)

1 Information Way
Bethesda, MD 20892-3560
Toll-Free: 800-860-8747
Toll-Free TTY: 866-569-1162
Fax: 703-738-4929
Website: http://www.diabetes.niddk.nih.gov
E-mail: ndic@info.niddk.nih.gov

Mission: To serve as a diabetes information, educational, and referral resource for health professionals and the public. NDIC is a service of the NIDDK.

Materials: Diabetes education materials are available free or at little cost. Literature searches on myriad subjects related to diabetes are provided. NDIC publishes *Diabetes Dateline,* a quarterly newsletter.

About This Chapter: Information in this chapter is from "Directory of Diabetes Organizations," National Institute of Diabetes and Digestive and Kidney Diseases, May 2009. All contact information was updated and verified in August 2011.

National Digestive Diseases Information Clearinghouse (NDDIC)

2 Information Way
Bethesda, MD 20892-3570
Toll-Free: 800-891-5389
Toll-Free TTY: 866-569-1162
Fax: 703-738-4929
Website: http://digestive.niddk.nih.gov
E-mail: nddic@info.niddk.nih.gov

Mission: To serve as a digestive disease informational, educational, and referral resource for health professionals and the public. NDDIC is a service of the NIDDK.

Materials: Educational materials about digestive diseases, available free or at little cost. Literature searches on a myriad of subjects related to digestive diseases are also provided. NDDIC publishes *Digestive Diseases News*, a quarterly newsletter.

National Kidney And Urologic Diseases Information Clearinghouse (NKUDIC)

3 Information Way
Bethesda, MD 20892-3580
Toll-Free: 800-891-5390
Toll-Free TTY: 866-569-1162
Fax: 703-738-4929
Website: http://www.kidney.niddk.nih.gov
E-mail: nkudic@info.niddk.nih.gov

Mission: To serve as a kidney and urologic disease informational, educational, and referral resource for health professionals and the public. NKUDIC is a service of NIDDK.

Materials: Educational materials on kidney and urologic diseases are available free or at little cost. Literature searches on a myriad of subjects related to kidney and urologic diseases are provided. NKUDIC publishes *Kidney Disease Research Updates* and *Urologic Diseases Research Updates*, quarterly newsletters.

National Diabetes Education Program (NDEP)

1 Diabetes Way
Bethesda, MD 20814-9692
Toll-Free: 888-693- NDEP (888-693-6337) (Publications by phone)
Phone: 301-496-3583

Website: http://www.ndep.nih.gov

Mission: To improve the treatment and outcomes for people with diabetes, to promote early diagnosis, and to prevent or delay the onset of diabetes.

Materials: Diabetes education materials are available free or at little cost.

National Kidney Disease Education Program (NKDEP)

3 Kidney Information Way
Bethesda, MD 20892
Toll-Free: 866-4-KIDNEY (866-454-3639)
Fax: 301-402-8182
Website: http://www.nkdep.nih.gov
E-mail: nkdep@info.niddk.nih.gov

Mission: NKDEP is an initiative of the National Institutes of Health, designed to reduce the morbidity and mortality caused by kidney disease and its complications. NKDEP aims to raise awareness of the seriousness of kidney disease, the importance of testing those at high risk (those with diabetes, high blood pressure, or a family history of kidney failure), and the availability of treatment to prevent or slow kidney failure.

Materials: Educational materials about kidney disease, available free or at little cost.

Weight-control Information Network (WIN)

1 WIN Way
Bethesda, MD 20892-3665
Toll-Free: 877-946-4627
Phone: 202-828-1025
Fax: 202-828-1028
Website: win.niddk.nih.gov
E-mail: win@info.niddk.nih.gov

Mission: To address the health information needs of individuals through the production and dissemination of educational materials. In addition, WIN is developing communication strategies for a pilot program to encourage at-risk individuals to achieve and maintain a healthy weight by making changes in their lifestyle.

Materials: Fact sheets, brochures, reprints, consensus statements, and literature searches on weight control, obesity, and weight-related nutritional disorders. WIN's semiannual newsletter, WIN Notes, provides health professionals with the latest research findings and progress in the WIN program.

Diabetes Research And Training Centers (DRTCs) And Diabetes Endocrinology Research Centers (DERCs)

Mission: The NIDDK supports two types of centers to foster diabetes research: Diabetes Research and Training Centers and Diabetes Endocrinology Research Centers. These centers facilitate progress in research by providing shared resources to enhance the efficiency of biomedical research and foster collaborations within and among institutions with established, comprehensive bases of research relevant to diabetes mellitus. They focus on basic and clinical research. In addition, the DRTCs provide substantial support for cores and pilot and feasibility projects directed at prevention and control of diabetes and translation of research advances into clinical practice.

Materials: Individual centers produce a variety of diabetes education materials. For information about publications and programs, contact the individual centers listed below.

DRTCs

Albert Einstein College of Medicine DRTC

Jack and Pearl Resnick Campus
1300 Morris Park Avenue
Belfer Building, Room 705
Bronx, NY 10461
Phone: 718-430-2908
Fax: 718-430-8557
Website: http://www.einstein.yu.edu/centers/
diabetes-research/default.aspx?id=1066

University of Chicago DRTC

Howard Hughes Medical Institute
University of Chicago
Bell Laboratory
5801 South Ellis Street
Chicago, IL 60637
5841 South Maryland Avenue, AMB N216
Chicago, IL 60637
Phone: 773-702-1234
Fax: 773-702-4292
Website: http://drtc.bsd.uchicago.edu

Indiana University DRTC

Indiana University School of Medicine
The National Institute for Fitness and Sport
250 North University Boulevard
Room 122
Indianapolis, IN 46202
Phone: 317-278-0905
Fax: 317-278-0911

University of Michigan DRTC

Michigan Diabetes Research and Training Center
Room 6107, Brehm Tower
1000 Wall Street
Ann Arbor, MI 48105-5714
Phone: 734-763-5730
Website: http://www.med.umich.edu/mdrtc

Vanderbilt University DRTC

Vanderbilt Diabetes Center
802 Light Hall
Nashville, TN 37232-0202
Phone: 615-322-7004
Fax: 615-343-0172
Website: http://www.mc.vanderbilt.edu/
diabetes/drtc

Washington University DRTC

Division of Health Behavior Research
Washington University School of Medicine
Suite 6700, Box 8504
4444 Forest Park Avenue
St. Louis, MO 63108
Phone: 314-286-1904
Fax: 314-286-1919
Website: http://dhbr.im.wustl.edu

DERCs

Joslin Diabetes Center DERC

Harvard Medical School
One Joslin Place
Boston, MA 02215
Toll-Free: 800-JOSLIN-1 (800-567-5461)
Phone: 617-732-2400
Fax: 617-732-2444
Website: http://www.joslinresearch.org/
cores/derc_fl.asp

Massachusetts General Hospital DERC

Department of Molecular Biology
Simches Research Center
185 Cambridge Street, CPZN7250
Boston, MA 02114
Phone: 617-726-5944
Fax: 617-726-6893
Website: http://molbio.mgh.harvard.edu/
index.htm
E-mail: info@molbio.mgh.harvard.edu

University of Colorado DERC

Barbara Davis Center for Childhood
Diabetes
1775 Aurora Court
Aurora, CO 80045
Phone: 303-724-6836
Fax: 303-724-6838
Website: http://www.ucdenver.edu/
academics/colleges/medicalschool/centers/
BarbaraDavis/DERC/Pages/default.aspx

University of Iowa DERC

Iowa Diabetes and Endocrinology
Research Center
111 6th Avenue, Suite 450
Des Moines, IA 50314
Phone: 515-643-5122
Fax: 515-643-5150
Website: http://www.ideciowa.org/
clinicaltrials
E-mail: diabetes.research@iderc.org

University of Massachusetts Medical School DERC
Biotech 2, Suite 218
373 Plantation Street
Worcester, MA 01605
Phone: 508-856-3800
Fax: 508-856-4093
Website: http://www.umassmed.edu/diabetes

University of Pennsylvania DERC
Division of Endocrinology, Diabetes and Metabolism
Perelman Center for Advanced Medicine
3400 Civic Center Boulevard
Philadelphia, PA 19104
Phone: 215-898-0210
Fax: 215-898-5408
Website: www.uphs.upenn.edu/endocrin

University of Washington DERC
Box 358285
DVA Puget Sound Health Care System
1660 South Columbian Way
Seattle, WA 98108
Phone: 206-764-2688
Fax: 206-764-2693
Website: depts.washington.edu/diabetes
E-mail: derc@u.washington.edu

Yale University School of Medicine DERC
Department of Internal Medicine
P.O. Box 208020
300 Cedar Street, TAC S141
Section of Endocrinology
New Haven, CT 06520-8020
Phone: 203-737-5071
Fax: 203-737-5558
Website: http://derc.yale.edu/index.aspx

Other Resources At The National Institutes Of Health (NIH)

National Eye Institute (NEI)
Information Office
31 Center Drive MSC 2510
Bethesda, MD 20892-2510
Phone: 301-496-5248
Website: http://www.nei.nih.gov
E-mail: 2020@nei.nih.gov

Mission: To promote public and professional awareness of the importance of early diagnosis and treatment of diabetic eye disease. NEHEP is a partnership with various public and private organizations that plan and implement eye health education programs targeted to a variety of high-risk audiences.

Materials: NEI produces patient and professional education materials related to diabetic eye disease and its treatment, including literature for patients, guides for health professionals, and education kits for community health workers and pharmacists. The following titles focus on diabetic eye disease: Educating People with Diabetes (kit), Information Kit for Pharmacists, and Ojo con su Visión (Watch Out for Your Vision) (in Spanish).

National Heart, Lung, And Blood Institute (NHLBI) Information Center

Attention: Website
P.O. Box 30105
Bethesda, MD 20824-0105
Phone: 301-592-8573
TTY: 240-629-3255
Fax: 240-629-3246
Website: http://www.nhlbi.nih.gov
E-mail: nhlbiinfo@nhlbi.nih.gov

Mission: To provide information and respond to inquiries related to the prevention and treatment of heart, lung, blood, and sleep disorders.

Materials: Patient education and professional materials are available on numerous topics, including cholesterol, high blood pressure, asthma, blood disease, heart disease, heart attack, exercise, obesity, lung disease, and sleep disorders. Treatment guidelines for health professionals are available on cholesterol, high blood pressure, obesity, and asthma. Serial publications *Heart Memo*, which provides program updates about cholesterol, high blood pressure, and heart attack, and *Asthma Memo*, which describes the activities of the National Asthma Education and Prevention Program, are available only online.

National Institute Of Dental And Craniofacial Research

National Oral Health Information Clearinghouse (NOHIC)
1 NOHIC Way
Bethesda, MD 20892-3500
Toll-Free: 866-232-4528
Fax: 301-480-4098
Website: http://www.nidcr.nih.gov/OralHealth
E-mail: nidcrinfo@mail.nih.gov

Mission: To serve as a resource for patients, health professionals, and the public who seek information about general oral health topics and the oral health of special care patients: people with genetic or systemic disorders that compromise oral health, people whose medical treatment causes oral problems, and people with mental or physical disabilities that make dental hygiene difficult. A service of the National Institute of Dental and Craniofacial Research, NOHIC gathers and disseminates information from many sources, including voluntary health organizations, educational institutions, government agencies, and industry.

Materials: NOHIC provides a variety of services to help patients and professionals obtain information including patient and professional educational materials.

Other Resources At The U.S. Department of Health And Human Services

Centers For Disease Control And Prevention (CDC)

National Center for Chronic Disease Prevention and Health Promotion
Division of Diabetes Translation
Mail Stop K-10
4770 Buford Highway NE
Atlanta, GA 30341-3717
Toll-Free: 800-CDC-INFO (800-232-4636)
Toll-Free TTY: 888-232-6348
Website: www.cdc.gov/diabetes
E-mail: cdcinfo@cdc.gov

Mission: To eliminate the preventable burden of diabetes through leadership, research, programs, and policies that translate science into practice.

Materials: CDC distributes several publications including a patient guide for people with diabetes (available in English and Spanish) and the eight-page "National Diabetes Fact Sheet: National Estimates and General Information on Diabetes in the United States." State-based diabetes prevention and control programs develop and maintain local programs and produce materials on diabetes for the general public and health professionals. Internet home page includes fact sheets, statistics, publications, and information about state diabetes prevention and control programs.

Indian Health Service (IHS)

Indian Health Service National Diabetes Program
5300 Homestead Road
Albuquerque, NM 87110
Phone: 505-248-4182 or 505-248-4236
Fax: 505-248-4188

Website: http://www.ihs.gov/MedicalPrograms/Diabetes

E-mail: diabetesprogram@ihs.gov

Mission: To develop, document, and sustain a health effort to prevent and control diabetes in American Indian and Alaska Native communities.

Materials: IHS makes many diabetes resources available, including the Diabetes Curriculum Packet, nutrition education materials, general diabetes information, professional resources, training programs, posters, audiovisual materials, and other patient education materials. Educational materials are directed toward American Indian and Alaska Native populations, and some materials are available at a lower reading level. Materials can be obtained upon request from the IHS National Diabetes Office.

Office Of Minority Health Resource Center (OMH-RC)

Resource Center

P.O. Box 37337

Washington, DC 20013-7337

Toll-Free: 800-444-6472

Fax: 301-251-2160

Website: http://www.omhrc.gov

E-mail: info@minorityhealth.hhs.gov

Mission: To improve the health of racial and ethnic populations through the development of health policies and programs. OMH-RC is the largest resource and referral service on minority health in the nation.

Materials: OMH-RC offers information, publications, mailing lists, database searches, referrals, and more for African American, Asian, Hispanic/Latino, American Indian/Alaska Native, and Pacific Islander populations. OMH-RC publishes the newsletters *Closing the Gap* and *HIV Impact*.

Department Of Veterans Affairs

Veterans Health Administration (VHA)

Program Chief, Diabetes

810 Vermont Avenue NW

Washington, DC 20420

Phone: 202-273-5400

Fax: 202-273-9142

Website: http://www.va.gov

Mission: To decrease the prevalence of adverse health outcomes in veterans with diabetes by ensuring that each patient at each facility has access to preventive and treatment programs that meet national standards of care.

Materials: The VHA Diabetes Clinical Practice Guidelines is a comprehensive, evidence-based document that incorporates information from several existing, national consensus, evidence-based guidelines into a format that maximally facilitates clinical decision making. An algorithmic format was chosen because of evidence that such a format improves data collection and diagnostic and therapeutics decision making and changes patterns of resource use. Guidelines were developed in six major subject areas, including glycemic control, foot care, eye care, hypertension, lipids, and renal disease. A computer version of the algorithm is under discussion.

Professional And Consumer Health Care Associations

American Association Of Clinical Endocrinologists (AACE)

245 Riverside Avenue, Suite 200
Jacksonville, FL 32202
Phone: 904-353-7878
Fax: 904-353-8185
Website: http://www.aace.com

Mission: To provide an avenue for the study of the scientific, social, political, and economic aspects of endocrinology consistent with maintaining the highest levels of patient care and the highest standards of medical practice. AACE is an international organization representing physicians devoted to enhancing the field of clinical endocrinology.

Materials: AACE publishes a peer-reviewed scientific journal, *Endocrine Practice.* The organization also publishes *The First Messenger* newsletter and other timely publications, such as practice guidelines, to keep members abreast of scientific developments and news.

American Association Of Diabetes Educators (AADE)

200 West Madison Avenue, Suite 800
Chicago, IL 60606
Toll-Free: 800-338-3633
Phone: 312-424-2426
Fax: 312-424-2427
Website: http://www.diabeteseducator.org

E-mail: aade@aadenet.org

Mission: AADE is a multi-disciplinary organization of more than 10,000 health professionals dedicated to advocating quality diabetes education and care.

Materials: AADE publishes *The Diabetes Educator,* a bimonthly journal for multidisciplinary members of the diabetes health care team. The journal publishes the latest diabetes education research and provides valuable teaching tools and techniques. AADE also produces the most comprehensive diabetes education resource, "A Core Curriculum for Diabetes Education," now in its third edition. AADE members receive *AADE News,* providing association-related news and practice information, nine times per year. Call AADE for a complete listing of all educational products, including publications, videotapes, and patient materials, available through the association.

American Diabetes Association (ADA)

Attention: Center for Information
1701 North Beauregard Street
Alexandria, VA 22311
Toll-Free: 800-DIABETES (800-342-2383)
Phone: 703-549-1500
Fax: 703-549-6995
Website: http://www.diabetes.org
E-mail: askada@diabetes.org or Preguntas@diabetes.org (Spanish)

Mission: To prevent and cure diabetes and to improve the lives of everyone affected by diabetes.

Materials: The American Diabetes Association publishes many books and resources for health professionals and people with diabetes. In addition, it publishes *Diabetes Forecast,* a monthly magazine for people with diabetes, and *Diabetes, Diabetes Care,* and *Diabetes Spectrum,* which are professional journals.

The ADA National Call Center (800-DIABETES; 800-342-2383) is dedicated to answering thousands of calls and e-mails a day from people with diabetes, as well as their families, friends and health care professionals. The National Call Center is available Monday through Friday from 8:30 a.m. to 8:00 p.m. Eastern time to provide support, encouragement, and education on diabetes management through a variety of free pamphlets and brochures.

American Dietetic Association (ADA)

120 South Riverside Plaza, Suite 2000
Chicago, IL 60606-6995

Toll-Free: 800-877-1600

Phone: 312-899-0040

Website: http://www.eatright.org

E-mail: knowledge@eatright.org

Mission: To promote optimal nutrition and well-being for all people by advocating for its members.

Materials: The American Dietetic Association publishes a monthly professional journal, *The Journal of the American Dietetic Association*, and a monthly newsletter, *ADA Courier*. In addition, it publishes many books and other resources for consumers and professionals.

The Diabetes Care and Education Dietetic Practice Group (DCE) is a subgroup of the American Dietetic Association to promote quality nutrition care and education.

American Podiatric Medical Association (APMA)

9312 Old Georgetown Road

Bethesda, MD 20814-1621

Toll-Free: 800-FOOT-CARE (800-366-8227) (Foot Care Information Center)

Phone: 301-581-9200

Fax: 301-530-2752

Website: http://www.apma.org

Mission: To serve the professional needs and promote the standards and ethics of doctors of podiatric medicine and their services to the public.

Materials: The APMA's website has a "Find a Podiatrist" feature, which allows users to search for an APMA member podiatrist by zip code. The APMA also publishes a monthly magazine, *APMA News*; a monthly journal, *Journal of the American Podiatric Medical Association*; and a diabetes-specific booklet, "Your Podiatric Physician Talks About Diabetes," along with many other brochures on various foot health topics.

American Urological Association Foundation (AUAF)

1000 Corporate Boulevard

Linthicum, MD 21090

Toll-Free: 800-828-7866

Phone: 410-689-3990

Fax: 410-689-3998

Website: http://www.urologyhealth.org

E-mail: auafoundation@auafoundation.org

Mission: To provide research grants, patient and public education and awareness, Government relations, and patient support group activities.

Materials: Informational brochure about the American Urological Association Foundation, *Family Urology* (quarterly magazine), and patient education brochures.

Diabetes Action Research And Education Foundation

426 C Street NE
Washington, DC 20002
Phone: 202-333-4520
Fax: 202-558-5240
Website: http://www.diabetesaction.org
E-mail: info@diabetesaction.org

Mission: To support and promote education and scientific research to enhance the quality of life for everyone affected by diabetes.

Materials: The foundation publishes the booklet "Managing Your Diabetes: Basics and Beyond."

Diabetes Exercise And Sports Association (DESA)

310 West Liberty, Suite 604
Louisville, KY 40202
Toll-Free: 800-898-4322
Phone: 502-581-0207
Fax: 502-581-0206
Website: http://www.diabetes-exercise.org
E-mail: desa@diabetes-exercise.org

Mission: To enhance the quality of life for people with diabetes through exercise.

Materials: The Challenge is DESA's quarterly newsletter. DESA also provides pamphlets on diabetes and exercise.

Endocrine Society

8401 Connecticut Avenue, Suite 900
Chevy Chase, MD 20815-5817
Toll-Free: 888-363-6274
Phone: 301-941-0200
Fax: 301-941-0259
Website: http://www.endo-society.org

Mission: To promote excellence in research, education, and the clinical practice of endocrinology; foster a greater understanding of endocrinology among the general public and practitioners of complementary medical disciplines; and promote the interests of all endocrinologists at the national scientific research and health policy levels of government.

Materials: The Endocrine Society publishes four professional journals: *Endocrinology*, *The Journal of Clinical Endocrinology and Metabolism*, *Endocrine Reviews*, and *Molecular Endocrinology*. Another publication, *The Clinical Endocrinology Update Syllabus*, provides practicing endocrinologists with a review of the diagnosis and management of all major components of contemporary endocrinology.

Juvenile Diabetes Research Foundation International (JDRF)

26 Broadway, 14th Floor
New York, NY 10004
Toll-Free: 800-533-CURE (800-533-2873)
Fax: 212-785-9595
Website: http://www.jdrf.org
E-mail: info@jdrf.org

Mission: To support and fund research to find a cure for diabetes and its complications. The Juvenile Diabetes Research Foundation International (JDRF) is a nonprofit, voluntary health agency, and the world's leading charitable funder of research to find a cure for diabetes.

Materials: JDRF publishes the quarterly magazines *Countdown* and *Countdown for Kids*, as well as a series of patient education brochures about type 1 and type 2 diabetes and also a research e-newsletter to provide the latest information about research on type 1 diabetes and its complications.

National Certification Board For Diabetes Educators (NCBDE)

330 East Algonquin Road, Suite 4
Arlington Heights, IL 60005
Toll-Free: 877-239-3233
Phone: 847-228-9795
Fax: 847-228-8469
Website: http://www.ncbde.org
E-mail: info@ncbde.org

Mission: To promote excellence in the field of diabetes education through the development, maintenance, and protection of the Certified Diabetes Educator (CDE) credential and the certification process.

Materials: NCBDE publishes a brochure that contains information about eligibility requirements and the certification examination.

National Glycohemoglobin Standardization Program (NGSP)

Department of Child Health
University of Missouri Hospital and Clinics
1 Hospital Drive, DC0.5800
Columbia, MO 65212
Phone: 573-882-6882
Fax: 573-884-8823
Website: http://www.ngsp.org
E-mail: ngsp@missouri.edu

Mission: To standardize glycated hemoglobin test results so that clinical laboratory results are comparable to those reported in the Diabetes Control and Complications Trial (DCCT), where relationships to mean blood glucose and risk for vascular complications have been established.

National Kidney Foundation (NKF)

30 East 33rd Street
New York, NY 10016
Toll-Free: 800-622-9010
Phone: 212-889-2210
Fax: 212-689-9261
Website: http://www.kidney.org
E-mail: info@kidney.org

Mission: To prevent kidney and urinary tract diseases, improve the health and well-being of individuals and families affected by these diseases, and increase the availability of all organs for transplantation. Through its 51 affiliates nationwide, NKF conducts programs in research, professional education, patient and community services, public education, and donation. The work of NKF, a major voluntary health organization, is funded primarily by public donations.

Materials: NKF has several publications including *American Journal of Kidney Diseases*, *Journal of Renal Nutrition*, *Advances in Renal Replacement Therapy*, *Journal of Nephrology Social Work*, *Renalink*, *NKF MD*, *NKF Family Focus*, *Transplant Chronicles*, and *For Those Who Give and Grieve*. Additional patient and public education materials are also available.

Pedorthic Footwear Association (PFA)

2025 M Street NW, Suite 800
Washington, DC 20036
Toll-Free: 800-673-8447
Phone: 202-367-1145
Fax: 202-367-2145
Website: http://www.pedorthics.org
E-mail: info@pedorthics.org

Mission: To increase knowledge and understanding of pedorthics and its practice, encourage development of new pedorthic tools and techniques, and foster the professional development of pedorthic practitioners.

Materials: PFA publishes the bimonthly magazine *Current Pedorthics*, formerly called *Pedoscope*; the brochures "Pedorthics: Foot Care Through Proper Footwear" and "Diabetes and Pedorthics: Conservative Foot Care"; reference guides; and manuals.

Chapter 53

Finding Diabetes-Friendly Recipes And Cookbooks

Diabetes-Friendly Recipes Online

American Diabetes Association

http://www.diabetes.org/food-and-fitness/food/recipes
http://www.diabetes.org/assets/pdfs/winning-at-work/soul-recipes.pdf

Children with Diabetes

http://www.childrenwithdiabetes.com/recipes

ChooseMyPlate.gov

http://www.choosemyplate.gov/downloads/MyPlate/Recipes.pdf

Diabetes Action

http://www.diabetesaction.org/site/PageNavigator/recipe

Diabetes Daily

http://www.diabetesdaily.com/recipes

Diabetic Gourmet

http://diabeticgourmet.com/recipes

About This Chapter: This chapter includes recipes excerpted from "Tasty Recipes for People with Diabetes and Their Families," National Diabetes Education Program, 2008. Resources were compiled from other sources deemed accurate. Inclusion does not constitute endorsement and there is no implication associated with omission. All website information was verified in August 2011.

DiabeticLifestyle/Vertical Health

http://www.diabeticlifestyle.com/recipes

Diabetic Living Online/Meredith Corporation

http://www.diabeticlivingonline.com/diabetic-recipes

dLife/LifeMed Media

http://www.dlife.com/diabetes/diabetic-recipes

Eating Well

http://www.eatingwell.com/recipes_menus/collections/diabetic_diet
http://apps.nccd.cdc.gov/dnparecipe/recipesearch.aspx

Helpguide.org

http://helpguide.org/life/healthy_recipes.htm

Joslin Diabetes Center

http://www.joslin.org/phs/recipes.html

Juvenile Diabetes Research Foundation International

http://kids.jdrf.org/index.cfm?page_id=109765

Mayo Clinic

http://www.mayoclinic.com/health/diabetes-recipes/RE00091

National Kidney Foundation

http://www.kidney.org/patients/kidneykitchen/diabetes_ckd.cfm

Nemours Foundation

http://kidshealth.org/kid/recipes/diabetes/about_diabetes_recipes.html

U.S. Food and Drug Administration

http://www.fda.gov/ForConsumers/ByAudience/ForWomen/FreePublications/ucm136131.htm

Diabetes-Friendly Cookbooks And Meal Planning Guides

All-Natural Diabetes Cookbook

By Jackie Newgent
Published by the American Diabetes Association, 2007

The American Diabetes Association Month of Meals Diabetes Meal Planner

By the American Diabetes Association
Published by the American Diabetes Association, 2010

Betty Crocker 30-Minute Meals for Diabetes

By the Betty Crocker Editors
Published by Wiley Publishing, 2008

Betty Crocker's Diabetes Cookbook

By Richard M. Bergenstal, Diane Reader, and Maureen Doran
Published by Wiley Publishing, 2003

Biggest Book of Diabetic Recipes

By Better Homes and Gardens
Published by Meredith Books, 2005

Choose Your Foods: Exchange Lists for Diabetes

By Anne Daly and the American Diabetes Association
and the American Dietetic Association
Published by the American Dietetic Association, 2007

Diabetes and Heart Healthy Cookbook

By the American Diabetes Association and the American Heart Association
Published by the American Diabetes Association, 2004

Diabetes Cookbook for Dummies, Third Edition

By Alan L. Rubin and Cait James
Published by Wiley Publishing, 2009

Diabetes Diet Cookbook: Discover the New Fiber-FULL Eating Plan for Weight Loss

By Ann Fittante and the editors of *Prevention Magazine*
Published by Rodale Books, 2008

Diabetes Meal Planning Made Easy, Fourth Edition

By Hope Warshaw
Published by the American Diabetes Association, 2010

Diabetic Cooking: Snacks, Main Dishes and Desserts

By Favorite Name Brand™
Publisher: Publications International, 2007

Diabetic Living Quick and Easy Meals

By *Diabetic Living* Editors
Published by John Wiley and Sons, 2010

Diabetic Living: Slow Cooker Recipes

By Carrie E. Holcomb
Published by Meredith Books, 2005

Diabetic Meals in 30 Minutes—Or Less, Second Edition

By Robyn Webb
Published by American Diabetes Association, 2006

Joslin Cooks!

By the Joslin Diabetes Center Staff
Available from Joslin Diabetes Center: www.joslin.org

Joslin Diabetes Quick and Easy Cookbook

By Frances T. Giedt and Bonnie S. Polin
Published by Fireside, 1998

The Everything Diabetes Cookbook, Second Edition

By Gretchen Scalpi
Published by Adams Media, 2010

The New Family Cookbook for People with Diabetes, Revised and Updated

By the American Diabetes Association and the American Dietetic Association
Published by Simon and Schuster, 2007

No-Fuss Diabetes Recipes for 1 or 2

By Jackie Boucher, Marcia Hayes, and Jane Stephenson
Published by John Wiley and Sons, 1999

The Official Pocket Guide to Diabetic Exchanges, Second Edition

By the American Diabetes Association
Published by the American Diabetes Association, 2003

Real Food for People with Diabetes, Second Edition

By Doris Cross and Alice Williams

Published by Prima Health, 2001

Ultimate Diabetes Meal Planner: A Complete System for Eating Healthy with Diabetes

By Jaynie F. Higgins and David Groetzinger

Published by the American Diabetes Association, 2009

Some Recipes For You To Try

Diabetic exchanges are calculated based on the American Diabetes Association Exchange System. Percent Daily Values are based on a 2,000 calorie diet.

Spanish Omelet

This tasty dish provides a healthy array of vegetables and can be used for breakfast, brunch, or any meal. Serve with fresh fruit salad and a whole grain dinner roll.

Nutrition Facts

Serving Size: ⅓ of omelet

Amount Per Serving

     Calories 260

     Calories from Fat 90

% Daily Value (DV)

     Total Fat 10g, 15%

     Saturated Fat 3.5g, 18%

     Trans Fat 0g

     Cholesterol 135mg, 45%

     Sodium 240mg, 10%

     Total Carbohydrate 30g, 10%

     Dietary Fiber 3g, 12%

     Sugars 3g

     Protein 16g

     Vitamin A 8%

     Vitamin C 60%

     Calcium 15%

     Iron 8%

Ingredients

5 small potatoes, peeled and sliced

vegetable cooking spray

½ medium onion, minced

1 small zucchini, sliced

1½ cups green/red peppers, sliced thin

5 medium mushrooms, sliced

3 whole eggs, beaten

5 egg whites, beaten

pepper and garlic salt with herbs, to taste

3 ounces shredded part-skim mozzarella cheese

1 tablespoon low-fat parmesan cheese

Directions

- Preheat oven to 375° F.
- Cook potatoes in boiling water until tender.
- In a nonstick pan, add vegetable spray and warm at medium heat.
- Add onion and sauté until brown. Add vegetables and sauté until tender but not brown.
- In a medium mixing bowl, slightly beat eggs and egg whites, pepper, garlic salt, and low-fat mozzarella cheese. Stir egg-cheese mixture into the cooked vegetables.
- In a 10-inch pie pan or ovenproof skillet, add vegetable spray and transfer potatoes and egg mixture to pan. Sprinkle with low-fat parmesan cheese and bake until firm and brown on top, about 20–30 minutes.
- Remove omelet from oven, cool for 10 minutes, and cut into five pieces.

Exchanges

Meat 2

Bread 2

Vegetable ⅔

Fat 2

Beef Or Turkey Stew

This dish goes nicely with a green leaf lettuce and cucumber salad and a dinner roll. Plantains or corn can be used in place of the potatoes.

Nutrition Facts

Serving Size: 1½ cup

Amount Per Serving

      Calories: 320

      Calories from Fat: 60

% Daily Value (DV)

      Total Fat 7g, 11%

      Saturated Fat 1.5g, 8%

      Trans Fat 0g

      Cholesterol 40mg, 13%

      Sodium 520mg, 22%

      Total Carbohydrate 41g, 14%

      Dietary Fiber 8g, 32%

      Sugars 9g

      Protein 24g

      Vitamin A 340%

      Vitamin C 80%

      Calcium 6%

      Iron 15%

Ingredients

      1 pound lean beef or turkey breast, cut into cubes

      2 Tbsp. whole wheat flour

      ¼ tsp. salt (optional)

      ¼ tsp. pepper

      ¼ tsp. cumin

      1½ Tbsp. olive oil

      2 cloves garlic, minced

2 medium onions, sliced

2 stalks celery, sliced

1 medium red/green bell pepper, sliced

1 medium tomato, finely minced

5 cups beef or turkey broth, fat removed

5 small potatoes, peeled and cubed

12 small carrots, cut into large chunks

1¼ cups green peas

Directions

- Preheat oven to 375° F.

- Mix the whole wheat flour with salt, pepper, and cumin. Roll the beef or turkey cubes in the mixture. Shake off excess flour.

- In a large skillet, heat olive oil over medium-high heat. Add beef or turkey cubes and sauté until nicely brown, about 7–10 minutes.

- Place beef or turkey in an ovenproof casserole dish.

- Add minced garlic, onions, celery, and peppers to skillet and cook until vegetables are tender, about five minutes.

- Stir in tomato and broth. Bring to a boil and pour over turkey or beef in casserole dish. Cover dish tightly and bake for one hour at 375° F.

- Remove from oven and stir in potatoes, carrots, and peas. Bake for another 20–25 minutes or until tender.

Exchanges

Lean Meat 3

Vegetable 2½

Bread 2⅔

Fat 1

Two Cheese Pizza

Serve your pizza with fresh fruit and a mixed green salad garnished with red beans to balance your meal.

Nutrition Facts

Serving Size: 2 slices (¼ of pie)

Amount Per Serving

    Calories: 420

    Calories from Fat: 170

% Daily Value (DV)

    Total Fat 19g, 29%

    Saturated Fat 7g, 35%

    Trans Fat 0g

    Cholesterol 25mg, 8%

    Sodium 580mg, 24%

    Total Carbohydrate 44g, 15%

    Dietary Fiber 3g, 12%

    Sugars 5g

    Protein 20g

    Vitamin A 30%

    Vitamin C 90%

    Calcium 40%

    Iron 15%

Ingredients

2 Tbsp. whole wheat flour

1 can (10 ounces) refrigerated pizza crust

Vegetable cooking spray

2 Tbsp. olive oil

½ cup low-fat ricotta cheese

½ tsp. dried basil

1 small onion, minced

2 cloves garlic, minced

¼ tsp. salt (optional)

4 ounces shredded part-skim mozzarella cheese

2 cups mushrooms, chopped

1 large red pepper, cut into strips

Directions

- Preheat oven to 425° F.

- Spread whole wheat flour over working surface. Roll out dough with rolling pin to desired crust thickness.

- Coat cookie sheet with vegetable cooking spray. Transfer pizza crust to cookie sheet. Brush olive oil over crust.

- Mix low-fat ricotta cheese with dried basil, onion, garlic, and salt. Spread this mixture over crust.

- Sprinkle crust with part-skim mozzarella cheese. Top cheese with mushrooms and red pepper.

- Bake at 425° F for 13–15 minutes or until cheese melts and crust is deep golden brown.

- Cut into 8 slices.

Exchanges

Meat 2½
Bread 3
Vegetable 1
Fat 3¾

Rice With Chicken, Spanish Style

This is a good way to get vegetables into the meal plan. Serve with a mixed green salad and some whole wheat bread.

Nutrition Facts

Serving Size: 1½ cup

Amount Per Serving

Calories 400

Calories from Fat 60

% Daily Value (DV)

Total Fat 7g, 11%

Saturated Fat 1.5g, 8%

Trans Fat 0g

Cholesterol 85mg, 28%

Sodium 530mg, 22%

Total Carbohydrate 46g, 15%

Dietary Fiber 3g, 12%

Sugars 5g

Protein 37g

Vitamin A 30%

Vitamin C 70%

Calcium 4%

Iron 20%

Ingredients

2 Tbsp. olive oil

2 medium onions, chopped

6 cloves garlic, minced

2 stalks celery, diced

2 medium red/green peppers, cut into strips

1 cup mushrooms, chopped

2 cups uncooked whole grain rice

3 pounds boneless chicken breast, cut into bite-sized pieces, skin removed

1½ tsp. salt (optional)

2½ cups low-fat chicken broth

Saffron or Sazón™ for color

3 medium tomatoes, chopped

1 cup frozen peas

1 cup frozen corn

1 cup frozen green beans

Olives or capers for garnish (optional)

Directions

- Heat olive oil over medium heat in a non-stick pot. Add onion, garlic, celery, red/green pepper, and mushrooms. Cook over medium heat, stirring often, for three minutes or until tender.

- Add whole grain rice and sauté for two to three minutes, stirring constantly to mix all ingredients.

- Add chicken, salt, chicken broth, water, Saffron/Sazón™, and tomatoes. Bring water to a boil.

- Reduce heat to medium-low, cover, and let the casserole simmer until water is absorbed and rice is tender, about 20 minutes.

- Stir in peas, corn, and beans and cook for 8–10 minutes. When everything is hot, the casserole is ready to serve. Garnish with olives or capers, if desired.

Exchanges

Meat 5⅓
Bread 3
Vegetable 1
Fat 1⅓

Pozole

Nutrition Facts

Serving Size: 1 cup

Amount Per Serving
Calories: 220
Calories from Fat: 70

% Daily Value (DV)
Total Fat 7g, 11%
Saturated Fat 2g, 10%
Trans Fat 0g
Cholesterol 70mg, 23%
Sodium 390mg, 16%
Total Carbohydrate 17, g6%
Dietary Fiber 3g, 12%
Sugars 5g
Protein 21g
Vitamin A 4%

Vitamin C 10%

Calcium 4%

Iron 15%

Ingredients

2 pounds lean beef, cubed

1 Tbsp. olive oil

1 large onion, chopped

1 clove garlic, finely chopped

¼ tsp. salt

⅛ tsp. pepper

¼ cup fresh cilantro, chopped

1 can (15 ounces) stewed tomatoes

2 ounces tomato paste

1 can (1 pound 13 ounces) hominy

Directions

- In a large pot, heat olive oil. Add beef and sauté. Only a small amount of oil is needed to sauté meat.

- Add onion, garlic, salt, pepper, cilantro, and enough water to cover meat. Stir to mix ingredients evenly. Cover pot and cook over low heat until meat is tender.

- Add tomatoes and tomato paste. Continue cooking for about 20 minutes.

- Add hominy and continue cooking another 15 minutes, stirring occasionally. If too thick, add water for desired consistency.

Option: Skinless, boneless chicken breasts can be used instead of beef cubes.

Exchanges

Meat 3

Bread 1

Vegetable ½

Fat 1⅓

Avocado Tacos

These fresh tasting tacos are great for a light meal.

Nutrition Facts

Serving Size: 1 taco

Amount Per Serving

    Calories: 270

    Calories from Fat: 80

% Daily Value (DV)

    Total Fat 8g, 12%

    Saturated Fat 2g, 10%

    Trans Fat 0g

    Cholesterol 0mg, 0%

    Sodium 460mg, 19%

    Total Carbohydrate 43g, 14%

    Dietary Fiber 5g, 20%

    Sugars 4g

    Protein 7g

    Vitamin A 25%

    Vitamin C 100%

    Calcium 10%

    Iron1 5%

Ingredients

    1 medium onion, cut into thin strips

    2 large green peppers, cut into thin strips

    2 large red peppers, cut into thin strips

    1 cup fresh cilantro, finely chopped

    1 ripe avocado, peeled and seeded, cut into 12 slices

    1½ cups fresh tomato salsa (see ingredients below)

    12 flour tortillas

    Vegetable cooking spray

Fresh Tomato Salsa Ingredients

> 1 cup tomatoes, diced
> ⅓ cup onions, diced
> ½ clove garlic, minced
> 2 tsp. cilantro
> ⅓ tsp. jalapeño peppers, chopped
> ½ tsp. lime juice
> Pinch of cumin

Directions

- Mix together all salsa ingredients and refrigerate in advance.
- Coat skillet with vegetable spray.
- Lightly sauté onion and green and red peppers.
- Warm tortillas in oven and fill with peppers, onions, avocado, and salsa. Fold tortillas and serve. Top with cilantro.

Exchanges

> Bread 3
> Vegetable 1
> Fat 1½

Tropical Fruits Fantasia

The tropics offer a great variety of fruits that will make this delicious and colorful recipe stand out; it will also make your mouth water even before tasting it.

Nutrition Facts

Serving Size: ½ cup

Amount Per Serving

> Calories: 170
> Calories from Fat: 5

% Daily Value (DV)

> Total Fat 0.5g, 1%

Saturated Fat 0g, 0%

Trans Fat 0g

Cholesterol 0mg, 0%

Sodium 40mg, 2%

Total Carbohydrate 41g, 14%

Dietary Fiber 5g, 20%

Sugars 30g

Protein 4g

Vitamin A 50%

Vitamin C 230%

Calcium 15%

Iron 2%

Ingredients

8 ounces fat-free, sugar-free orange yogurt

5 medium strawberries, cut into halves

3 ounces honeydew melon, cut into slices (or ½ cup cut into cubes)

3 ounces cantaloupe melon, cut into slices (or ½ cup cut into cubes)

1 mango, peeled and seeded, cut into cubes

1 papaya, peeled and seeded, cut into cubes

3 ounces watermelon, seeded and cut into slices (or ½ cup cut into cubes)

2 oranges, seeded and cut into slices

½ cup unsweetened orange juice

Directions

- Add yogurt and all fruits to a bowl and carefully mix together

- Pour orange juice over fruit mixture.

- Mix well and serve ½ cup as your dessert.

Exchanges

Fruit 2¾

Milk ⅓

Index

Index

Page numbers that appear in *Italics* refer to tables or illustrations. Page numbers that have a small 'n' after the page number refer to information shown as Notes at the beginning of each chapter. Page numbers that appear in **Bold** refer to information contained in boxes on that page (except Notes information at the beginning of each chapter).

A

O